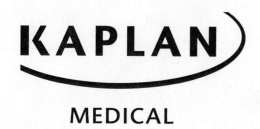

MEDICAL

USMLE® STEP 1 Lecture Notes 2017 | Immunology and Microbiology

USMLE® is a joint program of the Federation of State Medical Boards (FSMB) and the National Board of Medical Examiners (NBME), neither of which sponsors or endorses this product.

This publication is designed to provide accurate information in regard to the subject matter covered as of its publication date, with the understanding that knowledge and best practice constantly evolve. The publisher is not engaged in rendering medical, legal, accounting, or other professional service. If medical or legal advice or other expert assistance is required, the services of a competent professional should be sought. This publication is not intended for use in clinical practice or the delivery of medical care. To the fullest extent of the law, neither the Publisher nor the Editors assume any liability for any injury and/or damage to persons or property arising out of or related to any use of the material contained in this book.

© 2017 by Kaplan, Inc.

Published by Kaplan Medical, a division of Kaplan, Inc.
750 Third Avenue
New York, NY 10017

10 9 8 7 6 5 4 3 2 1

Course ISBN: 978-1-5062-0873-2

Retail ISBN: 978-1-5062-0836-7

Kaplan Publishing print books are available at special quantity discounts to use for sales promotions, employee premiums, or educational purposes. For more information or to purchase books, please call the Simon & Schuster special sales department at 866-506-1949.

IMMUNOLOGY

Editors

Tiffany L. Alley, Ph.D.
Former Associate Professor of Immunology and Microbiology
Chair of Molecular Sciences
Lincoln Memorial University
DeBusk College of Osteopathic Medicine
Harrogate, TN

Current Osteopathic Medical Student, III, and Anatomy Fellow
Lincoln Memorial University
DeBusk College of Osteopathic Medicine
Harrogate, TN

Kim Moscatello, Ph.D.
Professor of Microbiology and Immunology
Director of Curriculum and Student Achievement
Lake Erie College of Osteopathic Medicine
Erie, PA

MICROBIOLOGY

Editors

Tiffany L. Alley, Ph.D.
Former Associate Professor of Immunology and Microbiology
Chair of Molecular Sciences
Lincoln Memorial University
DeBusk College of Osteopathic Medicine
Harrogate, TN

Current Osteopathic Medical Student, III, and Anatomy Fellow
Lincoln Memorial University
DeBusk College of Osteopathic Medicine
Harrogate, TN

Christopher C. Keller, Ph.D.
Associate Professor of Microbiology and Immunology
Lake Erie College of Osteopathic Medicine
Erie, PA

Kim Moscatello, Ph.D.
Professor of Microbiology and Immunology
Director of Curriculum and Student Achievement
Lake Erie College of Osteopathic Medicine
Erie, PA

Previous contributions by Thomas F. Lint, Ph.D.

We want to hear what you think. What do you like or not like about the Notes?
Please email us at **medfeedback@kaplan.com**.

Contents

Section II: Microbiology

SECTION I

Immunology

The Immune System

1

Learning Objectives

❏ Define and describe the components of the immune system

❏ Discriminate between innate and acquired immunity

THE IMMUNE SYSTEM

The immune system is designed to recognize and respond to non-self antigen in a coordinated manner. Additionally, cells that are diseased, damaged, distressed or dying are recognized and eliminated by the immune system.

The immune system is divided into 2 complementary arms: the **innate** and the **adaptive** immune systems.

Innate Immunity

Innate immunity provides the body's first line of defense against infectious agents. It involves several defensive barriers:

- Anatomic and physical (skin, mucous membranes and normal flora)
- Physiologic (temperature, pH, anti-microbials and cytokines)
- Complement
- Cellular: phagocytes and granulocytes
- Inflammation

Innate immune defenses have the following characteristics in common:

- Are **present intrinsically** with or without previous stimulation
- Have **limited specificity** for shared microbe and cellular structures (pathogen-associated molecular patterns [PAMPs] and damage-associated molecular patterns [DAMPs])
- Have **limited diversity** as reflected by a limited number of pattern recognition receptors
- Are not enhanced in activity upon subsequent exposure—**no memory**

Adaptive Immunity

The components of the adaptive immune response are B and T lymphocytes and their effector cells.

Adaptive immune defenses have the following characteristics in common:

- Each B and T lymphocyte is **specific** for a particular antigen
- As a population, lymphocytes have extensive diversity
- Are enhanced with each repeat exposure—**immunologic memory**
- Are capable of **distinguishing self** from **non-self**
- Are **self-limiting**

The features of adaptive immunity are designed to give the individual the best possible defense against disease.

- **Specificity** is required, along with **immunologic memory,** to protect against persistent or recurrent challenge.
- **Diversity** is required to protect against the maximum number of potential pathogens.
- **Specialization** of effector function is necessary so that the most effective defense can be mounted against diverse challenges.
- The ability to **distinguish between self** (host cells) **and non-self** (pathogens) is vital in inhibiting an autoimmune response.
- **Self-limitation** allows the system to return to a basal resting state after a challenge to conserve energy and resources and to avoid uncontrolled cell proliferation resulting in leukemia or lymphoma.

Table I-1-1. Innate versus Adaptive Immunity

Characteristics	Innate	Adaptive
Specificity	For pathogen-associated molecular patterns (PAMPs)	For specific antigens of microbial and nonmicrobial agents
Diversity	Limited	High
Memory	No	Yes
Self-reactivity	No	No
Components		
Anatomic and physiologic barriers	Skin, mucosa, normal flora, temperature, pH, antimicrobials, and cytokines	Lymph nodes, spleen, mucosal-associated lymphoid tissues
Blood proteins	Complement	Antibodies
Cells	Phagocytes, granulocytes and natural killer (NK) cells	B lymphocytes and T lymphocytes

Function

The innate and adaptive arms of the immune response work in collaboration to stop an infection. Once a pathogen has broken through the anatomic and physiologic barriers, the innate immune response is immediately activated, oftentimes it is able to contain and eliminate the infection.

When the innate immune response is unable to control the replication of a pathogen, the adaptive immune response is engaged and activated by the innate immune response in an antigen-specific manner. Typically, it takes 1-2 weeks after the primary infection for the adaptive immune response to begin clearance of the infection through the action of effector cells and antibodies.

Once an infection has been cleared, both the innate and adaptive immune responses cease. Antibodies and residual effector cells continue to provide protective immunity, while memory cells provide long-term immunologic protection from subsequent infection.

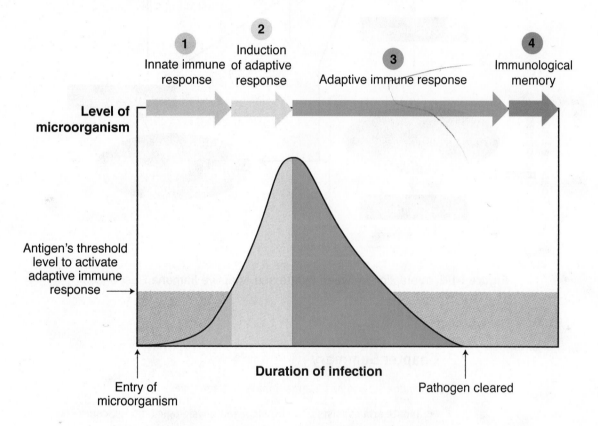

Figure I-1-1. Timeline of the Immune Response to an Acute Infection

The innate and adaptive immune responses do not act independently of one another; rather, they work by a positive feedback mechanism.

- Phagocytic cells recognize pathogens by binding PAMPs through various pattern-recognition receptors leading to phagocytosis.

- Phagocytic cells process and present antigen to facilitate stimulation of specific T lymphocytes with subsequent release of cytokines that trigger initiation of specific immune responses.

- T lymphocytes produce cytokines that enhance microbicidal activities of phagocytes.

- Cytokines released by phagocytes and T lymphocytes will drive differentiation of B lymphocytes into plasma cells and isotype switching.

- Antibodies will aid in the destruction of pathogen through opsonization, complement activation and antibody-dependent cellular cytotoxicity.

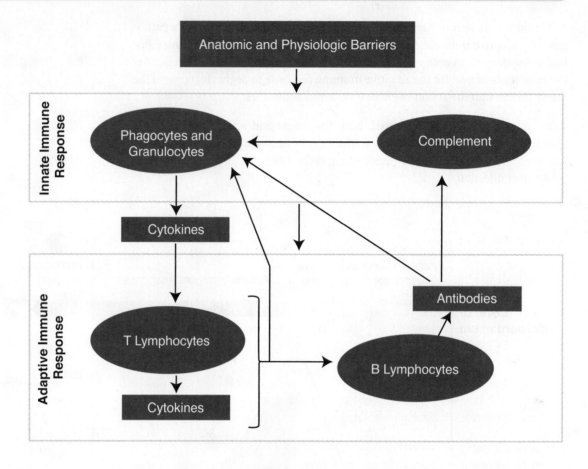

Figure I-1-2. Interaction between Innate and Adaptive Immune Responses

Chapter Summary

The immune system has 2 arms: innate and adaptive.

- **Innate arm** consists of anatomical and physiologic barriers, complement, phagocytes and granulocytes and inflammatory components

  - Innate arm is present intrinsically, has limited specificity and diversity, and is not enhanced by repeated exposure

- **Adaptive arm** consists of T and B lymphocytes

  - Adaptive immune responses are specific, diverse, self-limiting, capable of self- versus non-self-recognition, and display memory

Learning Objectives

❏ Explain information related to origin and function of cells of the immune system

❏ Explain information related to antigen recognition molecules of lymphocytes

❏ Answer questions about the generation of receptor diversity

ORIGIN

Hematopoiesis involves the production, development, differentiation, and maturation of the blood cells (erythrocytes, megakaryocytes and leukocytes) from **multipotent stem cells**. The site of hematopoiesis changes during development.

During embryogenesis and early fetal development, the yolk sac is the site of hematopoiesis. Once organogenesis begins, hematopoiesis shifts to the liver and spleen, and finally, to the bone marrow where it will remain throughout adulthood.

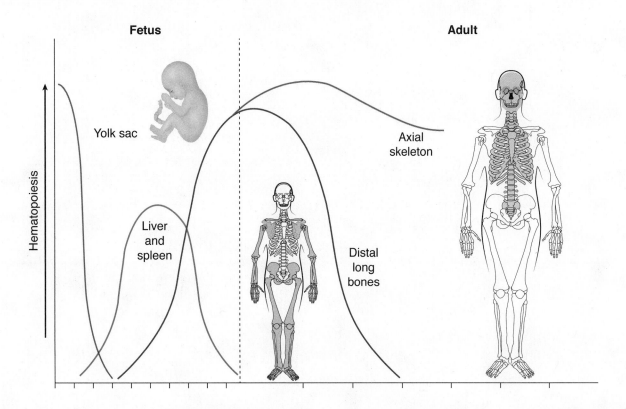

Figure I-2-1. Sites of Hematopoiesis during Development

These **multipotent stem cells** found in the bone marrow have the ability to undergo asymmetric division. One of the 2 daughter cells will serve to renew the population of stem cells (**self-renewal**), while the other can give rise to either a common lymphoid progenitor cell or a common myeloid progenitor cell (**potency**). The multipotent stem cells will differentiate into the various lymphoid and myeloid cells in response to various cytokines and growth factors.

- The **common lymphoid progenitor cell** gives rise to B lymphocytes, T lymphocytes and natural killer (NK) cells.

- The **common myeloid progenitor cell** gives rise to erythrocytes, megakaryocytes/thrombocytes, mast cells, eosinophils, basophils, neutrophils, monocytes/macrophages and dendritic cells.

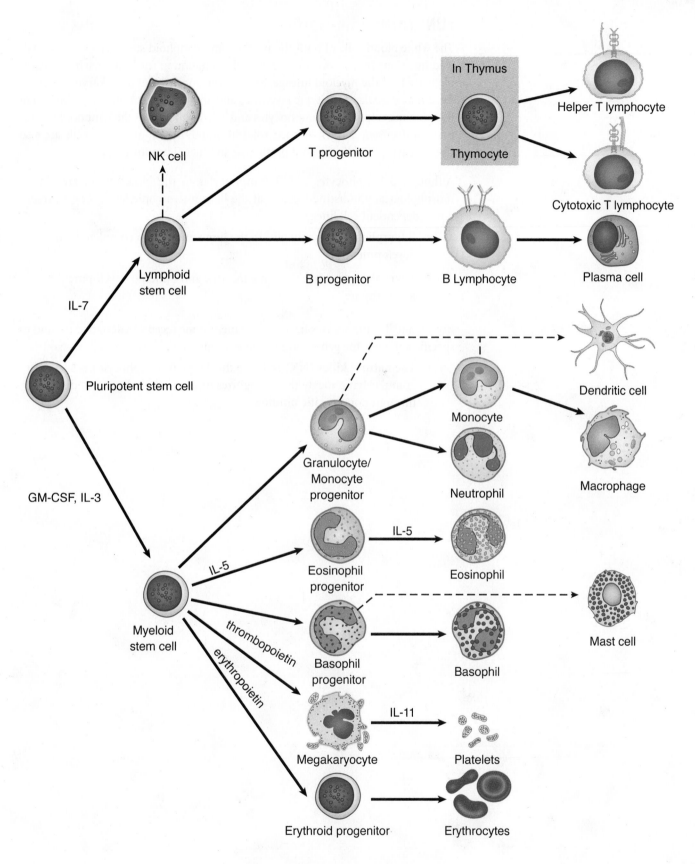

Figure I-2-2. Ontogeny of Immune Cells

FUNCTION

The white blood cells of both the myeloid and lymphoid stem cells have specialized functions in the body once their differentiation in the bone marrow is complete. Cells of the myeloid lineage, except erythrocytes and megakaryocytes, perform non-specific, stereotypic responses and are members of the innate branch of the immune response. B lymphocytes and T lymphocytes of the lymphoid lineage perform focused, antigen-specific roles in immunity. Natural killer cells are also from the lymphoid lineage but participate in innate immunity.

Although B lymphocytes and T lymphocytes in the bloodstream are almost morphologically indistinguishable at the light microscopic level, they represent 2 interdependent cell lineages.

- **B lymphocytes** remain within the **bone marrow** to complete their development.

- **T lymphocytes** leave the bone marrow and undergo development within the **thymus**.

Both B and T lymphocytes have surface membrane receptors designed to bind to specific antigens; the generation of these receptors will be discussed in chapter 4.

- The **natural killer (NK) cell** (the third type of lymphocyte) is a large granular lymphocyte that recognizes tumor and virally infected cells through non-specific binding.

Table I-2-1. White Blood Cells

(Order is based on relative percentages as they appear in the blood)

Myeloid Cell	Tissue Location	Physical Description	Function
Neutrophil or polymorpho-nuclear (PMN) cell	Most abundant circulating blood cell	Granulocyte with a segmented, lobular nuclei (3–5 lobes) and small pink cyto-plasmic granules	Phagocytic activity aimed at killing extracellular pathogens

Lymphoid Cell	Tissue Location	Physical Description	Function

Lymphocyte	Bloodstream, secondary lym-phoid tissues	Large, dark-staining nucleus with a thin rim of cytoplasm
		
		Surface markers:
		  B lymphocytes
		    – CD19, 20, 21
		  T lymphocytes
		    – CD3
		  Helper T cells
		    – CD4
		  CTLs
		    – CD8
			No function until activated in the secondary lymphoid tissues

Plasma cell	Bloodstream, sec-ondary lymphoid tissue and bone marrow	Small eccentric nucleus, intensely staining Golgi ap-paratus	Terminally differentiated B lymphocyte that secretes antibodies
Natural killer cell	Bloodstream	Lymphocyte with large cytoplasmic granules Surface markers: CD16, 56	Kills virally infected cells and tumor cells

(Continued)

Table I-2-1. White Blood Cells (*cont'd*)

Myeloid Cell	Tissue Location	Physical Description	Function
Monocyte	Circulating blood cell	Agranulocyte with a bean or kidney-shaped nucleus	Precursor of tissue macrophage
Macrophage	Resident in all tissues	Agranulocyte with a ruffled cytoplasmic membrane and cytoplasmic vacuoles and vesicles	• Phagocyte • Professional antigen presenting cell • T-cell activator
Dendritic cell	Resident in epithelial and lymphoid tissue	Agranulocyte with thin, stellate cytoplasmic projections	• Phagocyte • Professional antigen presenting cell • T-cell activator
Eosinophil	Circulating blood cell recruited into loose connective tissue of the respiratory and GI tracts	Granulocyte with bilobed nucleus and large pink cytoplasmic granules	• Elimination of large extracellular parasites • Type I hypersensitivity
Mast cell	Reside in most tissues adjacent to blood vessels	Granulocyte with small nucleus and large blue cytoplasmic granule	• Elimination of large extracellular parasites • Type I hypersensitivity
Basophil	Low frequency circulating blood cell	Granulocyte with bilobed nucleus and large blue cytoplasmic granules	• Elimination of large extracellular parasites • Type I hypersensitivity

Laboratory evaluation of patients commonly involves assessment of white blood cell morphology and relative counts by examination of a blood sample. Changes in the morphology and proportions of white blood cells indicate the presence of some pathologic state. A standard white blood cell differential includes neutrophils, band cells, lymphocytes (B lymphocytes, T lymphocytes, and NK cells), monocytes, eosinophils and basophils.

Table I-2-2. Leukocytes Evaluated in a WBC Differential

Cell Type	Adult Reference Range (%)
Neutrophils (PMNs)	50–70
Band cells	0–5
Lymphocytes	20–40
Monocytes	5–10
Eosinophils	0–5
Basophils	‹1

Chapter Summary

- Site of hematopoiesis changes location through development first in yolk sac, next shifting to the liver and spleen, and then finally to bone marrow

- Cells of the immune system arise from multipotent stem cell in bone marrow

- Common lymphoid progenitor will give rise to B lymphocytes, T lymphocytes, and NK cells

- Common myeloid progenitor will give rise to erythrocytes, megakaryocytes/platelets, monocytes/macrophage, dendritic cells, neutrophils, mast cells, eosinophils, and basophils

Lymphocyte Development and Selection

3

Learning Objectives

❏ Answer questions about selection of T and B lymphocytes

❏ Solve problems concerning innate immunity and components/barriers

ANTIGEN RECOGNITION MOLECULES OF LYMPHOCYTES

Each cell of the lymphoid lineage is clinically identified by the characteristic surface molecules that it possesses.

- The mature, naïve **B lymphocyte**, in its mature ready-to-respond form, expresses 2 isotypes of antibody or immunoglobulin called IgM and IgD within its surface membrane.

- The mature, naive **T cell** expresses a single genetically related molecule, called the **T-cell receptor (TCR)**, on its surface.

Both of these types of antigen receptors are encoded within the immunoglobulin superfamily of genes and are expressed in literally millions of variations in different lymphocytes as a result of complex and random rearrangements of the cells' DNA.

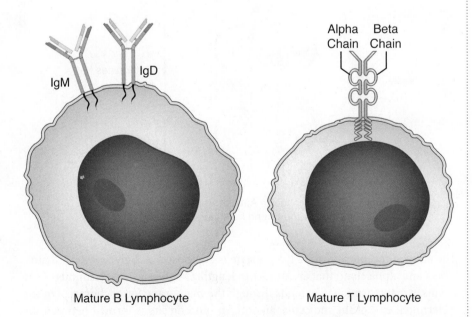

Figure I-3-1. Antigen Receptors of Mature Lymphocytes

The antigen receptor of the B lymphocyte, or **membrane-bound immunoglobulin**, is a 4-chain glycoprotein molecule that serves as the basic monomeric unit for each of the distinct antibody molecules destined to circulate freely in the serum. This monomer has 2 identical halves, each composed of a **heavy chain** and a **light chain**. A cytoplasmic tail on the carboxy-terminus of each heavy chain extends through the plasma membrane and anchors the molecule to the cell surface. The 2 halves are held together by disulfide bonds into a shape resembling a "Y." Some flexibility of movement is permitted between the halves by disulfide bonds forming a **hinge region**.

On the N-terminal end of the molecule where the heavy and light chains lie side by side, an antigen binding site is formed whose 3-dimensional shape will accommodate the noncovalent binding of one, or a very small number, of related antigens. The unique structure of the antigen binding site is called the **idiotype** of the molecule. Although 2 classes **(isotypes)** of membrane immunoglobulin (IgM and IgD) are coexpressed on the surface of a mature, naïve B lymphocyte, only one idiotype or **antigenic specificity** is expressed per cell (although in multiple copies). Each individual is capable of producing hundreds of millions of unique idiotypes.

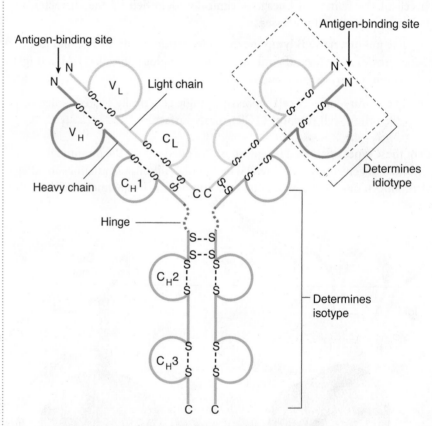

Figure I-3-2. B-Lymphocyte Antigen Recognition Molecule
(Membrane-Bound Immunoglobulin)

The antigen receptor of the T lymphocyte is composed of 2 glycoprotein chains, a beta and alpha chain that are similar in length. On the carboxy-terminus of the chains, a cytoplasmic tail extends through the membrane for anchorage. On the N-terminal end of the molecule, an antigen-binding site is formed between the 2 chains, whose 3-dimensional shape will accommodate the binding of a small antigenic **peptide complexed to an MHC molecule** presented on the surface of an antigen-presenting cell. This groove forms the idiotype of the TCR. There is no hinge region present in this molecule, and thus its conformation is quite rigid.

The membrane receptors of B lymphocytes are designed to bind **unprocessed antigens** of almost any chemical composition, i.e., polysaccharides, proteins, lipids, whereas the TCR is designed to bind only **peptides complexed to MHC**. Also, although the B-cell receptor is ultimately modified to be secreted **antibody**, the TCR is never released from its membrane-bound location.

In association with these unique antigen-recognition molecules on the surface of B and T cells, accessory molecules are intimately associated with the receptors that function in signal transduction. Thus, when a lymphocyte binds to an antigen complementary to its idiotype, a cascade of messages transferred through its **signal transduction complex** will culminate in intracytoplasmic phosphorylation events leading to activation of the cell.

- In the B cell, this signal transduction complex is composed of 2 invariant chains, Ig-alpha and Ig-beta, and a B-cell co-receptor consisting of CD19, CD21 and CD81.

- The B-cell co-receptor is implicated in the attachment of several infectious agents. CD21 is the receptor for EBV and CD81 is the receptor for hepatitis C and *Plasmodium vivax*.

- In the T cell, the signal transduction complex is a multichain structure called CD3.

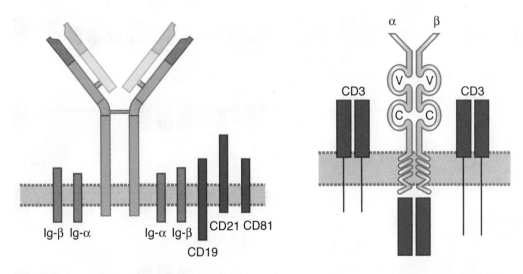

B-Cell Signal Transduction Complex   **T-Cell Signal Transduction Complex**

Figure I-3-3. Lymphocyte Signal Transduction

Table I-3-1. B- versus T-Lymphocyte Antigen Receptors

Property	B-Cell Antigen Receptor	T-Cell Antigen Receptor
Molecules/Lymphocyte	100,000	100,000
Idiotypes/Lymphocyte	1	1
Isotypes/Lymphocyte	2 (IgM and IgD)	1 (α/β)
Is secretion possible?	Yes	No
Number of combining sites/molecule	2	1
Mobility	Flexible (hinge region)	Rigid
Signal-transduction molecules	Ig-α, Ig-β, CD19, CD21	CD3

THE GENERATION OF RECEPTOR DIVERSITY

Because the body requires the ability to respond specifically to millions of potentially harmful agents it may encounter in a lifetime, a mechanism must exist to generate as many idiotypes of antigen receptors as necessary to meet this challenge. If each of these idiotypes were encoded separately in the germline DNA of lymphoid cells, it would require more DNA than is present in the entire cell. The generation of this necessary diversity is accomplished by a complex and unique set of rearrangements of DNA segments that takes place during the maturation of lymphoid cells.

It has been discovered that individuals inherit a large number of different segments of DNA which may be recombined and alternatively spliced to create unique amino acid sequences in the N-terminal ends (**variable domains**) of the chains that compose their antigen recognition sites. For example, to produce the **heavy chain variable domains** of their antigen receptor, B-lymphocyte progenitors select randomly and in the absence of stimulating antigen to recombine 3 gene segments designated variable (V), diversity (D), and joining (J) out of hundreds of germline-encoded possibilities to produce unique sequences of amino acids in the variable domains (VDJ recombination).

An analogous random selection is made during the formation of the beta-chain of the TCR.

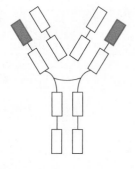

Note

VDJ rearrangements in DNA produce the diversity of heavy chain variable domains.

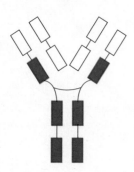

Note

mRNA molecules are created which join this variable domain sequence to μ or δ constant domains.

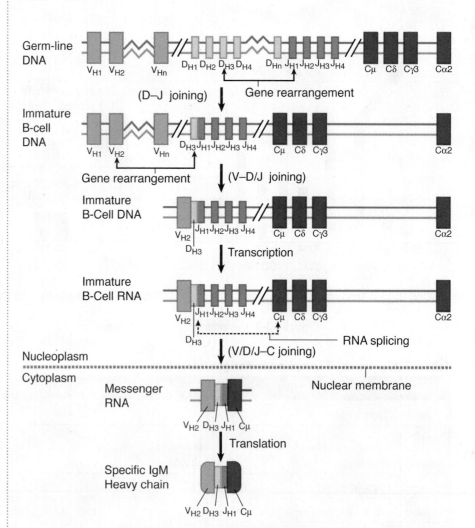

Figure I-3-4. Production of Heavy (B-Cell) or Beta (T-Cell) Chains of Lymphocyte Antigen Receptors

Next, the B-lymphocyte progenitor performs random rearrangements of 2 types of gene segments (V and J) to encode the **variable domain amino acids of the light chain.** An analogous random selection is made during the formation of the alpha-chain of the TCR. The enzymes responsible for these gene rearrangements are encoded by the genes *RAG1* and *RAG2*. The *RAG1* and *RAG2* gene products are 2 proteins found within the recombinase, a protein complex that includes a repair mechanism as well as DNA-modifying enzymes.

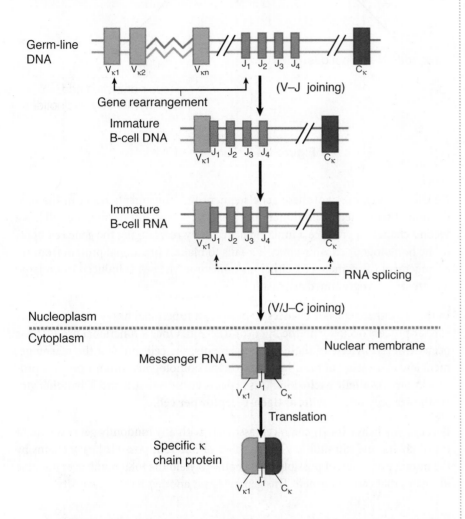

Figure I-3-5. Production of Light (B-Cell) or Alpha (T-Cell) Chain of a Lymphocyte Antigen Receptor

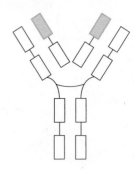

Note

VJ rearrangements in DNA produce the diversity of light chain variable domains.

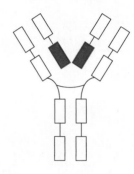

Note

K or λ constant domains are added to complete the light chain.

Bridge to Pathology

Tdt is used as a marker for early stage T- and B-cell development in acute lymphoblastic leukemia.

While heavy chain gene segments are undergoing recombination, the enzyme **terminal deoxyribonucleotidyl transferase** (Tdt) randomly inserts bases (without a template on the complementary strand) at the junctions of V, D, and J segments (**N-nucleotide addition**). The random addition of the nucleotide generates junctional diversity.

When the light chains are rearranged later, Tdt is not active, though it is active during the rearrangement of all gene segments in the formation of the TCR. This generates even more diversity than the random combination of V, D, and J segments alone.

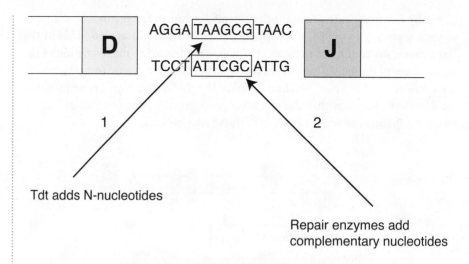

Figure I-3-6. Function of Tdt

Needless to say, many of these gene segment rearrangements result in the production of truncated or nonfunctional proteins. When this occurs, the cell has a second chance to produce a functional strand by rearranging the gene segments of the homologous chromosome. If it fails to make a functional protein from rearrangement of segments on either chromosome, the cell is induced to undergo **apoptosis** or programmed cell death.

In this way, the cell has 2 chances to produce a functional heavy (or β) chain. A similar process occurs with the light (or α) chain. Once a functional product has been achieved by one of these rearrangements, the cell shuts off the rearrangement and expression of the other allele on the homologous chromosome—a process known as **allelic exclusion**. This process ensures that B and T lymphocytes synthesize only **one specific antigen-receptor per cell**.

Because any heavy (or β) chain can associate with any randomly generated light (or α) chain, one can multiply the number of different possible heavy chains by the number of different possible light chains to yield the total number of possible idiotypes that can be formed. This generates yet another level of diversity.

Table I-3-2. Mechanisms for Generating Receptor Diversity

Mechanism	Cell in Which It Is Expressed
Existence in genome of multiple V, D, J segments	B and T cells
VDJ recombination	B and T cells
N-nucleotide addition	B cells (only heavy chain) T cells (all chains)
Combinatorial association of heavy and light chains	B and T cells
Somatic hypermutation	B cells only, after antigen stimulation (*see* Chapter 7)

Downstream on the germline DNA from the rearranged segments, are encoded the amino acid sequences of all the constant domains of the chain. These domains tend to be similar within the classes or isotypes of immunoglobulin or TCR chains and are thus called **constant domains**.

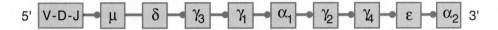

Figure I-3-7. Immunoglobulin Heavy Chain DNA

The first set of constant domains for the heavy chain of immunoglobulin that is transcribed is that of IgM and next, IgD. These 2 sets of domains are alternatively spliced to the variable domain product at the RNA level. There are only 2 isotypes of light chain constant domains, named κ and λ, and one will be combined with the product of light chain variable domain rearrangement to produce the other half of the final molecule. Thus, the B lymphocyte produces IgM and IgD molecules with identical idiotypes and inserts these into the membrane for antigen recognition.

Table I-3-3. Clinical Outcomes of Failed Gene Rearrangement

Clinical Syndrome	Genetics	Molecular Defect	Symptoms
Omenn syndrome	Autosomal recessive	Missense mutation in *RAG* genes The *RAG* enzymes have only partial activity	Lack of B cells (below limits of detection) Marked decrease in predominantly Th2 Characterized by early onset, failure to thrive, red rash (generalized), diarrhea, and severe immune deficiency
Severe combined immunodeficiency (SCID)	Autosomal recessive	Null mutations in *RAG1* or *RAG2* genes No *RAG* enzyme activity	Total lack of B and T cells Total defects in humoral and cell-mediated immunity

SELECTION OF T AND B LYMPHOCYTES

As lymphoid progenitors develop in the bone marrow, they make random rearrangements of their germline DNA to produce the unique idiotypes of antigen-recognition molecules that they will use throughout their lives. The bone marrow, therefore, is considered a **primary lymphoid organ** in humans because it supports and encourages these early developmental changes. B lymphocytes complete their entire formative period in the bone marrow and can be identified in their progress by the immunoglobulin chains they produce.

B Lymphocyte Development

In essence, the rearrangement of the gene segments and the subsequent production of immunoglobulin chains drive B-cell development.

Because these gene segment rearrangements occur randomly and in the absence of stimulation with foreign antigen, it stands to reason that many of the idiotypes of receptors produced could have a binding attraction or **affinity** for normal body constituents. These cells, if allowed to develop further, could develop into self-reactive lymphocytes that could cause harm to the host. Therefore, one of the key roles of the bone marrow stroma and interdigitating cells is to remove such potentially harmful products. Cells whose idiotype has too great an affinity for normal cellular molecules are either deleted in the bone marrow (**clonal deletion**) or inactivated in the periphery (**clonal anergy**). Anergic B cells express high levels of IgD on their surface rendering them inactive. The elimination of self-reactive cells in the bone marrow is intended to minimize the number of self-reactive B-lymphocytes released to the periphery, only those cells that are **selectively unresponsive** (**tolerant**) to self-antigens are allowed to leave the bone marrow.

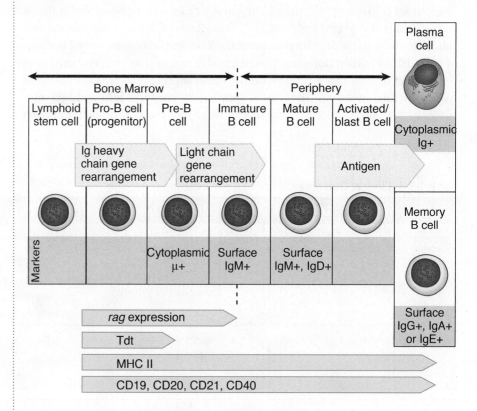

Figure I-3-8. B-Cell Differentiation

T Lymphocyte Development

Immature lymphocytes destined to the T-cell lineage leave the bone marrow and proceed to the **thymus**, the second **primary lymphoid organ** dedicated to the maturation of T cells. These pre-thymic cells are referred to as **double negative** T lymphocytes since they do not express CD4 or CD8 on their surface. The thymus is a bilobed structure located above the heart; it consists of an outer **cortex** packed with immature T cells and an inner **medulla** into which cells pass as they mature. Both the cortex and medulla are laced with a network of epithelial cells, dendritic cells, and macrophages, which interact physically with the developing thymocytes.

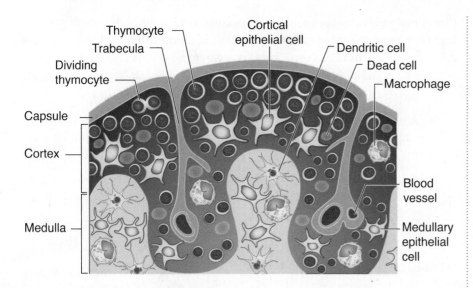

Figure I-3-9. Structure of the Thymus

Within the cortex, the thymocytes will begin to rearrange the beta and alpha chains of the T-cell receptor (TCR) while coexpressing the CD3 complex as well as the CD4 and CD8 co-receptors; these thymocytes are collectively referred to as being **double positive**. As the developing thymocytes begin to express their TCRs, they are subjected to a rigorous 2-step selection process. Because the TCR is designed to bind antigenic peptides presented on the surface of **antigen-presenting cells** (APCs) in the body, a selection process is necessary to remove those cells that would bind to normal self-antigens and cause **autoimmunity,** as well as those that have no attraction whatsoever for the surfaces of APCs. This is accomplished by exposure of developing thymocytes to high levels of a unique group of membrane-bound molecules known as **major histocompatibility complex** (MHC) antigens.

The MHC is a collection of highly polymorphic genes on the short arm of chromosome 6 in the human. There are 2 major classes of cell-bound MHC gene products: I and II. Both class I and class II molecules are expressed at high density on the surface of cells of the thymic stroma. MHC gene products are also called human leukocyte antigens (HLA).

- **Class I** MHC gene products: HLA-A, HLA-B, HLA-C

- **Class II** MHC gene products: HLA-DM, HLA-DP, HLA-DQ, HLA-DR

Table I-3-4. Class I and II Gene Products

Class I Gene Products			Class II Gene Products			
HLA-A	HLA-B	HLA-C	HLA-DM*	HLA-DP	HLA-DQ	HLA-DR

*HLA-DM is not a cell surface molecule but functions as a molecular chaperone to promote proper peptide loading.

Class I molecules are expressed on all nucleated cells in the body, as well as platelets. They are expressed in **codominant** fashion, meaning that each cell expresses 2 A, 2 B, and 2 C products (one from each parent).

- The molecules (A, B, and C) consist of an α heavy chain with 3 extracellular domains and an intracytoplasmic carboxy-terminus.

- A second light chain, β_2-microglobulin, is not encoded within the MHC and functions in peptide-loading and transport of the class I antigen to the cell surface.

- A groove between the first 2 extracellular domains of the α chain is designed to accommodate small peptides to be presented to the TCR.

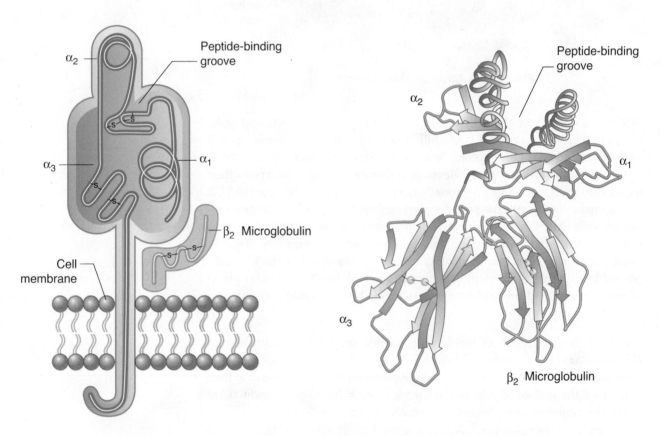

Figure I-3-10. Class I MHC Molecule (left) and X-Ray Crystallographic Image (right) of Class I MHC Peptide-Binding Groove

Class II MHC molecules are expressed (also **codominantly**) on the professional antigen-presenting cells of the body (primarily the macrophages, B lymphocytes, and dendritic cells).

- The molecules are 2 chain structures of similar length, called α and β, each possessing 2 extracellular domains and 1 intracytoplasmic domain.

- A groove that will accommodate peptides to be presented to the TCR is formed at the N-terminal end of both chains.

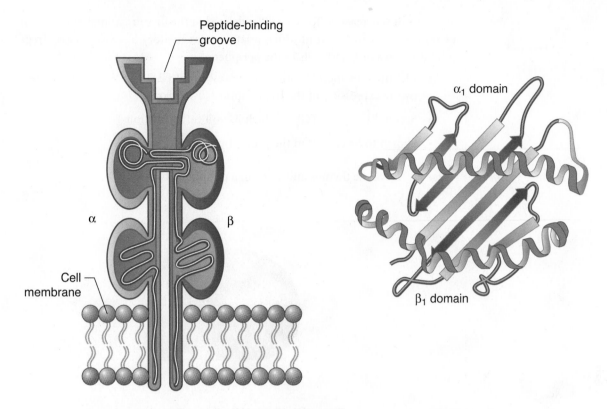

Figure I-3-11. Class II MHC Molecule (left), and X-ray Crystallographic Image (right) of Class II MHC Peptide-Binding Groove

Within the thymus, each of these MHC products, loaded with normal self-peptides, is presented to the developing double positive thymocytes.

- Those that have TCRs capable of binding with low affinity will receive a **positive selection** signal to divide and establish clones that will eventually mature in the medulla.

- Those that fail to recognize self-MHC at all will not be encouraged to mature (**failure of positive selection**).

- Those that bind too strongly to self MHC molecules and self-peptide will be induced to undergo apoptosis (**negative selection**) because these cells would have the potential to cause autoimmune disease.

Although double positive thymocytes co-express **CD4** and **CD8**, the cells are directed to express only CD8 if their TCR binds class I molecules, and only CD4 if their TCR binds class II molecules. At this point in T-cell development, the thymocytes are referred to as being **single positive**.

This selection process is an extraordinarily rigorous one. A total of 95–99% of all T-cell precursors entering the thymus are destined to die there. Only those with TCRs appropriate to protect the host from foreign invaders will be permitted to exit to the periphery: CD4+ cells that recognize class II MHC are destined to become **"helper" T cells** (Th), and CD8+ cells that recognize class I MHC are destined to become **cytotoxic T lymphocytes** (CTLs).

While most self-reactive T cells will be deleted in the thymus, a small population of these T cells will instead differentiate into regulatory T cells (Tregs). Tregs inhibit self-reactive Th1 cells in the periphery.

- Identified by their constitutive expression of CD25 on the surface and by the expression of the transcription factor FoxP3

- Secrete IL-10 and TGF-β which inhibit inflammation

- Shown to be critical in the prevention of autoimmunity

Tregs will leave the thymus and serve in a peripheral tolerance.

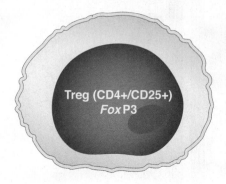

Figure I-3-12. Identification of Treg Cells

Markers	Pre-thymic	Thymic Cortex		Thymic Medulla	Circulating T Cells
Tdt					
rag expression					
CD2					
CD3					
TCR					
CD4					
+					
CD8					

Figure I-3-13. Human T-Cell Differentiation

Chapter Summary

- The antigen receptor of the B lymphocyte is membrane-bound IgM and IgD and is designed to bind unprocessed antigens of almost any chemical composition.

- The antigen receptor of the T lymphocyte is composed of two chains (α/β) and is designed to recognize cell-bound peptides.

- B-cell antigen receptors can be secreted, whereas T-cell receptors are always cell-bound.

- The antigen receptors of B and T cells are associated with signal transduction molecules: Igα, Igβ, CD19, CD21, and CD81 for B cells and CD3 for T cells.

- The diversity of idiotypes of antigen-combining sites is generated by rearrangements of gene segments coding for variable domain amino acids and is assisted by the action of the enzyme terminal deoxyribonucleotidyl transferase.

- Allelic exclusion is the process by which one chromosome of a homologous pair will be inactivated, ensuring that only one idiotype of antigen-recognition molecule will be produced per cell.

- The bone marrow and thymus are primary lymphoid organs in which the early development and selection of lymphocytes occurs (lymphopoiesis).

- Self-tolerance is induced by deletion of self-reactive β cells in the bone marrow (clonal deletion) or inactivation of self-reactive cells in the periphery (clonal anergy).

- T-cell precursors move from the bone marrow to the thymus where they are selected for self-tolerance by exposure to major histocompatibility complex (MHC) antigens on stromal cells.

- Class I MHC products are two chain structures: the α chain is encoded within the MHC and β_2-microglobulin is not.

- Class I MHC products are expressed on all nucleated cells of the body in a codominant fashion.

- Class II MHC products are 2 chain structures of which both α and β chains are encoded within the MHC.

- Class II MHC products are expressed on antigen-presenting cells in a codominant fashion.

- Thymocytes with antigen receptors that can recognize "altered" self are encouraged to clone themselves and mature (positive selection) and express CD4 molecules if their affinity is for MHC class II. These will become helper T cells.

- Thymocytes with antigen receptors that can recognize "altered" self are encouraged to clone themselves and mature (positive selection) and express CD8 molecules if their affinity is for MHC class I. These will become cytotoxic T lymphocytes.

- Thymocytes with antigen receptors that bind self-peptides presented in the groove of MHC I or II molecules will be induced to undergo apoptosis (negative selection).

- Thymocytes with antigen receptors that have no binding affinity whatsoever for classes I or II MHC are not directed to mature further (failure of positive selection).

Periphery: Innate Immune Response

4

Learning Objectives

❏ Describe the structure and function of secondary lymphoid organs

❏ Describe the structure of lymph nodes

❏ Answer questions about chemokines and adhesion molecules

INNATE IMMUNITY

The innate immune system is an important part of any immune response. It is responsible for reacting quickly to invading microbes and for keeping the host alive while the adaptive immune system is developing a very specific response. The innate immune defenses are all present at birth; they have a very limited diversity for antigen, and they attack the microbes with the same basic vigor no matter how many times they have seen the same pathogen.

The innate immune system handles pathogens in 2 general ways:

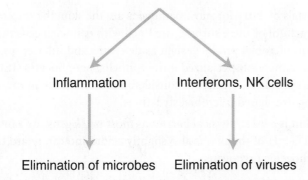

Figure I-4-1. Pathogen Clearance by the Innate Immune System

Microbes may gain access to the tissues if the physical barriers are breached. In the tissues, they come in contact with phagocytic cells such as neutrophils, macrophages and dendritic cells, which will produce chemical messengers called **cytokines** that can initiate an inflammatory response.

Many times the innate immune components are enough to eliminate the pathogen, but not always. The pathogens may gain access to the blood, in which the alternate pathway for complement activation may provide some additional help. But this is where the adaptive immune system may have to take over to resolve the infection and eliminate the pathogen.

Portals of entry for microbes (physical barriers)

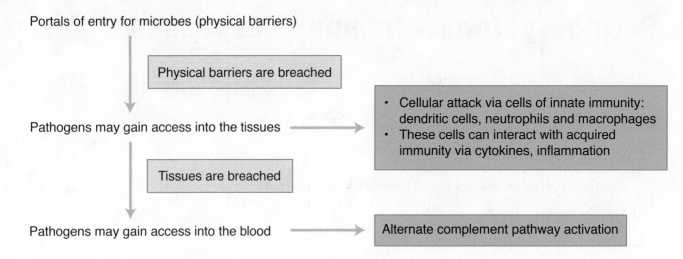

Figure I-4-2. Entry Sites for Pathogens

INNATE IMMUNE COMPONENTS/BARRIERS

There are several components to the innate immune response that are essential for this early defense against pathogens. They will be introduced here and discussed in more depth later in this chapter. They include **physical (anatomic) barriers, physiologic barriers, innate cellular response**, and **inflammation**.

Anatomic Barriers

The main portals of entry for most pathogens are the skin, the respiratory tract, and the GI tract. All of these surfaces are lined with epithelial cells that can produce a few antimicrobial products such as defensins and interferons. They may also contain a number of specialized intra-epithelial lymphocytes (IEL) called $\gamma\delta$ T cells. These specialized T cells are considered part of innate immunity as they can only recognize shared microbial structures.

- The skin is a great physical barrier as most pathogens can't invade intact skin. The pH of the skin is also slightly acidic and can retard the growth of pathogenic organisms.

- The respiratory tract is lined with cilia that physically attempt to remove microbes as they enter. Saliva and mucous are also difficult environments for microbes to live in, as there are many antimicrobial enzymes and chemicals within those entities.

- The GI tract is also a mucous membrane with similar properties to the respiratory tract; however, pathogens that enter here must first survive a trip through the stomach with a highly acidic pH that kills many microorganisms.

Physiologic Barriers

Physiologic barriers include the following components:

- **Temperature**
  - Many microbial pathogens can't survive much past human body temperature. When the inflammatory response is initiated in the local tissues, cytokines may act systemically to alter the temperature set point in the hypothalamus resulting in fever.

- **pH**
  - The acidic pH of the stomach impedes the growth and transmission to the gut of many pathogens.
  - The skin is also acidic and retards the growth of many microorganisms.

- **Chemical**
  - Lysozyme present in secretions such as tears, saliva, breast milk and mucous can break down the cell wall peptidoglycan of bacteria.
  - Defensins found within phagocytes can form pores in bacteria and fungi.

- **Interferons**
  - IFN-α and IFN-β are anti-viral interferons. They have a direct anti-viral effect by transiently inhibiting nascent protein synthesis in cells.

Innate Cellular Response

Phagocytic cells (monocytes/macrophages, neutrophils and dendritic cells) are part of the first line of defense against invading pathogens. They recognize pathogens via shared molecules that are not expressed on host cells. They are responsible for controlling the infections and sometimes are even capable of eradicating them.

Receptors of the innate immune system are referred to as **pattern recognition receptors (PRRs)**. PRRs recognize **pathogen-associated molecular patterns (PAMPs),** molecules that are shared by pathogens of the same type (bacterial LPS, n-formyl peptides etc.) or **damage-associated molecular patterns (DAMPs)** released from dying or damaged cells. These receptors are present intrinsically, encoded in the germline genes, and are not generated through somatic recombination as the lymphocyte receptors are generated.

The innate immune system can recognize <1,000 patterns on various pathogens, compared to the adaptive immune system (B and T cells) which can recognize over 1 billion specific sequences on pathogens.

Inflammasome

The inflammasome is an important part of the innate immune system. It is expressed in myeloid cells as a signalling system for detection of pathogens and stressors. Activation of the inflammasome results in the production of IL-1β and IL-18, which are potent inflammatory cytokines.

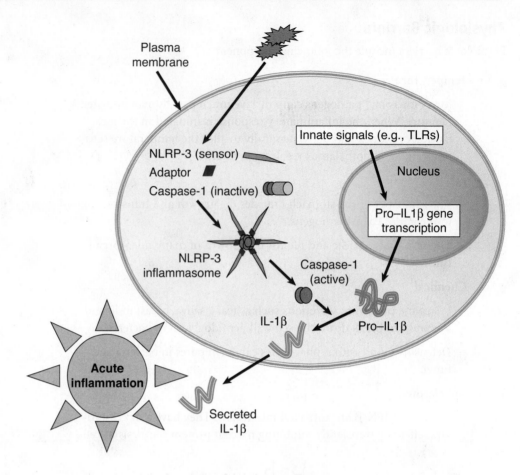

Figure I-4-3. Inflammasome

Table I-4-1. Receptors of the Innate Immune System

Receptor Type	Location in Cell	Receptor Name	Pathogen Target	Downstream Effects
Toll-like receptors (TLR)	Extracellular	TLR-1, 2, 6	Bacterial lipopeptides	Activation of transcription factors (including NF-κB) which results in the transcription of cytokines, adhesion molecules, and enzymes that are antimicrobial
		TLR-2	Bacterial peptidoglycan	
		TLR-4	Lipopolysaccharide (LPS)	
		TLR-5	Flagellin	
	Intracellular (endosomal)	TLR-3	DS RNA	
		TLR-7,8	SS RNA	
		TLR-9	Unmethylated CpG oligonucleotides	
NOD-like receptors (NLR)	Intracellular (cytosolic)	NOD1, NOD2	Components of bacterial PG	Signals via NF-κB result in macrophage activation
		NLRP-3	Microbial products and molecules from damaged or dying cells (ATP, uric acid crystals, reactive oxygen species)	Inflammasome NLRP-3 (sensor) + adaptor protein links procaspase 1 and activates it to caspase 1; it is the caspase that cleaves the pro-IL-1β to generate IL-1β
RIG-like receptors (RLR)	Cytoplasmic	RIG-1, MDA-5	Viral RNA	Interferon production

Clinical Correlate

Mutations in Innate Immune Receptors and Correlation with Disease

Mutation	Effect
Mutation in signaling molecules effecting TLRs	Recurrent, severe bacterial infections (pneumonia)
Gain of function mutations in inflammasome	• Gout • Atheroscleosis • Type II diabetes
NOD-2 mutations	IBD
• IL-12 receptor deficiency • IFN-γ receptor deficiency	Recurrent infections with intracellular bacteria (*Mycobacterium*)

Table I-4-2. Myeloid Cells

Myeloid Cell	Tissue Location	Identification	Function
Monocyte	Bloodstream, 0–900/μL	Kidney bean-shaped nucleus, CD14 positive	Phagocytic, differentiate into tissue macrophages
Macrophage	Tissues	Ruffled membrane, cytoplasm with vacuoles and vesicles, CD14 positive	Phagocytosis, secretion of cytokines
Neutrophil	Bloodstream, 1,800–7,800/μL	Multilobed nucleus; small light pink to purple granules CD14 positive	Phagocytosis and activation of bactericidal mechanisms

Cells of Innate Immunity

Neutrophils

- Circulating phagocytes
- Short lived
- Rapid response, not prolonged defense

Monocytes/Macrophages

- Monocytes circulate in the blood, become macrophages in the tissues
- Provide a prolonged defense
- Produce cytokines that initiate and regulate inflammation
- Phagocytose pathogens
- Clear dead tissue and initiate tissue repair
- Macophages will develop along one of 2 different pathways

Table I-4-3. Pathways for Macrophage Activation

Classical M1	Alternative M2
Induced by innate immunity (TLRs, IFN-γ)	Induced by IL-4, IL-13
Phagocytosis, initiate inflammatory response	Tissue repair and control of inflammation

Table I-4-4. Additional Myeloid Cells

Myeloid Cell	Tissue Location	Identification	Function
Dendritic Cells	Epithelia, tissues	Long cytoplasmic arms CD14 positive	Antigen capture, transport, and presentation, initiate inflammation
Mast Cells	Tissues, mucosa, epithelia	Small nucleus, cytoplasm packed with large blue granules	Release of granules containing histamine, etc., during allergic responses
Natural killer Lymphocyte	Lymph nodes, spleen, mucosal-associated lymphoid tissues, bone marrow	Lymphocytes with large cytoplasmic granules CD16 + CD56 positive	Kill tumor/virus cell targets or antibody-coated target cells, secretion of IFN-γ

Dendritic cells (DCs)

- Found in all tissues
- Antigen processing and presentation
- Two major functions: initiate inflammatory response and stimulate adaptive immune response

Mast cells

- Skin, mucosa
- 2 pathways for activation: innate TLRs and antibody-dependent (IgE)

Natural killer cells (NK cells)

- Blood, periphery
- Direct lysis of cells, secretion of IFN-γ

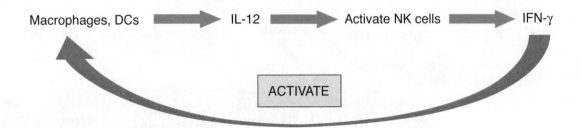

Figure I-4-4. Collaboration of Macrophages and NK Cells

INFLAMMATORY RESPONSE

Complement

The complement system is a set of interacting proteins released into the blood after production in the liver. The components act together as zymogens, activating one another in cascade fashion after initiation from a variety of stimuli. Three pathways of activation occur in the body and culminate similarly in the production of important split products that mediate inflammation, enhance phagocytosis by opsonization, and cause lysis of particles by membrane pore formation.

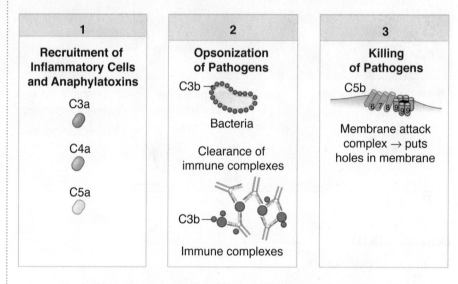

Figure I-4-5. Three Functions of the Complement System

Two of the pathways are considered part of the innate immune system: the alternate pathway and the lectin-binding or mannose-binding pathway (MBP). The alternate pathway for complement activation is shown below; the MBP activates the classical complement pathway but without the use of antibody, and is therefore considered part of innate immunity. The MBP is activated when mannose-binding lectin binds to carbohydrates on the pathogen.

The alternative pathway of complement activation is probably the more primitive of the pathways because it is initiated by simple attraction of the early factors to the surfaces of microbes. Bacterial polysaccharides and the lipopolysaccharide of the cell envelope of gram-negative bacteria both serve as potent, initiating stimuli.

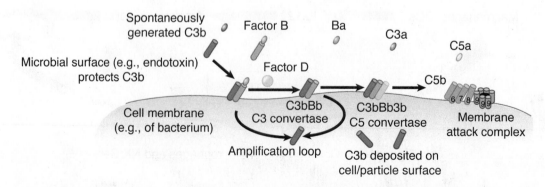

Figure I-4-6. The Alternative Complement Pathway

Acute Inflammatory Response

Antigens are normally introduced into the body across the mucosa or the epithelia. The **acute inflammatory response** is often the first response to this invasion and represents a response of the innate immune system to block the challenge.

The first step in the acute inflammatory response is activation of the vascular endothelium in the breached epithelial barrier. Cytokines and other inflammatory mediators released in the area as a result of tissue damage induce expression of selectin-type adhesion molecules on the endothelial cells. Neutrophils are the first cells to bind to the inflamed endothelium and extravasate into the tissues, peaking within 6 hours. Monocytes, macrophages, and even eosinophils may arrive 5–6 hours later in response to neutrophil-released mediators.

The extravasation of phagocytes into the area requires **4 sequential, overlapping steps**:

Step 1: Rolling

Phagocytes attach loosely to the endothelium by low-affinity, selectin-carbohydrate interactions. E-selectin molecules on the endothelium bind to mucin-like adhesion molecules on the phagocyte membrane and bind the cell briefly, but the force of blood flow into the area causes the cell to detach and reattach repeatedly, rolling along the endothelial surface until stronger binding forces can be elicited.

Step 2: Activation by chemo-attractants

Chemokines released in the area during inflammation, such as interleukin 8 (IL-8), complement split product C5a, and N-formyl peptides produced by bacteria bind to receptors on the phagocyte surface and trigger a G-protein–mediated activating signal. This signal induces a conformational change in integrin molecules in the phagocyte membrane that increases their affinity for immunoglobulin-superfamily adhesion molecules on the endothelium.

Step 3: Arrest and adhesion

Interaction between integrins and Ig-superfamily cellular adhesion molecules (Ig-CAMs) mediates the tight binding of the phagocyte to the endothelial cell. These integrin-IgCAM interactions also mediate the tight binding of phagocytes and their movement through the extracellular matrix.

Step 4: Transendothelial migration

The phagocyte extends pseudopodia through the vessel wall and extravasates into the tissues.

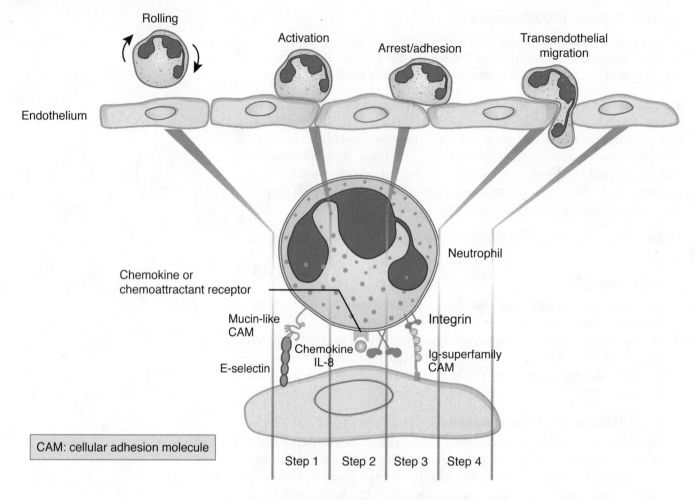

Figure I-4-7. Steps of Phagocyte Extravasation

Clinical Correlate

Leukocyte adhesion deficiency (LAD) is a rare autosomal recessive disease in which there is an absence of **CD18** (the common β_2 chain of a number of integrin molecules). A key element in the migration of leukocytes is integrin-mediated cell adhesion; patients suffer from an inability of their leukocytes to undergo adhesion-dependent migration into sites of inflammation. The first indication of this defect is often omphalitis, a swelling and reddening around the stalk of the umbilical cord.

- Patients are no more susceptible to viral infection than are normal controls, but they suffer recurrent, chronic bacterial infections.

- Patients frequently have abnormally high numbers of granulocytes in their circulation, but migration into sites of infection is not possible, so **abscess and pus formation do not occur**.

- One method for diagnosing LAD involves evaluating expression (or lack) of the β chain (CD18) of the integrin by flow cytometry.

- Bacterial infections in LAD patients can be treated with antibiotics but they recur. If a suitable bone marrow donor can be found, the hematopoietic system of the patient is destroyed with cytotoxic chemicals and a bone marrow transplant is performed.

Once in the tissues, neutrophils express increased levels of receptors for chemo-attractants and exhibit chemotaxis migrating up a concentration gradient toward the attractant. Neutrophils release chemoattractive factors that call in other phagocytes.

Table I-4-5. Chemoattractive Molecules

Chemoattractive Molecule	Origin
Chemokines (IL-8)	Tissue mast cells, platelets, neutrophils, **monocytes**, **macrophages**, eosinophils, basophils, lymphocytes
Complement split product C5a	Classical or alternative pathways
Leukotriene B$_4$	Membrane phospholipids of macrophages, monocytes, neutrophils, mast cells → arachidonic acid cascade → lipoxygenase pathway
Formyl methionyl peptides	Released from microorganisms

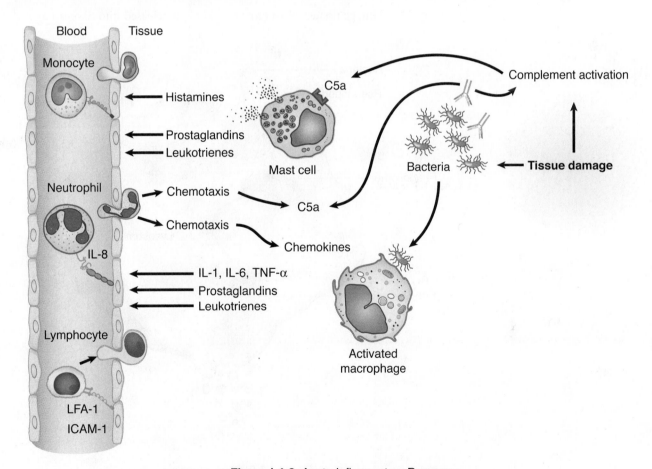

Figure I-4-8. Acute Inflammatory Response

Phagocytosis

Once chemotaxis of phagocytic cells into the area of antigen entry is accomplished, these cells ingest and digest particulate debris, such as microorganisms, host cellular debris, and activated clotting factors. This process, called phagocytosis, involves the following:

- Extension of pseudopodia to engulf attached material

- Fusion of the pseudopodia to trap the material in a phagosome

- Fusion of the phagosome with a lysosome to create a phagolysosome

- Digestion

- Exocytosis of digested contents

Neutrophils release granule contents into extracellular milieu during phagocytosis and inflammation in which the neutrophils die, forming what is known as pus. They extrude nuclear contents, histones, neutrophil extracellular traps (NETs) which function to:

- Trap and kill pathogens

- May damage tissues when enzymes, ROS get released into tissues

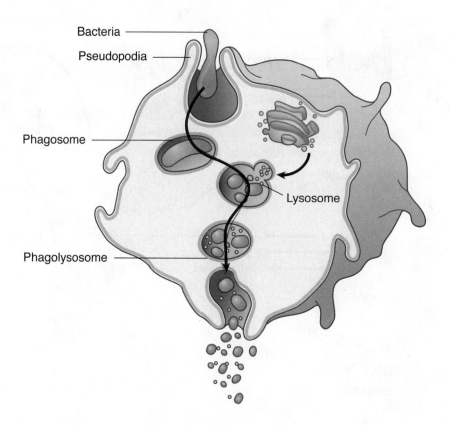

Figure I-4-9. Phagocytosis

Opsonization

Both macrophages and neutrophils have membrane receptors for certain types of antibody (IgG) and certain complement components (C3b). If an antigen is coated with either of these materials, adherence and phagocytosis may be enhanced by up to 4,000-fold. Thus, antibody and complement are called **opsonins**, and the means by which they enhance phagocytosis is called opsonization.

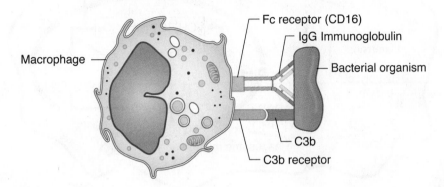

Figure I-4-10. Opsonization of Bacteria with Antibody and Complement C3b

Intracellular Killing

During phagocytosis, a metabolic process known as the respiratory burst activates a membrane-bound oxidase that generates oxygen metabolites, which are toxic to ingested microorganisms. Two oxygen-dependent mechanisms of intracellular digestion are activated as a result of this process.

- NADPH oxidase reduces oxygen to superoxide anion, which generates hydroxyl radicals and hydrogen peroxide, which are microbicidal.

- Myeloperoxidase in the lysosomes acts on hydrogen peroxide and chloride ions to produce hypochlorite (the active ingredient in household bleach), which is microbicidal.

Additionally, reactive nitrogen intermediates play an important role. Inducible nitric oxide synthase converts arginine to nitric oxide, which has potent antimicrobial properties.

The lysosomal contents of phagocytes contain oxygen-independent degradative materials:

- Lysozyme digests bacterial cell walls by cleaving peptidoglycan

- Defensins form channels in bacterial cell membranes

- Lactoferrin chelates iron

- Hydrolytic enzymes

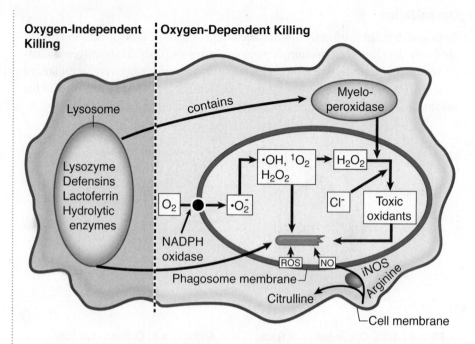

Oxygen-Independent Killing | **Oxygen-Dependent Killing**

Figure I-4-11. Metabolic Stimulation and Killing Within the Phagocyte

Systemic Inflammation

During the acute inflammatory response, pro-inflammatory cytokines such as IL-1, IL-6 and TNF-α are produced. These cytokines have systemic effects on the tissues, including fever, production of acute phase proteins, and leukocytosis.

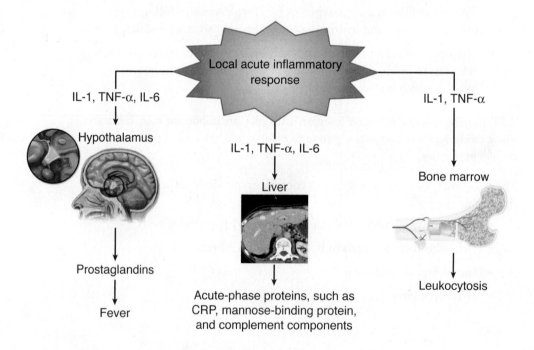

Figure I-4-12. Systemic Inflammatory Response

Clinical Correlate

When defects prevent phagocytes from performing their critical functions as first responders and intracellular destroyers of invading antigens, clinically important pathologic processes ensue. Such defects tend to make the patient susceptible to severe infections with **extracellular bacteria** and **fungi**.

Chronic granulomatous disease (CGD) is an inherited deficiency in the production of one of several subunits of **NADPH oxidase**. This defect eliminates the phagocyte's ability to produce many critical oxygen-dependent intracellular metabolites ($\cdot O_2^-$, $\cdot OH$, $^1O_2$, and H_2O_2). The 2 other intracellular killing mechanisms remain intact (myeloperoxidase + $H_2O_2 \rightarrow$ HOCl and lysosomal contents).

- If the patient is infected with a catalase-negative organism, the H_2O_2 waste product produced by the bacterium can be used as a substrate for myeloperoxidase, and the bacterium is killed.

- If the patient is infected with a catalase-positive organism (e.g., *Staphylococcus, Klebsiella, Serratia, Aspergillus*), the myeloperoxidase system lacks its substrate (because these organisms destroy H_2O_2), and the patient is left with the oxygen-independent lysosomal mechanisms that prove inadequate to control rampant infections. Thus, CGD patients suffer from chronic, recurrent infections with **catalase-positive** organisms.

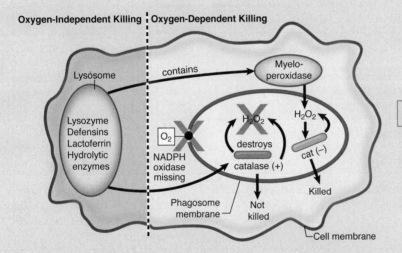

Intracellular Killing in CGD

Failures of phagocytic cells to generate oxygen radicals are easily detected by the nitroblue tetrazolium (NBT) reduction test or neutrophil oxidative index (NOI; a flow cytometric assay). The dihydrorhodamine test—a similar test using flow cytometry—may also be used.

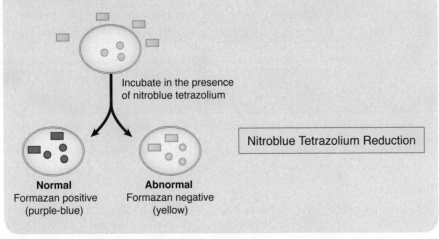

Nitroblue Tetrazolium Reduction

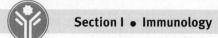

Table I-4-6. Cytokines Involved in Innate Immunity*

Cytokine(s)		Cell Secreted by	Target Cells/Tissues	Activity
Pro-inflammatory cytokines	IL-1	Macrophages	Hypothalmus	Fever
			Endothelial cells	Increases expression of ICAMs
			Liver	Stimulates production of acute phase proteins
	IL-6	Macrophages	Liver	Synthesis of acute phase proteins
	TNF-α	Macrophages	Hypothalamus	Fever
			Endothelial cells	Increases expression of ICAMs
			Liver	Stimulates production of acute phase proteins
			Neutrophils	Activation
			Tumor cells	Apoptosis
			Fat, muscle	Cachexia
Chemokine	IL-8	Macrophages	Leukocytes	Induces adherence to endothelium, chemotaxis, extravasation
IL-12		Macropages, dendritic cells	NK cells	IFN-γ production
IL-15		Macrophages	NK cells	Proliferation
IL-18		Macrophages		IFN-γ synthesis
Regulatory	IL-10	Macrophages, dendritic cells	Macrophages, dendritic cells	Inhibition of IL-12 production, decreased expression of co-stimulatory molecules, decreased class II MHC expression
Type I IFNs	IFN-α	Dendritic cells, macrophages	All cells	Transient inhibition of protein synthesis, increased class I MHC expression
			NK cells	Activation
	IFN-β	Fibroblasts	All cells	Transient inhibition of protein synthesis, increased class I MHC expression
			NK cells	Activation
TGF-β		Macrophages, lymphocytes, etc.		Anti-inflammatory

*Only the innate functions of these cytokines are described here. Many of these cytokines have important functions in the regulation of the adaptive immune response; those will be discussed in subsequent chapters.

Innate Response to Viruses

The innate response to viruses is unique in that it is geared toward eliminating these intracellular pathogens. The 2 major mechanisms for dealing with viral infections are IFN-α/β and NK cells.

Interferons

Interferons (IFNs) are a family of eukaryotic cell proteins classified according to the cell of origin. IFN-α and IFN-β are produced by a variety of virus-infected cells. They do the following:

- Act on target cells to inhibit viral replication, not the virus

- Are not virus-specific

Interferon inhibits viral protein synthesis:

- Activation of an RNA endonuclease, which digests viral RNA

- Phosphorylation of protein kinase, which inactivates eIF2, inhibiting viral protein synthesis

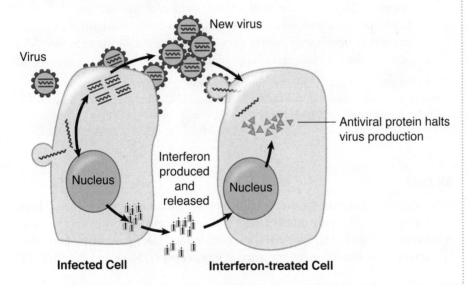

Figure I-4-13. Interferon Production

NK Cells

NK cells are members of the innate branch of the immune response. They exhibit the capacity to kill virally infected cells and tumor cells. They kill via the same mechanisms of inducing apoptosis observed with CTLs (granzymes, perforin). NK activity is increased in the presence of interferons (IFNs) α and β, and IL-12.

NK cells share a common early progenitor with T cells, but they do not develop in the thymus. They do not express antigen-specific receptors or CD3. The markers used clinically to enumerate NK cells include CD16 (FcRγ) and CD56 (CAM). Their recognition of targets is not MHC-restricted, and their activity does not generate immunologic memory.

NK cells employ 2 categories of receptor: **killer activating receptor (KAR)** and **killer inhibitory receptor (KIR)**. If only KARs are engaged, the target cells will be killed. If both the KIRs and the KARs are ligated, the target cell lives. Therefore the inhibitory signals trump the activation signals.

NKG2D is the major KAR expressed by NK cells. There are many ligands for KARs; the MIC glycoproteins are one type. MIC proteins are stress proteins that are expressed only when cells are infected or undergoing transformation. Upon the binding of KAR to a MIC protein, NK cells become cytotoxic, resulting in death of the target cell.

The KIRs activate protein tyrosine phosphatases which inhibit intracellular signaling and activation by removing tyrosine residues from various signaling molecules. The KIRs on the NK cell bind to a specialized type of MHC class I antigens called HLA-E. HLA-E has a ubiquitous tissue distribution, as do the other class I HLA molecules. The HLA-E molecules bind to peptides derived from the leader sequence of HLA-A, -B and –C. HLA-E requires a bound peptide for proper expression within a cell. Therefore, the amount of HLA-E expression on a cell is indicative of the overall well-being of the cell. During viral infections or in transformed cells, the amount of class I HLA expression may be decreased, which would prevent the leader sequences from binding to HLA-E. This would decrease the expression of HLA-E, and make cells susceptible to NK mediated killing.

Interestingly, when NK cells are activated through the FcR (CD16), only one signal is required because the antibody signals that there is an active infection. This occurs through a mechanism called antibody-dependent cell-mediated cytotoxicity (ADCC) (*see* chapter 8).

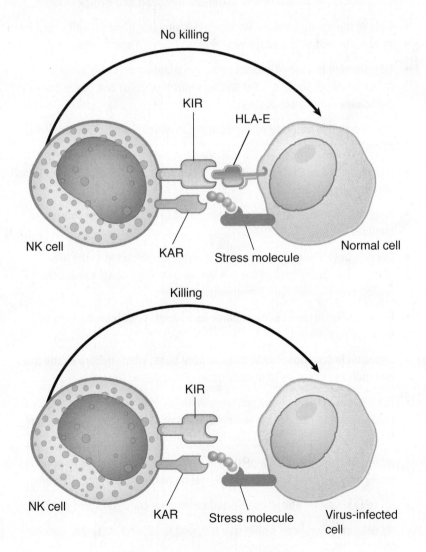

Figure I-4-14. Activation of NK Cells

Chapter Summary

- The innate immune system deals with pathogens in 2 general ways:
  - Inflammation for the elimination of bacteria and other extracellular pathogens
  - Interferons and NK cells for the elimination of viruses

- There are many sites of entry for pathogens to initiate infection. The innate immune system reacts when the physical barriers and tissues are breached with both a cellular attack and activation of the alternate complement pathway.

  - **Inflammasome:** a signaling system for detection of pathogens and stressors which result in the production of IL-1β and Il-18; these cytokines play a major role in the inflammatory response

    ○ The signals which trigger inflammasome activation recognize both microbial products and material from dead and dying cells.

- Cells of the innate immune system (macrophages, dendritic cells, etc.) help to activate cells of the adaptive immune system (B and T cells).

- Complement is a set of interacting serum proteins which enhance inflammation (C3a, C4a, C5a) and opsonization (C3b) and cause lysis of particulate substances (C5b-9).

- The alternative pathway of complement is activated by interaction with microbial surfaces.

- Important chemoattractants include IL-8, C5a, leukotriene B4, and N-formyl methionyl peptides.

- Integrins on the phagocyte membrane bind to Ig-CAMs on endothelia to mediate adhesion.

- Once through the endothelium, phagocytes are attracted to the area of injury by chemokines of the IL-8 family, complement split products, leukotriene B4, and formyl methionyl peptides.

- Opsonization is the coating of particles with IgG or C3b (or both) to enhance engulfment.

- Ingestion is accompanied by a respiratory burst, which generates the toxic metabolites necessary to destroy intracellular materials.

- The systemic inflammatory response is engaged by acute inflammation in the tissues and results in fever, production of acute phase proteins from the liver and leukocytosis via the bone marrow.

- Interferons alpha and beta (IFNα and IFNβ) are proteins released from virally infected cells that afford anti-viral properties to neighboring cells.

- NK cells kill tumor and virus-infected cells using granzymes and perforin.

- NK cells are stimulated by IFN-α, IFN-β, and IL-12, and kill targets lacking MHC I.

Secondary Lymphoid Tissue: Innate Immune Response Meets Adaptive

5

Learning Objectives

❏ Demonstrate understanding of inflammatory response

❏ Solve problems concerning structure of and migration to secondary lymphoid tissue

MIGRATION TO THE SECONDARY LYMPHOID TISSUE

Within a few hours of the initiation of the acute inflammatory response, the professional APCs that have phagocytosed and processed the invading antigen begin to leave the area via lymphatic vessels. Dendritic cells are probably the most efficient of these cells and retract their membranous processes to round up and begin the journey to the closest lymph node (Figure I-5-1).

As discussed earlier, dendritic cells and other phagocytes such as macrophages bind to antigens via PRRs, with a limited diversity, such as the TLRs. The activation of the TLRs induces an acute inflammatory response in the tissue, leading to the production of pro-inflammatory cytokines. These cytokines cause a change in the phenotype of the phagocyte which eventually alters their migration pattern and enhances their function.

Activated dendritic cells will begin to express a chemokine receptor called CCR7. CCR7 is activated by chemokines that are produced by the endothelium.

- Chemokines bind to CCR7 on DCs, allowing them to exit the tissue.

- Upon activation, DCs switch focus from antigen-capture to antigen-presentation.

- Activated DCs concentrate in draining lymph nodes and become trapped in the paracortex.

- Naive T cells expressing CCR7 bind to chemokines on HEVs and migrate to the paracortex.

Considering the vast number of pathogens that enter the body, it would be a nearly impossible task for the lymphoid cells to travel to all body sites to protect the host. Thus, the antigens are taken to the secondary lymphoid tissues where the lymphocytes constantly recirculate in order to come into contact with their specific antigen.

If the initial tissue damage is sufficient, these cells can also be flushed into blood vessels, ultimately becoming trapped in the vascular sinusoids of the spleen. Regardless, the secondary lymphoid organs (lymph nodes and spleen) are the sites where naive, mature lymphocytes will first be exposed to their specific antigens.

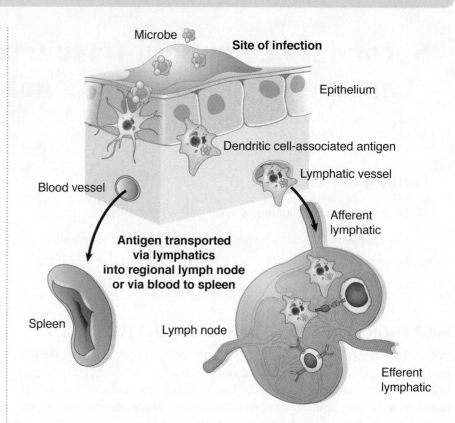

Figure I-5-1. Transportation of Antigen
to the Secondary Lymphoid Organs

STRUCTURE OF THE SECONDARY LYMPHOID TISSUE

Lymph nodes are small nodular aggregates of secondary lymphoid tissue found along the lymphatic channels of the body. They are designed to initiate immune responses to tissue-borne antigens.

- Each lymph node is surrounded by a fibrous capsule that is punctured by afferent lymphatics, which bring lymph into the subcapsular sinus.

- The fluid percolates through an outer cortex area that contains aggregates of cells called follicles.

- The lymph then passes into the inner medulla and the medullary sinus before leaving the node through the hilum in an efferent lymphatic vessel.

- Ultimately, lymph from throughout the body is collected into the thoracic duct, which empties into the vena cava and returns it to the blood.

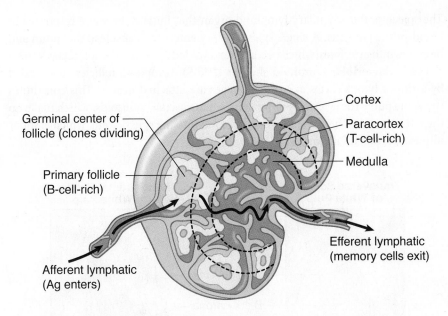

Figure I-5-2. Compartmentalization of a Lymph Node

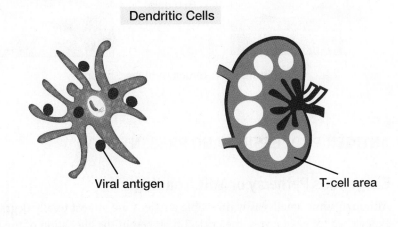

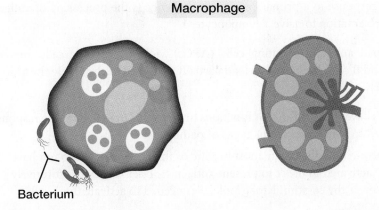

Figure I-5-3. Location of Macrophages and DCs in Secondary Lymphoid Tissue

The spleen is the secondary lymphoid organ that initiates immune responses to blood-borne antigens. A single splenic artery enters the capsule at the hilum and branches into arterioles, which become surrounded by cuffs of lymphocytes known as the **periarteriolar lymphoid sheaths (PALS)**. Lymphoid follicles surrounded by a rim of lymphocytes and macrophages are attached nearby. This constitutes the white pulp. The arterioles ultimately end in vascular sinusoids, which make up the red pulp. From here, venules collect blood into the splenic vein, which empties into the portal circulation.

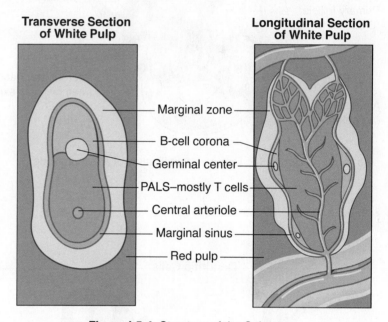

Figure I-5-4. Structure of the Spleen

ANTIGEN PROCESSING AND PRESENTATION

Exogenous Pathway of MHC Loading

Although some small, easily digestible antigens are almost totally degraded and exocytosed by phagocytes, the critical first step in the elicitation of the adaptive immune response to a primary antigenic challenge is the processing of antigen for the presentation to naive T lymphocytes.

Professional antigen-presenting cells (APCs) include dendritic cells, macrophages, and B cells; their job is to load partially degraded peptides into the groove of the MHC class II molecules.

The APCs have slightly different functions to help elicit unique immune responses required to eliminate various types of pathogens.

- **Dendritic cells** are the most prolific of the APCs, as they do not have to be activated in order to present antigen to T cells. They constitutively express the co-stimulatory molecules needed to activate the T cells.

- **Macrophages** help activate the Th1 response by digesting microbes and presenting them to the T cells to elicit a cell-mediated immune response (*see* chapter 8).

- **B cells** present specific protein antigens to T cells to help elicit a humoral immune response or a Th2 response (*see* chapter 7). B cells are unique, as they are the only APCs that specifically recognize antigen via the B cell receptors (of surface bound antibody).

Table I-5-1. APC Expression of Co-stimulatory Molecules, Class II MHC, and Function

APC	Expression of Co-stimulatory Molecules		Expression of HLA Class II	Major Function
Dendritic cells	Constitutive: B7 (B7.2)*, CD40		Constitutive but upregulated by IFN-γ	Activation of naïve Th cells
	Inducible: IFN-γ, TLR's			
Macrophages	Constitutive: B7 (B7.2), CD40		Negative or low level expression but induced by IFN-γ	Initiation and effector phase of the T_h1 response for cell mediated immunity
	Inducible: IFN-γ, TLR's			
B cells	Constitutive: CD40		Constitutive but upregulated by IL-4	Initiation of the T_h2 response for humoral immunity
	Inducible: T cells, B7			

*B7.2 is also called CD86.

When MHC class II molecules are produced in the endoplasmic reticulum of an APC, a protein called the invariant chain (Ii) is synthesized at the same time. The Ii has a class II invariant chain peptide (CLIP) that binds with high affinity to the peptide binding cleft of newly synthesized MHC class II molecule. The Ii with its associated CLIP blocks the peptide-binding groove so no normal cellular peptides can accidentally be attached. The CLIP + Ii is transported in a vesicle to the location of endocytic vesicles containing the ingested, internalized peptides.

A molecule called HLA-DM is found within the late endosome (lysosomal compartment). It is the job of HLA-DM to exchange the CLIP for a phagocytosed peptide that will bind to the MHC class II molecule with even higher affinity than the CLIP. Once exchanged for the CLIP, the peptide is loaded on the MHC class II molecule and the complex is transported to the cell surface, where it will be accessible for interaction with any T lymphocyte with a complementary TCR. If, however, the class II molecule does not find a peptide that it can bind with even higher affinity than the CLIP, the empty class II molecule is unstable and degraded, and will thus never make it to the cell surface.

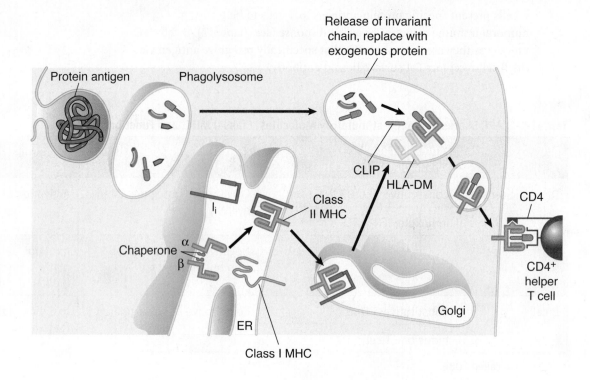

Figure I-5-5. Exogenous Pathway of Antigen Presentation

Endogenous Pathway of MHC Loading

The endogenous pathway of antigen-processing handles threats to the host which are intracellular. These might include viruses, altered/mutated genes (from tumors), or even peptides from phagocytosed pathogens that may escape or be transported out of phagosomes into the host cell cytoplasm. Intracellular proteins are routinely targeted by ubiquitin and degraded in proteasomes.

The peptides from these proteins are transported through a peptide transporter known as the **TAP complex (transporter of antigen processing)**, and into the endoplasmic reticulum, where they have the opportunity to bind to freshly synthesized MHC class I molecules.

- The TAP complex includes the TAP proteins that form the tunnel through which the proteins travel and a bridging protein called tapasin.

- Tapasin bridges the TAP transporter to the MHC class I molecule so that as these peptides enter the endoplasmic reticulum, they are easily bound by the newly synthesized and empty class I molecules.

- The peptide-MHC class I complexes are then transported to the cell membrane where they may be presented to CD8+ T lymphocytes (*see* chapter 8).

Just as with the MHC class II molecules, MHC class I is unstable without the addition of peptide and will not be expressed at the cell surface without the addition of peptide.

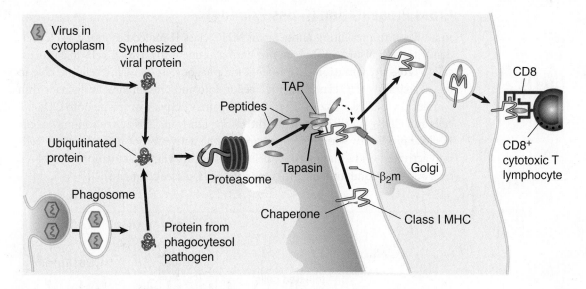

Figure I-5-6. Endogenous Pathway of Antigen Presentation

Clinical Correlate

Proteasome Inhibitors in the Treatment of Cancer

By their very nature, oncogenic cells are overly proliferative, requiring a higher rate of protein synthesis than their normal cell counterparts. A majority of cellular proteins are degraded via the ubiquitin proteasome pathway, including many proteins that play a role in maintaining cellular homeostasis. These include proteins that regulate the cell cycle, apoptosis, etc.

- Proteasome inhibitors induce apoptosis in tumor cells by interfering with the degradation of these regulatory proteins. For example, proteins that regulate the cell cycle such as p53 may be inactivated in transformed cells. This leads to a dysregulation of cell cycle control and a progression of the tumorigenesis.

- Proteasome inhibitors will produce an accumulation of p53 as well as other regulatory proteins, and therefore eventual cell death via apoptosis.

Table I-5-2. FDA-Approved Proteasome Inhibitors in Clinical Use

Drug Name	Use
Bortezomib	Currently approved to treat multiple myeloma and mantle cell lymphoma (clinical trials for leukemia)
Carfilzomib	Currently approved to treat multiple myeloma (clinical trials for leukemia and lymphomas)

Cross Presentation (Cross Priming)

In addition to presenting antigens on MHC class II molecules to CD4+ T cells, dendritic cells also have a role in presenting antigens to CD8+ T cells in a process called **cross presentation**. As professional phagocytes, dendritic cells are able to ingest a virally MHC class I infected cell in toto and present viral antigens within a molecule to CD8+ T cells. Therefore, DCs may activate or prime both CD4+ T cells and CD8+ T cells specific for the same pathogen. This activation may occur in close proximity, which is important for the activation of naïve CD8+ T cells into activated CTLs and memory cells. This occurs via the activation of CD4+ T cells and the production of cytokines such as IL-2 (*see* chapter 8).

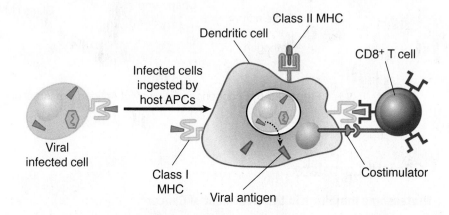

Figure I-5-7. Cross-Priming

Chapter Summary

- APCs migrate to the secondary lymphoid organs, where they present this processed antigen to recirculating naive lymphocytes.

- Lymph nodes are designed to filter antigens from the tissue fluids.

- Lymph enters through afferent lymphatics and percolates through an outer cortex and inner medulla before leaving through the efferent lymphatic in the hilus.

- The spleen is designed to filter antigens from blood; blood enters through a single splenic artery, which branches into arterioles that become surrounded by cuffs of lymphocytes (periarteriolar lymphoid sheaths) with follicles and macrophages nearby.

- MHC class I molecules are loaded with peptides via the endogenous pathway.

- Partially digested peptides are loaded into the groove of class II MHC molecules on antigen-presenting cells by the endosomal (exogenous) pathway.

- Dendritic cells may activate both CD4+ T cells and CD8+ T cells (cross priming) which is essential in the development of CTL's and CD8+ memory cells.

Secondary Lymphoid Tissue: B and T Lymphocyte Activation

6

Learning Objectives

❏ Answer questions about antigen processing and presentation

❏ Explain activation of T and B lymphocytes

ACTIVATION OF T LYMPHOCYTES

Once antigen is processed and presented to a T cell, the adaptive immune response is initiated. These interactions occur within the secondary lymphoid tissue. The purpose of these interactions is to generate effector cells, which will ultimately result in the elimination of the infection.

In order to generate specific effector cells, the activation of T cells via the TCR must go through several checkpoints to ensure antigen specificity and eventual T-cell activation.

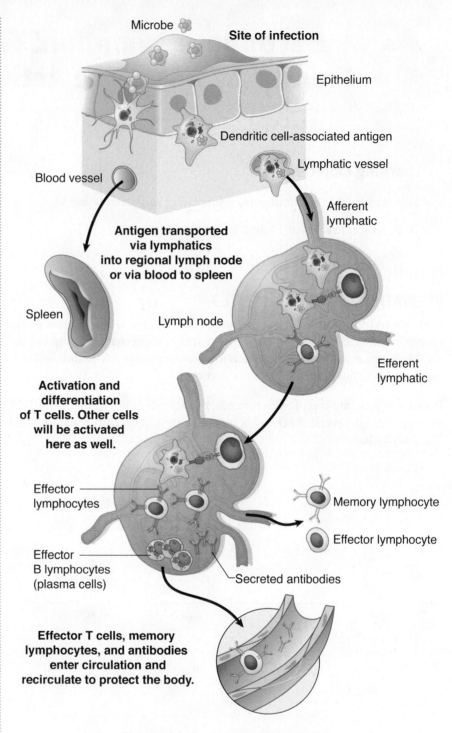

Figure I-6-1. Production of Effector Cells in the Secondary Lymphoid Organs

The binding of the TCR of the mature, naive T cell to the MHC peptide complex of the APC provides the first signal to the T cell to begin its activation. This provides the antigenic specificity of the response. The interaction is stabilized by the coreceptors CD4 and CD8 which bind to MHC class II and MHC class I molecules, respectively.

Intimately associated with the T cell receptor is the CD3 signal transduction complex. Interaction of cell adhesion molecules on the surface of the APCs and T cells allows for the formation of the immune synapse.

The costimulatory molecules B7-1 (CD80) and B7-2 (CD86) on APCs bind to CD28 on the mature, naïve T cells, providing the second signal necessary for successful activation. Under normal conditions, B7 is expressed at low levels on APCs. In the presence of infection or inflammation, the expression will increase, enhancing activation of the mature, naïve T cells. Later in the immune response, B7 will preferentially bind to CTLA-4 or PD-1, effectively turning off the T-cell response.

Cytokines secreted by APCs and the activating T cells themselves induce the proliferation (**clonal expansion**) and differentiation of the T cells into **effector cells** and **memory cells**.

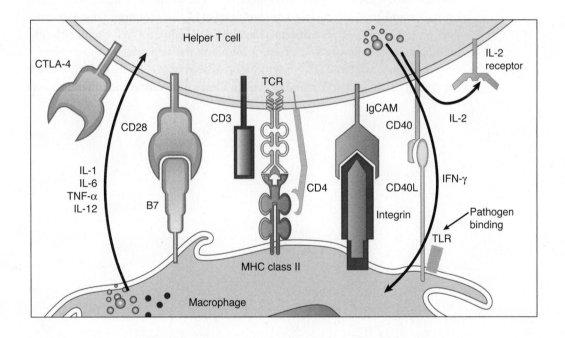

Figure I-6-2. Helper T Cell and Macrophage Adhesion

Several surface molecules are involved in the activation of mature, naive T lymphocytes:

- **First (primary) signal**: recognition of the MHC:peptide complex by the T cell receptor and coreceptors (CD4 and CD8)

- **Second (costimulatory) signal**: recognition of B7 by CD28

Clinical Correlate

CTLA-4 is an important immunoregulatory molecule in the immune system. Expressed on both activated Th and Tregs, CTLA-4 is responsible for downregulating the immune response by competitive binding to B7-1 and B7-2 on APCs.

The manipulation of CTLA-4 has important clinical implications first elucidated by the creation of CTLA-4 knockout mice that resulted in a fatal lymphoproliferative disorder. These deletions may also result in several autoimmune disorders.

Type of Regulation of CTLA-4	Drug Name	Clinical Use
Agonists	Abatacept	Rheumatoid arthritis
	Belatacept	Renal transplants
Antagonists	Ipilimumab	Melanoma and in clinical trials for several other types of cancer

The activated CD4+ (helper) T lymphocytes will begin to produce and secrete cytokines and increase surface expression of cytokine receptors. The first cytokine produced is IL-2, an autocrine signal, which induces T-cell proliferation by binding to a high affinity IL-2 receptor found on the same cells. Unlike helper T lymphocytes, activated CD8+ T lymphocytes secrete low levels of IL-2 and are dependent on the helper T lymphocytes for their proliferation and differentiation.

Clinical Correlate

Superantigens are viral and bacterial proteins that cross-link the variable β domain of a T-cell receptor to an α chain of a class II MHC molecule outside the normal peptide-binding groove. This cross-linkage provides an activating signal that induces T-cell activation and proliferation, in the absence of antigen-specific recognition of peptides in the MHC class II groove.

Because superantigens bind outside of the antigen-binding cleft, they activate any clones of T cells expressing a particular variable β sequence and thus cause polyclonal activation of T cells, resulting in the over-production of IFN-γ. This, in turn, activates macrophages, resulting in overexpression of proinflammatory cytokines (IL-1, IL-6 and TNF-α). Excess amounts of these cytokines induce systemic toxicity. Molecules produced during infectious processes and known to act as superantigens include staphylococcal enterotoxins, toxic-shock syndrome toxin-1 (TSST-1), and streptococcal pyrogenic exotoxins.

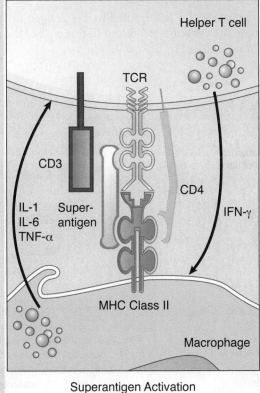

Superantigen Activation

Note that there is no complementarity between the TCR and MHC/peptide complex.

Development of the Th1, Th2, and Th17 Subsets

Helper T lymphocytes serve as the orchestrators of virtually all the possible **effector mechanisms** that will arise to destroy the pathogen. The effector mechanisms that are controlled by Th cells include antibody synthesis, macrophage activation and CTL killing. The "decision" as to which of these mechanisms should be engaged is based on the characteristics of the invading pathogen and is controlled by the differentiation of specialized classes of helper T cells. All CD4+ T cells require recognition of their specific antigen complexed to MHC class II by their TCR (first signal) and costimulation through the binding of B7 on the professional APC by CD28 (costimulatory signal).

There are 3 major classes of helper T (Th) cell that arise from the same precursor, the naive Th lymphocyte (or Th0 cell):

- Th1
- Th2
- Th17

The pattern of differentiation is determined by the antigen or type of pathogen causing the infection, the cytokines produced in response to the antigen, and the transcription factors stimulated by the cytokines.

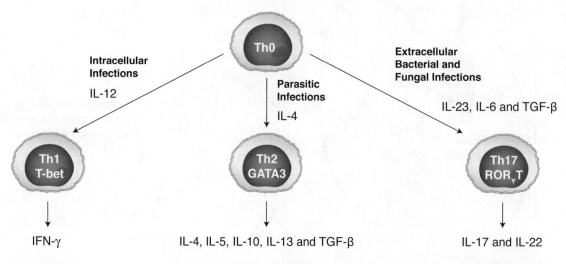

*Mucosal cells at the site of infection and T$_{regs}$ can also secrete TGF-β, causing isotype switching to IgA.

Figure I-6-3. Subsets of Helper T Cells

Differentiation of a Th0 cell into a Th1 cell is stimulated by intracellular pathogens (e.g., viruses and intracellular bacteria). These pathogens induce a strong innate immune response with the resultant production of **IL-12** by macrophages and **IFN-γ** by NK cells increasing the expression of the transcription factor T-bet.

In turn, Th1 cells secrete high levels of the inflammatory cytokine IFN-γ which does the following:

- Amplifies the Th1 response

- Inhibits the Th2 response

- Activates classical macrophage

- Enhances isotype switching to IgG

Differentiation of a Th0 cell into a Th2 cell seems to be encouraged in response to large extracellar parasites such as helminths or allergens. Due to the inability to phagocytose these pathogens, there is not significant macrophage or NK-cell stimulation. In this way, naive Th0 cells seem to produce IL-4 constitutively, and in the absence of IL-12 stimulation, these cells will upregulate their production of IL-4 to encourage differentiation into Th2 cells by induction of the transcription factor GATA-3. Additional IL-4 is produced by the activation of mast cells and eosinophils by the helminths or allergens further driving differentiation into Th2 cells.

Several cytokines are produced by Th2 cells, including IL-4, IL-5, IL-10, IL-13 and TGF-β.

- IL-4 causes B lymphocytes to isotype switch predominantly to IgE, which will bind to mast cells, eosinophils and basophils.

- In collaboration with IL-13, IL-4 enhances alternative macrophage activation for tissue repair and increased intestinal mucus secretion and peristalsis.

- The combination of IL-4, IL-10, and IL-13 together promotes a Th2 response while inhibiting the Th1 response.

- IL-5 drives maturation and activation of eosinophils.

Differentiation of a Th0 cell into a Th17 cell occurs in the presence of extracellular bacterial and fungal infections. Local cells react to the infection by secreting IL-1, IL-6, IL-23, and TGF-β, inducing the expression of the transcription factor RORγ-T in the Th17 cells. The activated Th17 cells will in turn secrete the cytokines IL-17 and IL-22.

- IL-17 induces local cells to increase chemokine production recruiting neutrophils.

- IL-22 stabilizes interactions between cells in the endothelium decreasing permeability.

- IL-17 and IL-22 induce secretion of anti-microbials by the endothelium.

Another population of T cells that arises from the Th0 is the T regulatory cell (T_{Reg} cell). T_{Reg} cells regulate (inhibit) Th1 cell function.

- Identified by their constitutive expression of CD25 on the surface and by the expression of the transcription factor FoxP3

- Secrete inflammation inhibiting cytokines such as IL-10 and TGF-β

- Have been shown to be critical for the prevention of autoimmunity

Development of Cytotoxic T Lymphocytes

Like CD4+ T cells, CD8+ T cells require both a primary and a costimulatory signal to become activated. The main difference between them is that CD8+ T cells recognize their specific antigen presented by MHC class I molecules and rely upon the cytokines produced by T helper cells to proliferate and ultimately differentiate into cytotoxic T lymphocytes (CTLs).

Clinical Correlate

Tuberculoid vs. Lepromatous Leprosy

The progression of disease with *Mycobacterium leprae* in humans is a well-documented example of the crucial balance between Th1 and Th2 subsets. Leprosy is not a single clinical entity, but rather a spectrum of diseases, with tuberculoid and lepromatous forms at the far poles.

- In **tuberculoid leprosy,** the patient has a strong Th1 response, which eradicates the intracellular pathogens by granuloma formation. There is some damage to skin and peripheral nerves, but the disease progresses slowly, if at all, and the patient survives.

- In **lepromatous leprosy,** the Th2 response is turned on, and because of reciprocal inhibition, the cell-mediated response is depressed. Patients develop antibodies to the pathogen that are not protective, and the mycobacteria multiply inside macrophages, sometimes reaching levels of 1010 per gram of tissue. Hypergammaglobulinemia may occur, and these cases frequently progress to disseminated and disfiguring infections.

ACTIVATION OF B LYMPHOCYTES

As mature naive B lymphocytes leave the bone marrow following successful rearrangement of their membrane immunoglobulin receptor genes, they recirculate throughout the body, attracted to **follicular areas** of the lymph nodes and spleen. If antigen entering these secondary lymphoid organs binds to and cross-links the idiotypes of the immunoglobulin, this provides the first signal for the activation of the B lymphocyte.

The antigens that B lymphocytes encounter are divided into 2 categories: **thymus-independent** (TI) antigens and **thymus-dependent** (TD) antigens.

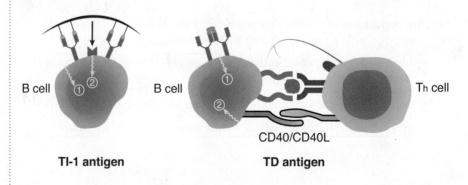

Figure I-6-4. TI versus TD Antigens

TI-Antigen Activated B Lymphocytes

Certain mature, naïve B lymphocytes are capable of being activated by macromolecules such as lipids, polysaccharides, and lipopolysaccharides without having to interact with helper T cells. These antigens are called **thymus-independent (TI)** antigens, and they directly stimulate B cells to proliferate and differentiate into plasma cells.

- The response to TI antigens is generally **weaker** than the response to TD antigens, resulting primarily in the **secretion of IgM antibodies** and the **absence of immunologic memory**.

- TI antigens may also act as B-cell **mitogens**, directly causing mitosis regardless of the cell's antigenic specificity.

- B lymphocytes activated by TI antigens are found in the spleen and mucosa.

- The marginal zone B cells are found in the periphery of the splenic white pulp and the B-1 cells in association with the mucosa and peritoneum.

TD-Antigen Activated B Lymphocytes

Most antigens introduced in the body fall into the category of **thymus-dependent (TD) antigens**. Response to such molecules requires the direct contact of B cells with helper T cells and are influenced by **cytokines** secreted by these cells. After the cross-linking of receptors on the B-cell surface with antigen, the material is endocytosed and processed via the exogenous pathway to generate an MHC class II:peptide complex, which is then inserted into the membrane of the professional APCs.

Simultaneously, expression of B7 is upregulated on the B lymphocytes, making the cells effective presenters of antigen to CD4+ T cells in the area. Once a CD4+ T cell recognizes its specific peptide displayed on MHC class II molecules, the 2 cells form a **conjugate**.

- The CD4+ T cell is activated and differentiates into a helper T cell.

- The helper T cells rearrange their Golgi apparatus toward the junction with the B cell leading to the directional release of cytokines.

- Expression of CD40L on the surface of the helper T cell is upregulated and interacts with CD40 on the B cell to provide the second signal for B-cell activation.

- The B cells respond by proliferating and differentiating into plasma cells and memory B cells.

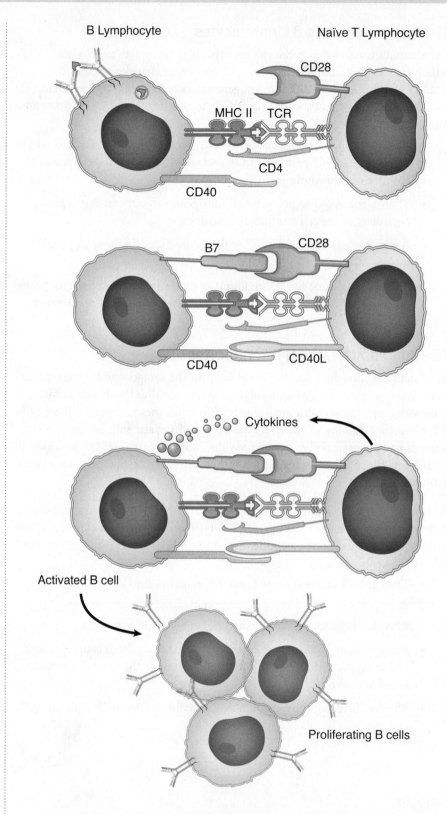

Figure I-6-5. Steps in T-Cell-Dependent B-Cell Activation

B lymphocytes activated by TD antigens are released in 2 subsequent waves.

- The primary wave of activated B lymphocytes is comprised of strictly IgM-secreting plasma cells which leave the secondary lymphoid tissue shortly after being activated.

- The second wave of activated B lymphocytes remains within the follicles of the secondary lymphoid tissue undergoing clonal expansion producing the germinal center. During the expansion, the clones will undergo affinity maturation and isotype switching.

Affinity Maturation

During the activation of B lymphocytes by helper T cells, intense proliferation of the B cells results in the formation of **germinal centers** in the follicles of the secondary lymphoid tissues. These are clones of proliferating, antigen-specific cells. During the intense proliferative response of the B cell, random mutations in the coding of the variable domain region may occur. This is called **somatic hypermutation** and creates single point mutations in the antibody idiotype. If these slightly altered idiotypes have increased affinity for the antigen, then the cell expressing them will be at a selective advantage in competing to bind antigen.

Because binding antigen serves as the first signal for proliferation, over time clones of cells with higher receptor affinity will begin to predominate in the germinal center. This **clonal selection** results in the predominance of clones capable of producing antibodies with increasing affinity for the antigen, a process known as **affinity maturation**.

This means that although isotype switching will necessarily **decrease the avidity** of the preponderance of antibody molecules as the immune response evolves, this will be substituted by an **increase in antibody affinity** over time.

Isotype Switching

Although all of the antibody molecules secreted by a clone of B lymphocytes will have an identical idiotype (*see* chapter 3), the B cell is induced to make new classes (**isotypes**) of immunoglobulin in response to cytokine-directed instruction from the helper T cells.

As the B lymphocyte receives cytokine signals from the helper T cells in the secondary lymphoid organs, it is induced to undergo **isotype switching**, changing the heavy-chain constant domains to classes of antibodies with new and different effector functions. It does this by rearranging the DNA encoding the constant regions of the heavy chain by activating switch regions that cause the intervening DNA to be looped out, excised, and degraded. The idiotype is then joined to a new constant region domain, resulting in an antibody molecule with identical antigenic specificity but a new effector function. This isotype switch is **one-way**; the excised DNA is degraded so a cell that has begun to produce an isotype downstream from IgM coding can never produce IgM again.

This is why IgM is the principal immunoglobulin of the **primary immune response** when antigen is first encountered, and it is replaced in later responses by antibodies of different isotypes. Although IgM antibodies are occasionally produced at low levels during secondary and later immunologic responses, they are always produced by cells encountering that antigen for the first time; namely, mature, naive B cells newly emerging from the bone marrow.

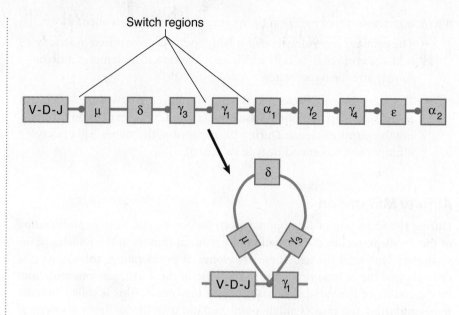

Figure I-6-6. Immunoglobulin Heavy Chain Switching

Chapter Summary

- Professional APCs migrate to the secondary lymphoid organs, where they present this processed antigen to recirculating naive lymphocytes.

- The binding of the TCR to the peptide/MHC class II complex provides the first signal in T-cell activation.

- Costimulatory interactions between CD28 and B7 provide the second T-cell activation signal.

- Superantigens are viral or bacterial proteins that cross-link the variable â domain of a T-cell receptor to an á chain of a class II MHC molecule and thereby cause polyclonal activation of T cells, overproduction of cytokines, and systemic toxicity.

- Activated Th cells act as the orchestrators of the effector mechanisms of the immune response (antibody synthesis, macrophage activation, cytotoxic T cell killing, and NK cell killing).

- Cytokines produced in response to various pathogens drive the differentiation of the T-cell subsets

- Naive Th cells (Th0) differentiate into Th1 cells when IL-12 from macrophages or IFN-γ from NK cells is present in response to intracellular infections. Th1 cells secrete the signature cytokine IFN-γ.

- Naive Th0 cells differentiate into Th2 cells in response to parasite infection or allergens. Th2 cells secrete IL-4, IL-5, IL-6, IL-10, IL-13 and TGF-β.

- Naive Th0 cells differentiate into Th17 cells in response to extracellular infection. Th17 cells secrete IL-17, IL-1, IL-6, and TGF-β driving a strong neutrophil and monocyte response.

- The cytokines produced by Th subsets are cross-regulatory: IFN-γ produced by Th1 cells inhibits Th2 cells, and IL-4 and IL-10 produced by Th2 cells inhibit Th1 cells.

- T_{Reg} cells are CD25+ and express the FoxP3 transcription factor. They develop from Th0 cells and are believed to be important in the prevention of autoimmunity.

- Humoral immunity is mediated by antibodies synthesized by B cells and secreted by plasma cells.

- Humoral immunity is the major defense mechanism against extracellular pathogens and toxins.

- Thymus-independent antigens, such as bacterial lipopolysaccharide, cross-link the receptors of B lymphocytes and cause them to proliferate and secrete IgM antibodies. These antigens *do not* create "immunologic memory."

- Most naturally occurring antigens are thymus-dependent: They require collaboration of helper T cells and B cells.

- Contact between specific B and Th cells involves MHC class II/peptide presentation, costimulatory molecules (B7/CD28), CD40/CD40L binding, and cytokine production

- Helper T cells direct isotype switching by B cells, which changes the effector function of the antibody produced.

- Helper T-cell activation of B lymphocytes causes intense proliferation in the germinal centers, and somatic hypermutation may cause slight variation in the shape of the idiotype. Clonal selection of the idiotype with the highest affinity for antigen results in "affinity maturation": a general improvement in the "goodness-of-fit" for the antigen as the immune response progresses.

Learning Objectives

❏ Explain information related to the primary humoral response

❏ Answer questions about antibodies of secondary immune responses

PRIMARY HUMORAL RESPONSE

The first isotype of immunoglobulin that can be produced by a B cell with or without T-cell help is IgM. This is because coding for the constant domains of the heavy chain of IgM (μ chains) are the first sequences downstream from the coding for the idiotype of the molecule.

The IgM molecule on the surface of the B cell is a monomer, but the secreted form of this molecule is a **pentamer**, held together in an extremely compact form by a **J chain** synthesized by the cell.

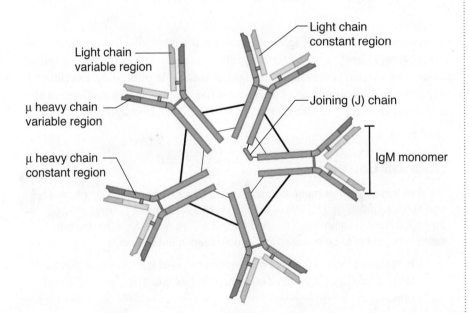

Light chain variable region

Light chain constant region

μ heavy chain variable region

Joining (J) chain

μ heavy chain constant region

IgM monomer

Figure I-7-1. IgM Pentamer

The design of the IgM pentamer maximizes its effect critical to the body early during antigenic challenge. Because of its multimeric structure (5 of the Y-shaped monomers joined into one unit), plasma IgM has 5 times the capacity for binding antigenic epitopes. The valence of the molecule is therefore 10. In other words, 10 identical epitopes can be simultaneously bound, as compared with 2 for the monomeric structure.

This design makes IgM the most effective immunoglobulin isotype at "sponging" the free antigen out of the tissues, and proves critical—as the humoral response evolves—in trapping antigen so it can be presented to the lymphocytes that will ultimately refine the choice of effector mechanism. Although the affinity (binding strength) of the idiotype for the epitope may not be strong early in the immune response, the IgM molecule possesses the highest avidity (number of antigen-binding sites available to bind epitopes) of any immunoglobulin molecule produced in the body.

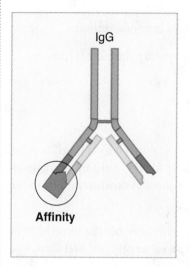 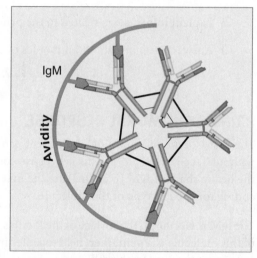

Figure I-7-2. Affinity and Avidity

The multimeric structure of IgM also makes it the most effective antibody at activating complement, a set of serum proteases important in mediating inflammation and antigen removal. Serum IgM is incapable of binding to cellular Fc receptors and thus cannot act as an opsonin (*see* chapter 4) or a mediator of antibody-dependent cell-mediated cytotoxicity (ADCC) (*see* chapter 8).

Clinical Correlate

X-linked hyper-IgM syndrome is characterized by a deficiency of IgG, IgA, and IgE and elevated levels of IgM. IgM levels can reach 2,000 mg/dL (normal 45–250 mg/dL). It is most commonly inherited as an X-linked recessive disorder, but some forms seem to be acquired and can be seen in both sexes.

- Peripheral blood of patients has high numbers of IgM-secreting plasma cells, as well as autoantibodies to neutrophils, platelets, and red blood cells.

- Patients fail to make germinal centers during a humoral immune response.

- Children with this condition suffer recurrent respiratory infections, especially those caused by *Pneumocystis jirovecii*.

The defect in this syndrome is in the gene encoding the CD40 ligand, which maps to the X chromosome. Therefore, Th cells in these patients will fail to express functional CD40L on their membrane, failing to give the costimulatory signal needed for the B-cell response to T-dependent antigens. As a result, only IgM antibodies are produced. The B-cell response to T-independent antigens is unaffected.

ANTIBODIES OF SECONDARY IMMUNE RESPONSES

Class Switching to IgG

The preponderant isotype of immunoglobulin that begins to be produced after IgM during the primary immune response is IgG. IgG is a monomeric molecule with a γ **heavy chain** and a new set of effector functions. A majority of IgG is produced in response to IFN-γ produced by the Th1 cells.

IgG exists in 4 different **subisotypes** (subclasses) in humans, IgG1, IgG2, IgG3, and IgG4, each of which exhibits a slightly different capacity in effector function. In general, however, IgG has the following characteristics:

- Activates complement
- Acts as an opsonin, enhancing phagocytosis
- Neutralizes pathogen and toxins
- Mediates ADCC

IgG is also actively transported across the placenta by receptor-mediated transport and thus plays a crucial role in protection of the fetus during gestation.

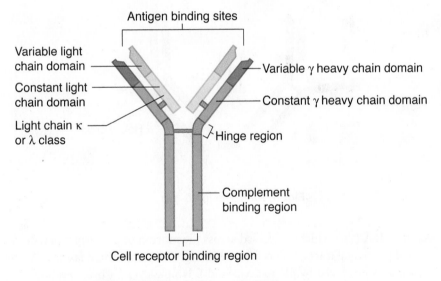

Figure I-7-3. Basic Structure of IgG

Class Switching to IgA

Another isotype of antibody that can be produced following class switching is IgA, though it is more commonly produced in the submucosa than in the lymph nodes and spleen. IgA generally exists as a **dimer**, held together by a J chain similar to that produced with IgM. IgA has the following characteristics:

- Serves as a major protective **defense of the mucosal surfaces of the body**
- Any pathogen that infects the mucosa will induce IgA production by the secretion of TGF-β by infected cells and to a lesser extent, IL-5.
- Functions as a neutralizing antibody by inhibiting the binding of toxins or pathogens to the mucosa of the digestive, respiratory, and urogenital systems (sole function)

- Does not activate complement, act as an opsonin, or mediate ADCC
- Exists in 2 isotypes, IgA1 and IgA2

The **classical pathway** is activated by antigen-antibody complexes and is probably the more phylogenetically advanced system of activation. Both IgG and IgM can activate the system by this pathway, although IgM is the more efficient.

Although the complement cascade is considered a component of the innate immune response, its overlapping stimulation of effector functions of cells of the adaptive immune response, as well as its role in enhancement of inflammation, make it a critical effector system for removal of extracellular invaders and concentration of antigens into the secondary lymphoid organs, where the adaptive immune responses are elicited.

The homing of specific memory cells to epithelial and mucosal surfaces leads to the production of specialized lymphoid aggregations along these barriers. Collectively referred to as **mucosal-associated lymphoid tissues** (MALT), they include the tonsils and Peyer patches, as well as numerous, less well-organized lymphoid accumulations in the lamina propria. Th2 cells in these sites are dedicated to providing help for class switching to IgA. Most IgA-secreting B lymphocytes and plasma cells in the body will be found in these locations.

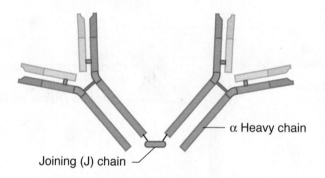

Figure I-7-4. The IgA Dimer

Secretory IgA (that which is released across the mucosa of the respiratory, digestive, and urogenital tracts) differs from serum IgA in an important fashion. As the IgA dimer is produced by plasma cells and B lymphocytes, it becomes bound to poly-Ig receptors on the basolateral side of the epithelia, is endocytosed, and is released into the lumen bound to a secretory piece that is the residue of the receptor. The **secretory component** thus serves an important function in transepithelial transport, and once in the lumen of the tract, has a function in protecting the molecule from proteolytic cleavage.

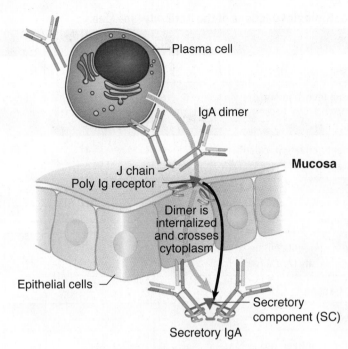

Figure I-7-5. Secretory IgA

Class Switching to IgE

IgE binds directly to Fcε receptors present on mast cells, eosinophils and basophils, and is involved in elicitation of protective immune responses against parasites and allergens (*see* chapter 12). It does not activate complement or act as an opsonin. Its heavy chain is called the ε chain.

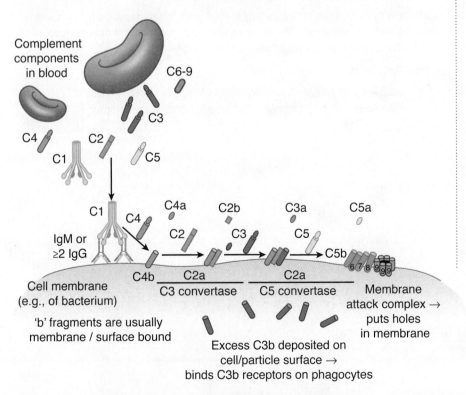

Figure I-7-6. The Classical Complement Pathway

Table I-7-1. Biologic Functions of the Antibody Isotypes

	IgM	IgG	IgA	IgD	IgE
Heavy chain	μ	γ	α	δ	ε
Adult serum levels (in mg/dL)	45–250	620–1,400	80–350	Trace	Trace
Functions					
Complement activation, classic pathway	+	+	−	−	−
Neutralization	+/−	+	+	−	−
Opsonization	−	+	−	−	−
Antibody-dependent cell-mediated cytotoxicity (ADCC)	−	+	−	−	+/−
Placental transport	−	+	−	−	−
Naive B-cell antigen receptor	+	−	−	+	−
Memory B-cell antigen receptor (one only)	−	+	+	−	+
Trigger mast cell granule release	−	−	−	−	+

Clinical Correlate

Immunodeficiencies Involving B Lymphocytes

Patients with B-cell deficiencies usually present with recurrent pyogenic infections with extracellular pathogens. The absence of immunoglobulins for opsonization and complement activation is a major problem (*see* chapter 11).

- T-cell immune system is intact.
- T-cell activities against intracellular pathogens, delayed-type hypersensitivity, and tumor rejection are normal (*see* chapter 8).

Chapter Summary

- IgM is the first isotype of antibody that can be produced. It exists in serum as a pentamer held together by a joining (J) chain.

- The functions of IgM are (as a monomer) receptor on B cells, antigen capture in the secondary lymphoid organs, and (as a pentamer) in plasma, activation of complement.

- IgG is the major isotype produced after IgM. It exists in 4 subisotypes. It activates complement, opsonizes, mediates ADCC, and is actively transported across the placenta.

- IgA is the major isotype produced in the submucosa, colostrum, and breast milk. It is a dimer with a J chain holding it together. It functions in inhibiting the bind- ing of substances to cells or mucosal surfaces. It does not activate complement or mediate opsonization.

- Secretory IgA is transported into the lumen of the gastrointestinal, respiratory, or genitourinary tracts by binding to a polyimmunoglobulin receptor.

- This receptor (now called a secretory component) is retained for protection of IgA from proteolytic cleavage.

- IgE is the antibody that binds to mast cells and is responsible for antihelminthic and allergic responses.

Learning Objectives

❏ Describe the role of macrophages, B cells, cytotoxic T lymphocytes, and NK cells

❏ Demonstrate understanding of antibody dependent cell-mediated cytotoxicity

❏ Demonstrate understanding of agglutination

❏ Answer questions about ABO testing

❏ Demonstrate understanding of lab tests, including labeled antibody systems, fluorescent antibody tests, enzyme-linked immunosorbent assay, and fluorescence activated cell sorting

CELL-MEDIATED IMMUNITY

Cell-mediated immunity has evolved to battle 2 different types of pathogens:

- **Facultative intracellular pathogens**, which have adapted to living inside of phagocytic cells that are designed to kill them

- **Obligate intracellular pathogens**, which can't replicate outside of host cells

Cell-mediated immunity is dictated by the Th1 response and is mediated primarily via macrophages and CD8+ T cells. While the Th1 response is geared toward eliminating intracellular pathogens, Th cells—in general—direct all aspects of the immune system.

The primary mechanism by which Th cells direct all aspects of immunity is the secretion of cytokines. NK cells also have a role in this type of immunity; they were covered in chapter 4 and will be reviewed here.

MACROPHAGES/B CELLS

The Th1 response activates both macrophages and B cells via the cytokine IFN-γ. IFN-γ activates classical M1 macrophages to eradicate intracellular pathogens and induces B cells to class switch to produce opsonizing IgG antibodies that can assist the macrophages with phagocytosis.

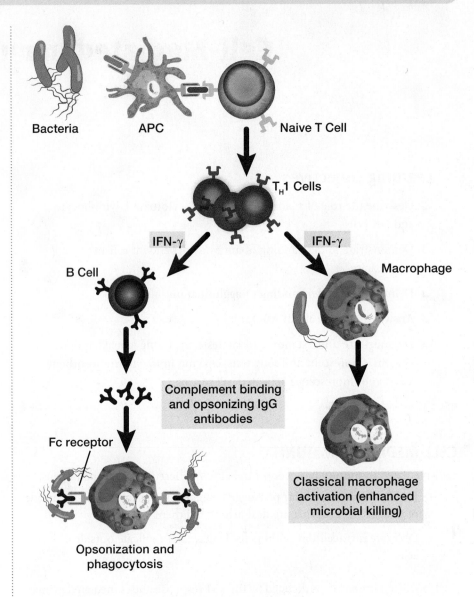

Figure I-8-1. Cell-Mediated Immunity

Macrophage-Th Cell Interaction

The binding of the TCR of the naive Th cell to the MHC class II–peptide complex of the macrophage provides the first signal to the T cell to begin its activation. This provides the antigenic specificity of the response. Co-stimulatory molecules on macrophage provide the second signal, and cytokines secreted by the macrophage and the activating T cells themselves induce the proliferation (clonal expansion) and differentiation of the T cells into effector cells and memory cells. Effector cells leave the secondary lymphoid tissue, enter into circulation, and travel to the site of the infection.

Table I-8-1. Summary of Macrophage Molecules and Function

Cell	CD Markers	MHC class I	Effector Mechanisms
Macrophage	CD14 (LPS receptor)	yes	Nitric oxide, oxygen radicals, TNF-α

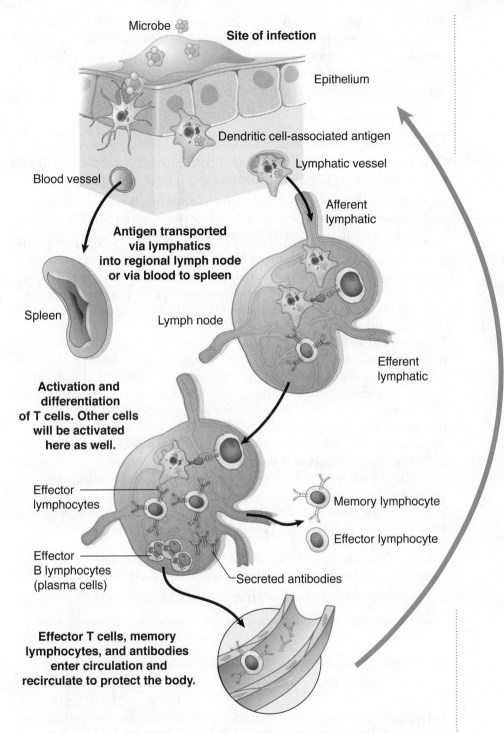

Site of infection

Microbe

Epithelium

Dendritic cell-associated antigen

Lymphatic vessel

Blood vessel

Afferent lymphatic

Antigen transported via lymphatics into regional lymph node or via blood to spleen

Spleen

Lymph node

Efferent lymphatic

Activation and differentiation of T cells. Other cells will be activated here as well.

Effector lymphocytes

Memory lymphocyte

Effector lymphocyte

Effector B lymphocytes (plasma cells)

Secreted antibodies

Effector T cells, memory lymphocytes, and antibodies enter circulation and recirculate to protect the body.

Figure I-8-2. Migration of Effector Cells to the Site of Infection

The proliferation of naïve T cells in response to antigen recognition is mediated principally by an autocrine growth pathway, in which the responding T cell secretes its own growth-promoting cytokines and also expresses receptor molecules for these factors. IL-2 is the most important growth factor for T cells and stimulates the proliferation of clones of T cells specific to that antigen. Additionally, the T cells provide IFN-γ, which promotes macrophage activation that also helps to activate Th cells. The production of IL-12 by the macrophage also helps to activate the Th cells. Together, IL-12 and IFN-γ also help to promote the differentiation of the naïve Th cell into a Th1 cell.

The reaction mediated by the Th1 cell via macrophage and CD8+ T cell activation is often referred to as the delayed-type hypersensitivity (DTH) reaction. Although this is the normal response of the body to intraceullular pathogens, it is the exact same mechanism of cellular interactions and cytokine production as a hypersensitivity to poison ivy or nickel (*see* chapter 12).

CYTOTOXIC T LYMPHOCYTES (CTLS)

CTLs recognize the cell they will ultimately kill by interaction between their TCR and the MHC class I peptide complex on the surface of the target cell.

- If the cell in question is performing **normal functions** and therefore producing normal "self" peptides, there should be no CD8+ T cells that have a complementary TCR structure.

- If the cell is **infected with an intracellular pathogen or is expressing neoantigens reflective of tumor transformation**, some small proportion of those CD8+ T cells generated from the thymus should be capable of binding their TCRs to this MHC class I/non-self-peptide complex.

Unfortunately, because of the extreme polymorphism of the HLA (MHC) system in humans, when tissues are transplanted between nonidentical individuals, cells of the transplant are often targeted by CTLs as abnormal. In spite of the fact that they may only be presenting normal cellular peptides, in these cases the HLA molecules themselves are different enough to elicit an immune response (*see* chapter 13). CTLs are capable of differentiation and cloning by themselves in the presence of the appropriate MHC class I non-self peptide complex stimulus, but are much more effective in so doing if they are assisted by signals from Th1 cells. The Th1 cell secretes IL-2, which acts on CD8+ cells to enhance their differentiation and cloning. This occurs via cross priming as discussed in chapter 5. Additionally, interferons produced in the area will increase the expression of MHC molecules to make target cells more susceptible to killing.

CTLs kill their target cells by the delivery of toxic granule contents that induce the apoptosis of the cell to which they attach. This process occurs in 4 phases:

- Attachment to the target cell (mediated by TCR, CD8, and LFA-1 integrin)

- Activation (cytoskeletal rearrangement to concentrate granules against attached target cell)

- Exocytosis of granule contents (perforin and granzymes)

- Detachment from the target cell

The death of the target cell may be mediated in distinct fashions. First, perforin present in the CTL granules creates pores in the membrane of the target cell through which granzymes (serine proteases) enter the cell, inducing the activation of caspases, which activate the "death domain." Second, cytokines such as IFN-γ with TNF-α or TNF-β can induce apoptosis. Furthermore, activated CTLs express a membrane protein called Fas ligand (FasL), which may bind to its complementary structure, Fas, on the target cell. When this occurs, caspases are induced and death results.

Table I-8-2. Summary of Cytotoxic T-Cell Markers and Function

Cell	CD Markers	MHC class I	Effector Mechanisms
CTL	CD8, CD3, TCR, CD2	Yes	Perforin, granzymes, cytokines

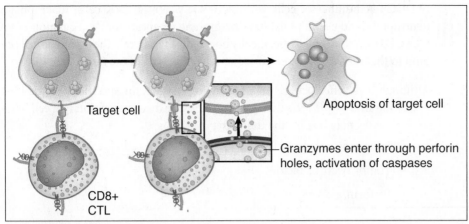

A: Perforin and Granzymes

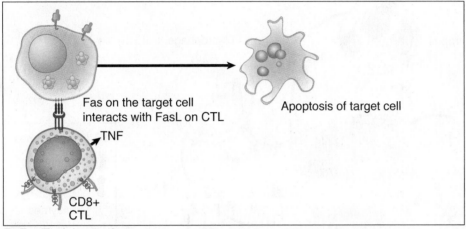

B: Fas/FasL Interaction

Figure I-8-3. Mechanisms of Cytotoxic T-Cell Killing

NK CELLS

Another cell-mediated effector mechanism enhanced by the action of Th1 cells is NK cell-killing. Since the innate function of NK cells was discussed in chapter 4, the table below summarizes that information.

Table I-8-3. Summary of NK Cell Markers and Function

Cell	CD Markers	MHC class I	Effector Mechanisms
NK	CD16 (FcR)* CD56 (CAM)	Inhibited by the normal expression of class I MHC via HLA-E.	Perforin, granzymes, cytokines (identical to CTL)**

*Keep in mind that CD16 is an FcR and is present on cells other than NK cells.

**The effector mechanisms of NK cell killing are identical to CTLs; the only difference between them is how they recognize the antigen.

ADCC

A final mechanism of cytotoxicity which bridges humoral and cell-mediated effector systems in the body is antibody-dependent cell-mediated cytotoxicity

(ADCC). A number of cells with cytotoxic potential (NK cells, macrophages, neutrophils, and eosinophils) have membrane receptors for the Fc region of IgG (aka CD16). When IgG is specifically bound to a target cell, the cytotoxic cells can bind to the free Fc "tail" and subsequently cause lysis of the target cell.

Although these effectors are not specific for antigen, the specificity of the idiotype of the antibody directs their cytotoxicity. The mechanism of target cell killing in these cases may involve the following:

- Lytic enzymes
- Tumor necrosis factor
- Perforin/granzymes

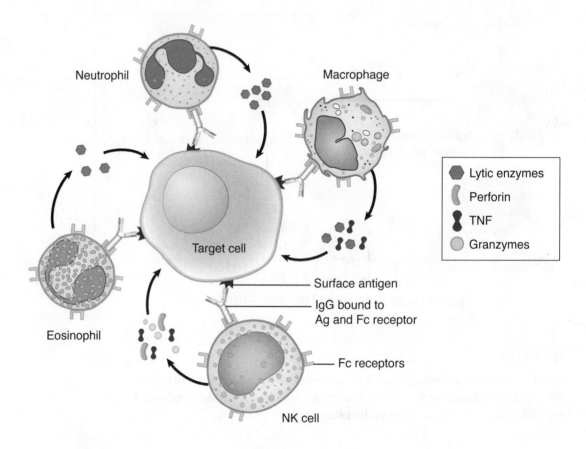

Figure I-8-4. Antibody-Dependent Cell-Mediated Cytotoxicity

Chapter Summary

- The cell-mediated immune response protects against intracellular pathogens.

- TH1 cells activate macrophages, B cells, CTLs, and NK cells.

- Macrophages kill intracellularly in response to TNF-α, TNF-β, and IFN-γ activation; the DTH skin test measures Th1 function.

- CTLs kill targets expressing MHC class I/altered-self peptides, using perforin, cytokines, granzymes, and Fas ligand.

- CTLs are stimulated by IL-2 from Th1 cells. IFNs increase MHC expression on targets.

Immunodiagnostics 9

Learning Objectives

❏ Describe the recirculation pattern of memory B and T lymphocytes

❏ Differentiate between primary and secondary immune response

SEROLOGY

Serology is an important diagnostic tool for many diseases including infections and autoimmune disorders. The interaction of antigen and antibody that occurs in vivo and in clinical laboratory settings provides the basis for all serologically based tests.

IgM and IgG

IgM is the principal immunoglobulin of the primary immune response when antigen is first encountered. It is replaced in later responses by antibodies of different isotypes, mostly IgG in the serum. Although IgM antibodies are occasionally produced at low levels during secondary and later immunologic responses, they are always produced by cells encountering that antigen for the first time.

IgM is extremely important in diagnosis of recent infections and infections in neonates or fetuses. For example, a patient with IgM antibodies to the core antigen of HBV (HBcAb) is an important diagnostic tool because it suggests a recent or acute infection and may also be found in the window period when other antibodies may not be detectable.

Also, we can make certain assumptions based on serology using IgM in the diagnoses of neonatal or fetal infections. For example, a neonate that is making IgM specific for a virus such as rubella is infected with the virus rather than immune or protected by maternal antibodies. This is because IgM does not cross the placenta. Therefore, the only way a neonate or fetus can be producing IgM specific for a certain pathogen is if the neonate or fetus were infected with that agent.

The predominant isotype of immunoglobulin that begins to be produced after IgM during the primary immune response is IgG.

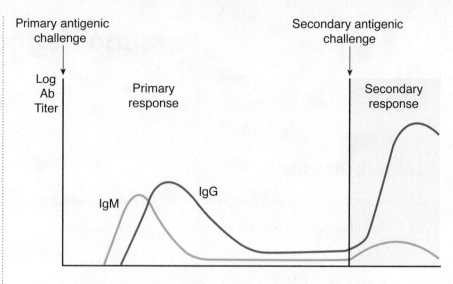

Figure I-9-1. Primary and Secondary Antibody Responses

Ideotype, Isotype, and Allotype

The unique pocket created by the variable regions of the light chain and the heavy chain is called the **idiotype** of the antibody. It is the region that is specific for antigen. It is both extremely diverse and specific. Each individual is capable of producing hundreds of millions of unique idiotypes.

The **isotype** of the antibody is determined by the constant region and is encoded by the heavy chain genes. The isotype of the antibody determines its function.

The **allotype** of an antibody is an allelic difference in the same antibody isotypes that differ between people. For example, 2 individuals with the same IgG have subtle differences in their immunoglobulins due to heterogeneity which tends to be specific for individuals. A patient receiving pooled gamma globulins might react to these allotypic differences in the constant regions which may result in type III hypersensitivity reactions.

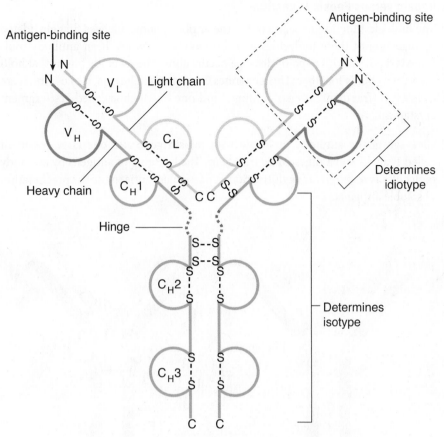

Figure I-9-2. B-Lymphocyte Antigen Recognition Molecule
(Membrane-Bound Immunoglobulin)

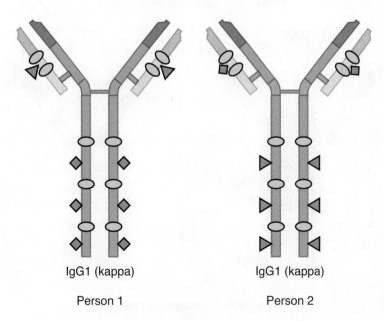

Figure I-9-3. Allotypes

Papain versus Pepsin Digestion

The biologic function of segments of the antibody molecule was first elucidated by digestion of these molecules with proteolytic enzymes. If an antibody molecule is digested with papain, cleavage occurs above the disulfide bonds that hold the heavy chains together. This generates 3 separate fragments, two of which are called Fab (fragment antigen binding), and one of which is called Fc (fragment crystallizable).

Cleavage of the antibody molecule with pepsin generates one large fragment called F(ab´)2 and a digested Fc fragment. The bridging of antigens by antibody molecules is required for agglutination of particulate antigens or the precipitation of soluble antigens.

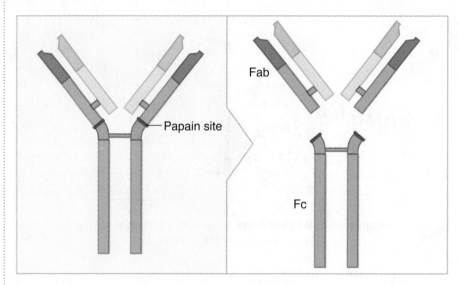

Proteolytic Cleavage with Papain

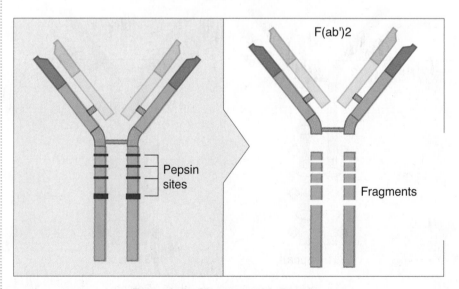

Proteolytic Cleavage with Pepsin

Figure I-9-4. Proteolytic Cleavage of Immunoglobulin by Papain/Pepsin

Zone of Equivalence

Interaction of antigen and antibody occurs in vivo, and in clinical settings it provides the basis for all serologically based assays. The formation of immune complexes produces a visible reaction that is the basis of precipitation and agglutination assays. Agglutination and precipitation are maximized when multiple antibody molecules share the binding of multiple antigenic determinants, a condition known as **equivalence**.

In vivo, the precipitation of such complexes from the blood is critical to the trapping of pathogens and the initiation of the immune response in the secondary lymphoid organs, as well as the initiation of the pathologic phase of many immune complex-mediated diseases. In vitro, the kinetics of such reactions can be observed by titration of antigen against its specific antibody.

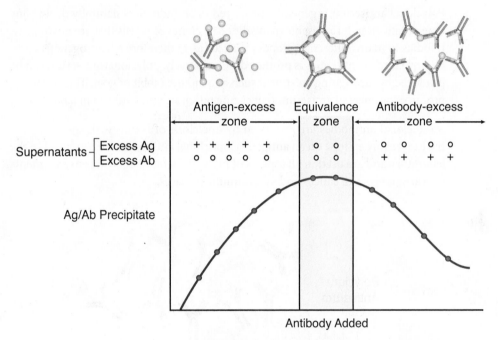

Figure I-9-5. Precipitation of Ag–Ab Complexes during Titration of Ag with Ab

Figure I-9-5 demonstrates the normal progression of the antibody response during many infectious diseases.

- At the **start of the infection**, the patient is in a state of antigen excess; the pathogen is proliferating in the host and the development of specific antibodies has not yet begun.

- As the patient begins to make an **adequate antibody response**, he enters the equivalence zone; all available antigen is complexed with antibody, and neither free antigen nor free antibody can be detected in the serum.

- Finally, as the **infection is resolved**, the patient enters the antibody excess zone, when more antibody is being produced than is necessary to precipitate all available antigen.

The clinical demonstration of this phenomenon is most easily seen in our use of the serologic diagnosis of hepatitis B infection.

- Early in the course of this infection, HBsAg is easily detectable in the blood. The patient is in the antigen excess zone for this antigen.

- As the patient enters the window period (the equivalence zone), the HBsAg disappears from the circulation because it is being removed by antibody precipitation.

- Finally, antibody titers (HBsAb) rise in the serum as the patient enters the antibody excess zone and resolves the infection.

Although the "window period" in the hepatitis B infection is used exclusively to note the absence of HBsAg and HBsAb from the serum (only antigen–antibody response that has a clinical significance in the prognosis of disease). An equivalence zone is a universal stage in the development of any antibody–antigen interaction.

Monoclonal versus Polyclonal Antiserum

Polyclonal antiserum is generally produced in an individual naturally during any type of infection. It represents many different clones of B cells that are making antibodies to many different epitopes on an antigen; therefore a heterogenous complex mixture of antibodies is produced. Alternatively, polyclonal antiserum can be produced by inoculating an animal such as a mouse, rabbit or goat. This is done to produce commercial antiserum that can be purchased and utilized in laboratories.

Monoclonal antibodies are produced by one clone of B cells with specificity for the exact same epitope on an antigen. Monoclonal antibodies are produced in the laboratory and are used in all aspects of medicine from diagnostics to treatments for various types of cancer and autoimmune diseases.

Polyclonal Antiserum

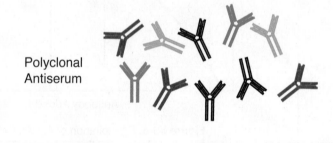

Monoclonal Antiserum

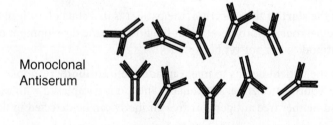

Figure I-9-6. Polyclonal versus Monoclonal Antibodies

Direct versus Indirect Serologic Tests

Direct serologic testing utilizes a known antiserum in order to detect an unknown antigen, either foreign or self. Direct tests are qualitative and provide results relatively quickly. They are used mostly for screening purposes.

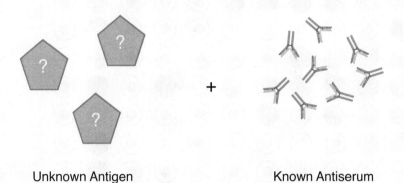

Unknown Antigen   Known Antiserum

Figure I-9-7. Direct Serologic Test

Indirect serologic testing utilizes antibodies from the patient that may be specific for either self or foreign antigen. This test is based on the concept that antibodies are produced in response to a specific disease state. Indirect tests may be qualitative and used for screening purposes or quantitative, which provides the amount of antibody in the patient's serum. Quantitative tests are also called antibody titers. A titer is often done to follow the progression of disease in a patient by looking for an increase or decrease in the level of antibodies. A titer involves diluting the patient's serum out to see how dilute the serum can be and still detect antigens in a solution.

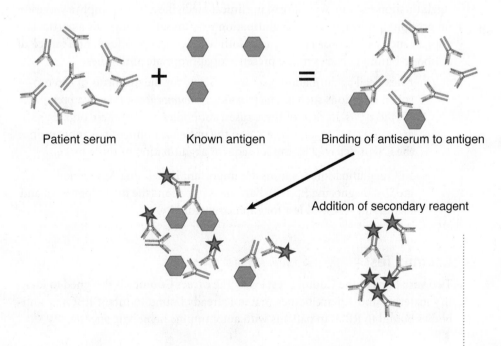

Patient serum   Known antigen   Binding of antiserum to antigen

Addition of secondary reagent

Figure I-9-8. Indirect Serologic Test

Patient	1/2	1/4	1/8	1/16	1/32	1/64	1/128	1/256	1/512	1/1024	Pos.	Neg.	Titer
1	●	●	●	●	●	●	●	◉	◉	◉	●	◉	128
2	●	●	◉	◉	◉	◉	◉	◉	◉	◉	●	◉	4
3	●	●	●	●	◉	◉	◉	◉	◉	◉	●	◉	32
4	●	●	●	●	●	●	●	●	●	◉	●	◉	512
5	●	●	●	●	●	●	◉	◉	◉	◉	●	◉	64
6	●	●	●	◉	◉	◉	●	●	●	●	●	◉	8
7	◉	◉	◉	◉	●	●	●	●	●	●	●	◉	<2
8	●	●	●	●	●	◉	◉	◉	◉	◉	●	◉	32

Figure I-9-9. Antibody Titers

Most immunologic tests can be performed using direct or indirect measures. Indirect tests are generally more specific, resulting in fewer false-positives. The Coombs, ELISA, and fluorescent antibody tests are all examples of tests that can be utilized in either a direct or indirect manner.

AGGLUTINATION

Agglutination tests are widespread in clinical medicine and are simply a variation on precipitation reactions. In agglutination reactions, the antigen is a particulate antigen such as RBCs or latex beads. Both will clump up to form of a lattice of antibody-bound particles in the presence of appropriate antibodies.

- Latex bead agglutination tests are available for the diagnosis of cerebrospinal infections such as *Haemophilus, pneumococcus, meningococcus, and Cryptococcus*. In each of these cases, antibodies against these organisms are conjugated to latex beads, and the presence of microbial antigens in the CSF is detected by the subsequent agglutination of those beads.

- RBC agglutination reactions are important in defining ABO blood groups, diagnosing Epstein-Barr virus infection (the monospot test), and identifying Coombs test for Rh incompatibility.

Coombs Test

Two variations of the Coombs test exist. The **direct Coombs** is designed to identify maternal anti-Rh antibodies that are already bound to infant RBCs or antibodies bound to RBCs in patients with autoimmune hemolytic anemia.

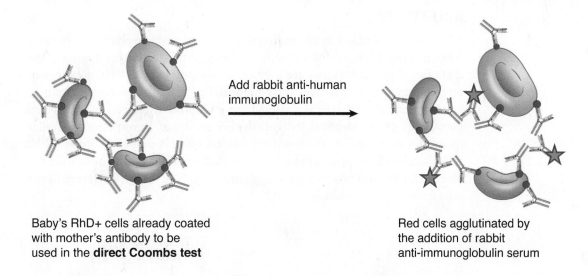

Baby's RhD+ cells already coated with mother's antibody to be used in the **direct Coombs test**

Red cells agglutinated by the addition of rabbit anti-immunoglobulin serum

Figure I-9-10. Direct Coombs Test

The **indirect Coombs test** is designed to identify Rh-negative mothers who are producing anti-Rh antibodies of the IgG isotype, which may be transferred across the placenta harming Rh-positive fetuses. The indirect Coombs is also used in the diagnosis of transfusion reactions.

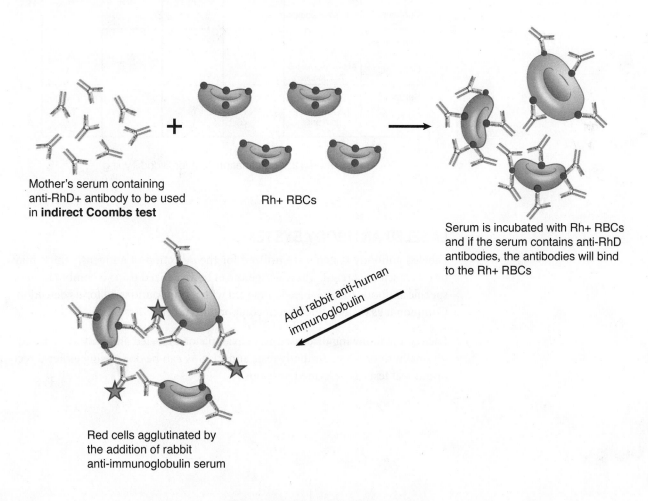

Mother's serum containing anti-RhD+ antibody to be used in **indirect Coombs test**

Rh+ RBCs

Serum is incubated with Rh+ RBCs and if the serum contains anti-RhD antibodies, the antibodies will bind to the Rh+ RBCs

Add rabbit anti-human immunoglobulin

Red cells agglutinated by the addition of rabbit anti-immunoglobulin serum

Figure I-9-11. Indirect Coombs Test

ABO TESTING

ABO blood typing is a uniform first step in all tissue transplantation because ABO incompatibilities will cause hyperacute graft rejection in the host. The ABO blood group antigens are a group of glycoprotein molecules expressed on the surface of erythrocytes and endothelial cells. Natural isohemagglutinins (IgM antibodies that will agglutinate the glycoprotein molecules on the red blood cells of nonidentical individuals) are produced in response to similar molecules expressed on the intestinal normal flora. A person is protected by self-tolerance from producing antibodies that would agglutinate his own red blood cells, but will produce those agglutinins that will react with the red blood cells from other individuals.

A: agglutination

N: no agglutination

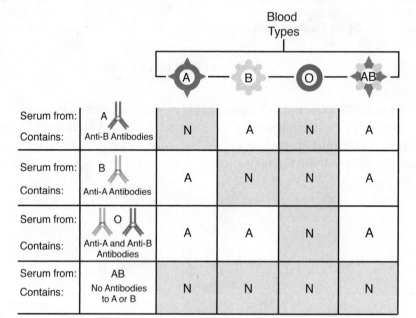

Figure I-9-12. Agglutination Test for Blood Typing

LABELED ANTIBODY SYSTEMS

Labeled antibody systems are utilized for the detection of antigens, which may be either self or foreign. These antigens can be visualized using a combination of specific antibody that is labeled or tagged with a compound used for its detection. Common tags include fluorescent compounds and enzymes.

Each of the following discussed is an example of a labeled antibody system. Additionally, fluorescent antibody tests and ELISAs can be done using either direct or indirect tests as described previously.

Fluorescent Antibody Tests

The **direct fluorescent antibody test (DFA)** is used to detect and localize antigen in the patient. The tissue sample to be tested is treated with antibodies against that particular antigen that have been labeled with a fluorescent dye. If the antigen is present in the tissues, the fluorescent-labeled antibodies will bind, and their binding can be detected with a microscope. Variations of this test are used to diagnose respiratory syncytial virus, herpes simplex 1 and 2, rabies in animal tissues, and *Pneumocystis* infections.

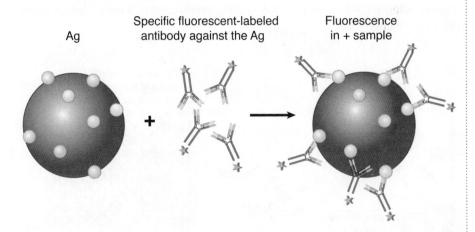

Figure I-9-13. Direct Fluorescent Antibody (DFA) Test

The **indirect fluorescent antibody test (IFA)** is used to detect pathogen-specific antibodies in the patient. In this case, a laboratory-generated sample of infected tissue is mixed with serum from the patient. A fluorescent labeled anti-immunoglobulin is then added. If binding of antibodies from the patient to the tissue sample occurs, then the fluorescent antibodies can be bound and detected by microscopy. This technique can be used to detect autoantibodies in various autoimmune diseases.

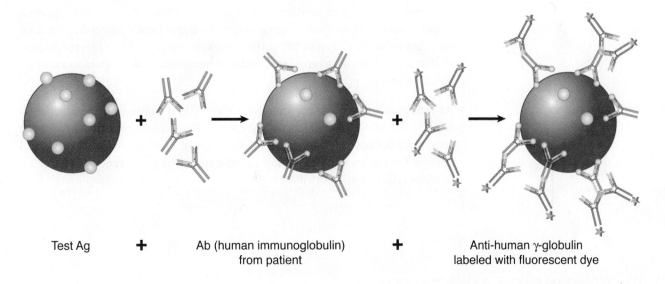

Test Ag **+** Ab (human immunoglobulin) from patient **+** Anti-human γ-globulin labeled with fluorescent dye

If the test Ag is fluorescent following these steps, then the patient's serum had antibody against this antigen.

Figure I-9-14. Indirect Fluorescent Antibody (IFA) Test

Enzyme-linked Immunosorbent Assay (ELISA)

The ELISA is an extremely sensitive test (as little as 10^{-9} g of material can be detected). It can be used to detect the presence of hormones, drugs, antibiotics, serum proteins, infectious disease antigens, and tumor markers. It does so by utilizing a chromogenic substrate that undergoes an enzyme-mediated color change.

In the screening test for HIV infection, the ELISA is used with the p24 capsid antigen coated onto microtiter plates. The serum from the patient is then added, followed by addition of an enzyme-labeled antihuman immunoglobulin. Finally, the chromogenic substrate is added, and the production of a color change in the well can be observed.

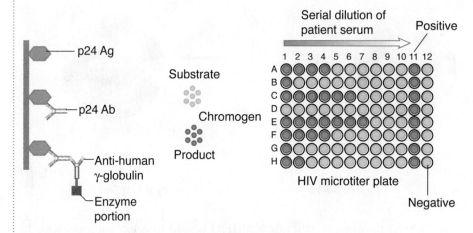

Figure I-9-15. ELISA Test

Fluorescence Activated Cell Sorting (FACS)

Fluorescence activated cell sorting (FACS) is a procedure used to rapidly analyze cell types in a complex mixture. This is done by sorting the cells into different populations based on their binding to specific fluorescently labelled antibodies. By using antibodies against cell-surface markers conjugated to different fluorescent dyes, it is possible to analyze the relative numbers of cells present in a specific tissue location.

As cells pass through the apparatus in a single file, a computer-generated graph is produced, plotting the intensity and color of fluorescence of each cell along the axes. Each dot on the graph reflects the passage of a cell with a certain level and color of fluorescence, so the darkly dotted areas of the graph reflect the presence of many cells of similar attributes.

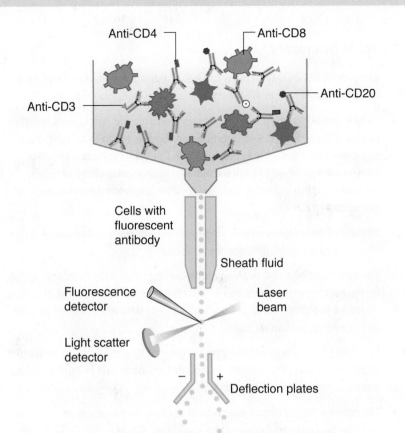

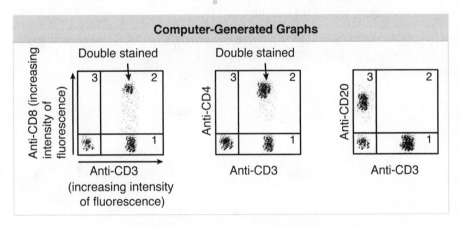

Figure I-9-16. Flow Cytometric Analysis

Chapter Summary

- Antigen–antibody interactions can be visualized in vitro and serve as the basis of many medical diagnostic tests.

- Early in infection when antigen is in excess, only the pathogen's antigens can be detected in patient serum. As antibodies begin to be produced, complexes are formed that precipitate out of the circulation, and the patient enters the equivalence zone. Rising titers of antibody are measured as the patient progresses into the antibody excess zone, and convalescence.

- Agglutination tests are used to measure antibodies that can cause clumping of particles (RBCs and latex beads).

- The direct Coombs test is an agglutination test that detects infants at risk for developing erythroblastosis fetalis; the indirect Coombs test is used to diagnose the presence of antibody in mothers who are at risk of causing this condition in their children.

- The direct fluorescent antibody test is used to detect and localize antigen in patient tissues; the indirect fluorescent antibody test is used to detect antibody production in a patient.

- The enzyme-linked immunoabsorbent assay is an extremely sensitive test that can be modified to detect antigens or antibodies. The ELISA is used as a screening test for HIV infection.

- Flow cytometry is used to analyze and separate cell types out of complex mixtures.

Immunizations 10

Learning Objectives

❏ Explain information related to vaccinations and secondary/subsequent responses

❏ Differentiate between killed, live, and component of vaccines

❏ Differentiate between bacterial and viral vaccines

❏ Answer questions about acquisition of immunoglobulins in the fetus and neonate

❏ Explain information related to childhood vaccine schedule

VACCINATION

Vaccination is a true milestone of medicine and has saved countless lives from preventable diseases. The concept dates back into the 1100s when the Chinese practiced the art of variolation. However, the practice is credited to Edward Jenner in 1798, when he used a strain of cowpox virus to protect a child from smallpox.

This chapter will discuss the science behind vaccination as well as a summary of the types of vaccine currently used in medicine.

SECONDARY AND SUBSEQUENT RESPONSES

When an antigen is introduced into the system a second time, the response of lymphocytes is accelerated and the result amplified over that of the primary immune response. The increased speed of this response is due to the presence of the memory-cell progeny of the primary response throughout the body. The increased amplitude of effector production is due to the fact that activation and cloning begin from a much larger pool of respondents.

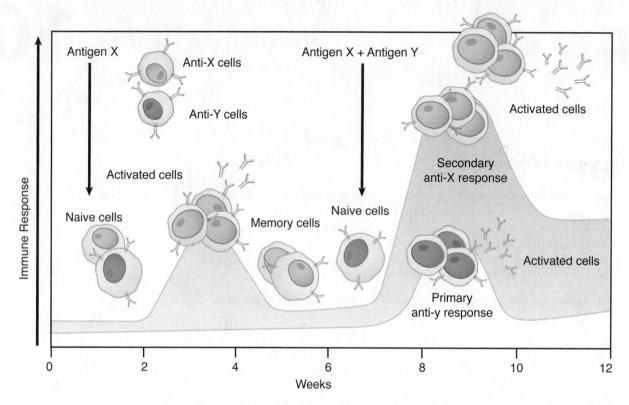

Figure I-10-1. Primary and Secondary Immune Responses

Table I-10-1. Primary versus Secondary Immune Response

Feature	Primary Response	Secondary Response
Time lag after immunization	5–10 days	1–3 days
Peak response	Small	Large
Antibody isotype	IgM, then IgG	Increasing IgG, IgA, or IgE
Antibody affinity	Variable to low	High (affinity maturation)
Inducing agent	All immunogens	**Protein** antigens
Immunization protocol	High dose of antigen (often with adjuvant)	Low dose of antigen (often without adjuvant)

TYPES OF IMMUNITY

Immunity to infectious organisms can be achieved by active or passive immunization. The goal of passive immunization is transient protection or alleviation of an existing condition, whereas the goal of active immunization is the elicitation of protective immunity and immunologic memory. Active and passive immunization can be achieved by both natural and artificial means.

Table I-10-2. Types of Immunity

Type of Immunity	Acquired Through	Examples
Natural	Passive means	Placental IgG transport, colostrum
Natural	Active means	Recovery from infection
Artificial	Passive means	Horse antivenin against black widow spider bite, snake bite
		Horse antitoxin against botulism, diphtheria
		Pooled human immune globulin versus hepatitis A and B, measles, rabies, varicella zoster or tetanus
		"Humanized" monoclonal antibodies versus RSV*
Artificial	Active means	Hepatitis B component vaccine
		Diphtheria, tetanus, pertussis toxoid vaccine
		Haemophilus capsular vaccine
		Polio live or inactivated vaccine
		Measles, mumps, rubella attenuated vaccine
		Varicella attenuated vaccine

*Monoclonal antibodies prepared in mice but spliced to the constant regions of human IgG

Passive Immunotherapy

Passive immunotherapy may be associated with several risks:

- Introduction of antibodies from other species can generate IgE antibodies, which may cause systemic anaphylaxis. The generation of IgE after infusion with even human gamma globulins is particularly an issue in persons with selective IgA deficiency (1:700 in population) as IgA is a molecule they have not encountered before. These patients can, however, be given IgA depleted globulins.

- Introduction of antibodies from other species can generate IgG or IgM anti-isotype antibodies, which form complement-activating immune complexes, leading to possible type III hypersensitivity reactions.

- Introduction of antibodies from humans can elicit responses against minor immunoglobulin polymorphisms or allotypes.

TYPES OF VACCINE

Live Vaccines

- **Attenuated** (attenuated = weak)

  - Comprised of **live** organisms which lose capacity to cause disease but still replicate in the host

  - Best at stimulating both a humoral and cell mediated immune response, as they mimic the natural infection and typically elicit lifelong immunity

  - Typically, 1 dose provides immunity but 2 doses are used to ensure seroconversion in most individuals

  - Dangerous for immunocompromised patients because even attenuated viruses can cause them significant disease; since attenuated vaccines are comprised of live organisms, there is slight potential to revert back to a virulent form

  - Live viral vaccines:

    ○ Recommended in the United States:

      ▪ Measles, mumps and rubella (MMR)

      ▪ Varicella zoster (VZV) (for both chicken pox and zoster [shingles])

      ▪ Rotavirus

      ▪ Influenza (flu-mist)

    ○ Available in the United States but recommended only under special circumstances:

      ▪ Polio (sabin)

      ▪ Smallpox

      ▪ Yellow fever

- **Non-attenuated**

  - Used by U.S. military against adenovirus types 4 and 7

  - Enteric coated, live, non-attenuated virus preparation

  - Produces an asymptomatic intestinal infection, thereby inducing mucosal IgA memory cells; these cells then populate the mucosal immune system throughout the body

  - Vaccine recipients are thus protected against adenovirus acquired by aerosol, which could otherwise produce pneumonia (this is the **only example** of a live non-attenuated vaccine that is used)

Killed Vaccines

- Utilize organisms that are killed so they can **no longer** replicate in the host

- Inactivated by chemicals rather than heat, as heat will often denature the immunogenic epitopes

- Typically require several doses to achieve desired response

- Predominantly produce humoral immunity

- Killed (inactivated) vaccines:
  - Rabies
  - Influenza
  - Polio (Salk)
  - Hepatitis A

Toxoid Vaccines

- Made from inactivated exotoxins from toxigenic bacteria
- Prevent disease but not infection
- Toxoid vaccines:
  - Diphtheria, tetanus, and acellular pertussis (DTaP)*

*The DTaP vaccine prep is composed of toxoids from both diphtheria and tetanus, while the pertussis is comprised of whole inactivated pertussis. The DTaP vaccine is considered safe with few side effects, and is the vaccine currently used in the United States.

Polysaccharide Vaccines

- Comprised of the capsular polysaccharide found in many bacteria
- Are only capable of producing IgM because of the inability of polysaccharide to activate Th cells (which require protein to become activated)
- Have largely been replaced with conjugate vaccines (see below)
- Polysaccharide vaccine(s):
  - *Streptococcus pneumoniae*, pneumococcal polysaccharide (PPSV23)
    ○ Comprised of 23 capsular serotypes of the most invasive and common strains of *S. pneumoniae*
    ○ Indicated for use in adults age >65 or special circumstances, i.e., splenectomy, COPD

Conjugate Vaccines

- Comprised of capsular polysaccharide conjugated to protein (usually a toxoid (see figure I-10-3); this creates a T cell-dependent immune response with class switching
- Creates a booster response to multiple doses
- Conjugate vaccines:
  - *Haemophilus influenzae type b* (Hib)
  - *Streptococcus pneumoniae*, Pneumococcal conjugate (PCV13)
    ○ Comprised of 13 capsular serotypes
    ○ Indicated for use in infants
  - *Neisseria meningitidis*

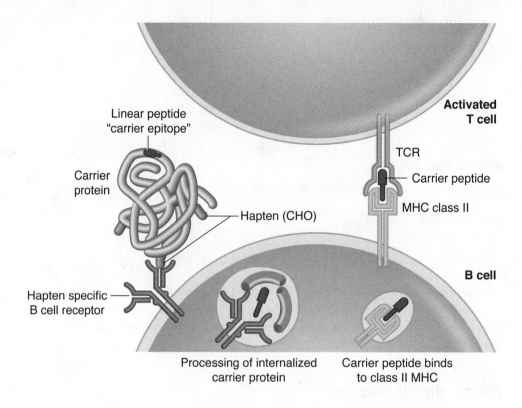

Figure I-10-2. Example of Conjugate Vaccine

Component Vaccines

- Comprised of an immunodominant protein from the virus that is grown in yeast cells

  - For example, in the hepatitis B vaccine, the gene coding for the HBsAg is inserted into yeast cells, which then releases this molecule into the culture medium; the molecule is then purified and used as the immunogen in the vaccine

- Component vaccines:

  - HBV

    - Hepatitis B surface antigen

  - HPV

    - Quadrivalent vaccine with serotypes 6, 11, 16 and 18

    - 9-valent vaccine (Gardasil 9) to prevent >90% of cancers, as opposed to the quadrivalent vaccine which can protect up to 70% of cancers; contains serotypes 6, 11, 16, 18, 31, 33, 45, 52 and 58

      - Released in February 2015

ACQUISITION OF IMMUNOGLOBULINS IN THE FETUS AND NEONATE

Persistence of maternal Ab affects vaccinations.

- Live attenuated virus vaccines are given only age >12 months because residual maternal antibodies would inhibit replication and the vaccine would fail.

- When children are at exceptionally high risk for exposure to a pathogen, this rule is sometimes broken, but administration of vaccine at age <6–9 months is almost always associated with the need for repeated booster inoculations.

- IgM is the only isotype useful in diagnosing infections in neonates.

- Normal infants have few infections during first few months because of maternal IgG.

- Children with immune deficiencies don't become ill until maternal IgG is low.

- Infants have 20% of adult IgA at age 12 months, so colostrum is important.

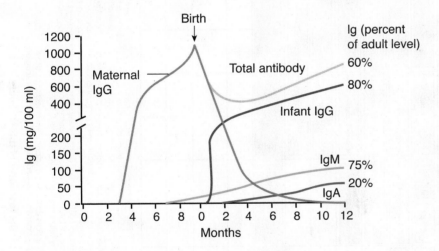

Figure I-10-3. Immunoglobulins in Serum of Fetus and Newborn Child

CHILDHOOD VACCINE SCHEDULE

The current recommended list of vaccines for children in the United States is listed below. The vaccines in this list are high yield.

Recommended immunization schedule for persons aged 0 through 18 years – United States, 2016.
(FOR THOSE WHO FALL BEHIND OR START LATE, SEE THE CATCH-UP SCHEDULE).
These recommendations must be read with the footnotes that follow. For those who fall behind or start late, provide catch-up vaccination at the earliest opportunity as indicated by the green bars in Figure 1. To determine minimum intervals between doses, see the catch-up schedule (Figure 2). School entry and adolescent vaccine age groups are shaded.

Vaccine	Birth	1 mo	2 mos	4 mos	6 mos	9 mos	12 mos	15 mos	18 mos	19–23 mos	2-3 yrs	4-6 yrs	7-10 yrs	11-12 yrs	13-15 yrs	16-18 yrs
Hepatitis B[1] (HepB)	1st dose	←— 2nd dose —→			←————————— 3rd dose —————————→											
Rotavirus[2] (RV) RV1 (2-dose series); RV5 (3-dose series)			1st dose	2nd dose	See footnote 2											
Diphtheria, tetanus, & acellular pertussis[3] (DTaP: <7 yrs)			1st dose	2nd dose	3rd dose		←————— 4th dose —————→					5th dose				
Haemophilus influenzae type b[4] (Hib)			1st dose	2nd dose	See footnote 4		3rd or 4th dose, See footnote 4									
Pneumococcal conjugate[5] (PCV13)			1st dose	2nd dose	3rd dose		←— 4th dose —→									
Inactivated poliovirus[6] (IPV: <18 yrs)			1st dose	2nd dose	←————————— 3rd dose —————————→							4th dose				
Influenza[7] (IIV; LAIV)					Annual vaccination (IIV only) 1 or 2 doses						Annual vaccination (LAIV or IIV) 1 or 2 doses			Annual vaccination (LAIV or IIV) 1 dose only		
Measles, mumps, rubella[8] (MMR)					See footnote 8		←— 1st dose —→					2nd dose				
Varicella[9] (VAR)							←— 1st dose —→					2nd dose				
Hepatitis A[10] (HepA)					See footnote 11		2-dose series, See footnote 10									
Meningococcal[11] (Hib-MenCY ≥6 weeks; MenACWY-D ≥9 mos; MenACWY-CRM ≥ 2 mos)					See footnote 11									1st dose		Booster
Tetanus, diphtheria, & acellular pertussis[12] (Tdap: ≥7 yrs)														(Tdap)		
Human papillomavirus[13] (2vHPV: females only; 4vHPV, 9vHPV: males and females)														(3-dose series)		
Meningococcal B[11]												See footnote 11				
Pneumococcal polysaccharide[5] (PPSV23)											See footnote 5					

Range of recommended ages for all children	Range of recommended ages for catch-up immunization
Range of recommended ages for certain high-risk groups	Range of recommended ages for non-high-risk groups that may receive vaccine, subject to individual clinical decision making
No recommendation	

This schedule includes recommendations in effect as of January 1, 2016. Any dose not administered at the recommended age should be administered at a subsequent visit, when indicated and feasible. The use of a combination vaccine generally is preferred over separate injections of its equivalent component vaccines. Vaccination providers should consult the relevant Advisory Committee on Immunization Practices (ACIP) statement for detailed recommendations, available online at http://www.cdc.gov/vaccines/hcp/acip-recs/index.html. Clinically significant adverse events that follow vaccination should be reported to the Vaccine Adverse Event Reporting System (VAERS) online (http://www.vaers.hhs.gov) or by telephone (800-822-7967). Suspected cases of vaccine-preventable diseases should be reported to the state or local health department. Additional information, including precautions and contraindications for vaccination, is available from CDC online (http://www.cdc.gov/vaccines/recs/vac-admin/contraindications.htm) or by telephone (800-CDC-INFO [800-232-4636]).

This schedule is approved by the Advisory Committee on Immunization Practices (http://www.cdc.gov/vaccines/acip), the American Academy of Pediatrics (http://www.aap.org), the American Academy of Family Physicians (http://www.aafp.org), and the American College of Obstetricians and Gynecologists (http://www.acog.org).

NOTE: The above recommendations must be read along with the footnotes of this schedule.

BACTERIAL VACCINES

Table I-10-3. Bacterial Vaccines

Organism	Vaccine	Vaccine Type
C. diphtheriae	**D**TaP	Toxoid
B. pertussis	DT**aP**	Toxoid plus filamentous hemagglutinin
C. tetani	D**T**aP	Toxoid
H. influenzae	Hib	Capsular polysaccharide and protein
S. pneumoniae	PCV Pediatric	13 capsular serotypes and protein
	PPV Adult	23 capsular serotypes
N. meningitidis	MCV-4	4 capsular serotypes (Y, W-135, C, A) and protein

VIRAL VACCINES

Table I-10-4. Viral Vaccines

Virus	Vaccine	Vaccine Type
Rotavirus	RV	Live
Polio	IPV	Killed (Salk)
	OPV	Live (Sabin)
Influenza	IIV	Inactivated (killed)
	LAIV	Live
Varicella zoster virus	VAR	Live
Hepatitis A	HepA	Inactivated (killed)
Human papilloma virus	HPV	Component
Hepatitis B virus	HepB	Component
Measles	MMR	Live
Mumps	MMR	Live
Rubella	MMR	Live

Chapter Summary

- **Active immunization** occurs when an individual is exposed (naturally or artificially) to a pathogen; **passive immunization** occurs when an individual receives preformed immune products (antibodies, cells) against a pathogen (naturally or artificially).

- Passive immunotherapy is useful in postexposure prophylaxis but runs the risk of eliciting adverse immune responses (hypersensitivity).

- Childhood vaccination protocols must take into account risk of exposure, presence of maternal antibodies, and the type of protective immune response needed.

- Live vaccines are not safe for use in immunocompromised patients.

- Live viral vaccines elicit both cellular and humoral responses, whereas killed viral vaccines elicit primarily antibody responses.

- The hepatitis B and human papilloma virus vaccines are component vaccines produced by recombinant DNA technology.

Primary Immunodeficiencies 11

Learning Objectives

❏ Solve problems concerning defects of phagocytic cells and humoral immunity

❏ Demonstrate understanding of deficiencies of complement or its egulation

❏ Use knowledge of defects of T lymphocytes to explain severe combined immunodeficiencies

Immunodeficiency diseases may occur with any aspect of immunity, including both the innate and adaptive branches. The symptoms of each disease highlight the importance of that aspect of the immune system on protecting the host. Most of these immune disorders are pediatric in nature and begin to appear around age 6 months. This highlights the importance of the protective immunity afforded by maternal IgG, which is nearly depleted by age 6 months and completely depleted by age 12-15 months.

Another important aspect of immunodeficiency diseases is that several are X-linked and therefore more common in males than females. Because these diseases reveal the importance of the immune system's basic function, they are often heavily tested.

DEFECTS OF PHAGOCYTIC CELLS

Table I-11-1. Defects of Phagocytic Cells

Disease	Molecular Defect(s)	Symptoms
Chronic granulomatous disease (CGD)	Deficiency of **NADPH oxidase** (any one of 4 component proteins); failure to generate super-oxide anion, other O_2 radicals	Recurrent infections with **catalase-positive** bacteria and fungi
Leukocyte adhesion deficiency	Absence of **CD18**—common β chain of the leukocyte integrins The 3 integrins that contain CD18: LFA-1, MAC-1 and gp150/95	Recurrent and chronic infections, failure to form pus, and delayed separation of umbilical cord stump
Chediak-Higashi syndrome	Nonsense mutation in the lysosomal trafficking regulator, CHS1/LYST protein, leads to aberrant fusion of vesicles	Recurrent infection with bacteria: chemotactic and degranulation defects; absent NK activity, partial **albinism**
Glucose-6-phosphate dehydrogenase (G6PD) deficiency	Deficiency of essential enzyme in hexose monophosphate shunt	Same as CGD, with associated **anemia**
Myeloperoxidase deficiency	Defect in MPO affects the ability to convert hydrogen peroxide to hypochlorite	Mild or none
Hyperimmunoglobulin E syndrome (formerly Job syndrome)	Defects in JAK-STAT signaling pathway leading to impaired Th17 function: decreased IFN-gamma production	Characteristic facies, severe, recurrent sinuso-pulmonary infections, pathologic bone fractures, retention of primary teeth, increased IgE, eczematous rash

DEFECTS OF HUMORAL IMMUNITY

Table I-11-2. Defects of Humoral Immunity

Disease	Molecular Defect	Symptoms/Signs	Treatment
Bruton (X-linked) agammaglobulinemia	Deficiency of the Bruton tyrosine kinase (btk) which promotes pre-B cell expansion; faulty B-cell development	Increased susceptibility to encapsulated bacteria and bloodborne viruses, low immunoglobulins of all isotypes, absent or low levels of circulating B-cells. B-cell maturation does not progress past the pre-B cell stage while maintaining cell-mediated immunity.	Monthly gamma-globulin replacement, antibiotics for infection
X-linked hyper-IgM syndrome	Deficiency of **CD40L** on activated T cells	**High serum titers of IgM without other isotypes,** normal B and T-cell numbers, susceptibility to encapsulated bacteria and opportunistic pathogens.	Antibiotics and gammaglobulins
Selective IgA deficiency	Multiple genetic causes	Decreased IgA levels and normal IgM and IgG with elevation of IgE. Repeated **sinopulmonary and gastrointestinal** infections, ↑ **atopy**	Antibiotics, not immunoglobulins
Common variable Immunodeficiency	Collection of syndromes; several associated genetic defects	Onsets in **late teens**, early twenties; B cells present in peripheral blood, immunoglobulin levels decrease with time; ↑ autoimmunity	Antibiotics
Transient hypogammaglob-ulinemia of infancy	Delayed onset of normal IgG synthesis	Detected in 5th to 6th month of life, resolves by 16–30 months; susceptibility to pyogenic bacteria	Antibiotics and in severe cases, gamma-globulin replacement

DEFICIENCIES OF COMPLEMENT OR ITS REGULATION

Table I-11-3. Deficiencies of Complement or Its Regulation

Deficiencies in Complement Components	Deficiency	Signs/Diagnosis
Classic pathway	C1q, C1r, C1s, C4, C2	Marked increase in immune complex diseases, increased infections with pyogenic bacteria
Both pathways	C3	Recurrent bacterial infections, immune complex disease
	C5, C6, C7, C8, or C9	Recurrent **meningococcal and gonococcal infections**
Deficiencies in complement regulatory proteins	C1-INH **(hereditary angioedema)**	Overuse of C1, C4, or C2, edema at mucosal surfaces

DEFECTS OF T LYMPHOCYTES AND SEVERE COMBINED IMMUNODEFICIENCIES

Although patients with defects in B lymphocytes can deal with many pathogens adequately, defects in T lymphocytes are observed globally throughout the immune system. Because of the central role of T cells in activation, proliferation, differentiation, and modulation of virtually all naturally occurring immune responses, abnormalities in these cell lines send shock waves throughout the system. It is often a Herculean clinical effort to dissect the cause-and-effect relationships in such inherited diseases, and their diagnosis is often one of trial-and-error, which takes years to unravel.

Although in some cases both B- and T-lymphocyte defects may occur, the initial manifestation of these diseases is almost always infection with agents such as **fungi and viruses** that are normally destroyed by T-cell–mediated immunity. The B-cell defect, if any, is usually not detected for the first few months of life because of the passive transfer of immunoglobulins from the mother through the placenta or colostrum. The immune system is so compromised that even attenuated vaccine preparations can cause infection and disease.

Table I-11-4. T-Cell Deficiencies and Combined Deficiencies

Category	Disease	Defect	Clinical Manifestations
Selective T-cell deficiency	**DiGeorge Syndrome**	Heterozygous deletion of chromosome 22q11 . Failure of formation of **3rd and 4th pharyngeal pouches**, thymic aplasia	Characteristic facies and a clinical triad of cardiac malformations, hypocalcemia and hypoplastic thymus
	MHC class I deficiency	Failure of TAP 1 molecules to transport peptides to endoplasmic reticulum	**CD8+ T cells deficient, CD4+ T cells normal,** recurring viral infections, normal DTH, normal Ab production
Combined partial B- and T-cell deficiency	**Wiskott-Aldrich Syndrome**	Defect in the WAS protein which plays a critical role in actin cytoskeleton rearrangement	Defective responses to bacterial polysaccharides and depressed IgM, gradual **loss of humoral and cellular responses, thrombocytopenia, and eczema** IgA and IgE may be elevated eczema ⟷ thrombocytopenia ⟷ immunodeficiency
	Ataxia telangiectasia	Defect in the ATM kinase involved in the detection of DNA damage and progression through the cell cycle	**Ataxia** (gait abnormalities), **telangiectasia** (capillary distortions in the eye), **deficiency of IgA and IgE** production
Complete functional B- and T-cell deficiency	Severe combined immunodeficiency (SCID)	Defects in common γ chain of IL-2 receptor (present in receptors for IL-4, −7, −9, −15), X-linked	Chronic diarrhea; skin, mouth, and throat lesions; opportunistic (**fungal**) infections; low levels of circulating lymphocytes; cells unresponsive to mitogens
		Adenosine deaminase deficiency (results in toxic metabolic products in cells)	Clinical overlap with X-linked SCID plus neurologic deficiency
		*rag*1 or *rag*2 gene nonsense mutations	Total absence B+ T cells
	Bare lymphocyte syndrome/**MHC class II deficiency**	Failure of MHC class II expression, defects in transcription factors	T cells present and responsive to nonspecific mitogens, no GVHD, **deficient in CD4+ T cells**, hypogammaglobulinemia. Clinically observed as a severe combined immunodeficiency

Chapter Summary

- B-cell, phagocyte, and complement defects predispose to infections with extra-cellular pathogens.

- T-cell defects predispose to infections with intracellular pathogens.

- Severe combined immunodeficiencies tend to manifest first as T-cell defects (especially fungal infections).

Hypersensitivity and Autoimmune Disease

12

Learning Objectives

❏ Differentiate type I (immediate), type II (antibody-mediated), type III (immune complex), and type IV (T-cell-mediated) hypersensitivity

❏ Answer questions about the pathogenesis of autoimmunity

Hypersensitivity diseases are conditions in which tissue damage is caused by immune responses. They may result from uncontrolled or excessive responses against **foreign** antigens or from a **failure of self-tolerance**, in which case they are called **autoimmune diseases**.

The 2 principal factors which determine the clinical and pathologic consequences of such conditions are the **type of immune response** elicited and the **nature and location of the inciting antigen**.

What the hypersensitivity reactions have in common:

- The first exposure to the antigen "sensitizes" lymphocytes.

- Subsequent exposures elicit a damaging reaction.

- The response is specific to a particular antigen or a cross-reacting substance.

Hypersensitivity diseases are classified on the basis of the effector mechanism responsible for tissue injury, and 4 types are commonly recognized.

Table I-12-1. Classification of Immunologic Diseases

Type of Hypersensitivity	Immune Mechanisms	Mechanisms of Tissue Injury
Immediate (type I)	Activation of Th2 cells resulting in the production of IgE which in turn binds to FcεR on mast cells, basophils and eosinophils	**Immediate reaction** • Degranulation and release of vasoactive amines (ie. histamine) and proteases **Late-phase reaction** • Synthesis and secretion of prostaglandins and leukotrienes • Cytokine-induced inflammation and leukocyte recruitment
Antibody-mediated (type II)	IgM and IgG against surface (cell surface or extracellular matrix)	**Complement-mediated (cytotoxic)** • Opsonization and enhances phagocytosis • Recruitment and activation of inflammatory cells **Non-cytotoxic** • Change in physiologic behavior of a cell
Immune complex–mediated (type III)	Deposition of immune complexes comprised of IgM or IgG and soluble antigen	Complement-mediated recruitment and activation of inflammatory cells resulting in some combination of arthritis, vasculitis and/or nephritis.
Delayed-type hypersensitivity (type IV)	Inflammatory cytokines, IFN-γ and IL-17, produced by CD4+ Th1 and Th17 cells, respectively.	**Cytokine-mediated tissue damage** • IFN-γ activation of macrophage • IL-17 recruitment and activation of neutrophil **Direct killing** • CTL-mediated cellular death
		CD8+ CTLs (T-cell-mediated cytolysis) Direct target cell killing, cytokine-mediated inflammation

TYPE I (IMMEDIATE) HYPERSENSITIVITY

Type I is the only type of hypersensitivity mediated by IgE antibodies and mast cells. It is manifested within minutes of the reexposure to an antigen. The IgE response is the normal protective response against many metazoan parasites, which are too large to be phagocytized or killed by other cytopathic mechanisms. Approximately 20% of all individuals in the United States, however, display this immune response against harmless environmental antigens, such as pet dander or pollen; these responses are called **atopic** or **allergic** responses.

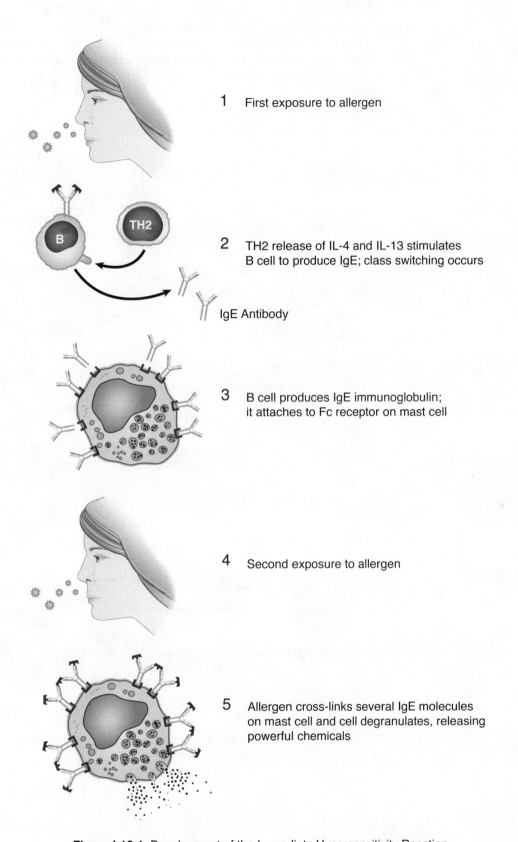

1 First exposure to allergen

2 TH2 release of IL-4 and IL-13 stimulates B cell to produce IgE; class switching occurs

IgE Antibody

3 B cell produces IgE immunoglobulin; it attaches to Fc receptor on mast cell

4 Second exposure to allergen

5 Allergen cross-links several IgE molecules on mast cell and cell degranulates, releasing powerful chemicals

Figure I-12-1. Development of the Immediate Hypersensitivity Reaction

The effector cells of the immediate hypersensitivity reaction are mast cells, basophils, and eosinophils. The soluble substances they release into the site cause the symptoms of the reaction. Approximately 2-4 hours after the immediate response to release of these mediators, a **late-phase reaction** is mediated by products of the arachidonic acid cascade.

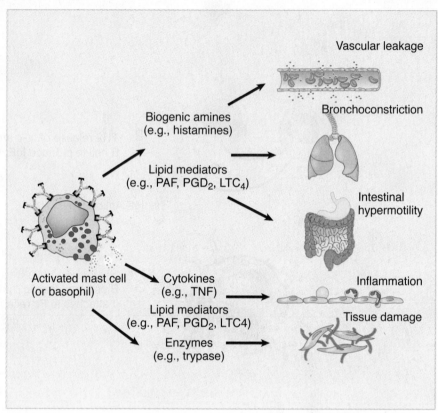

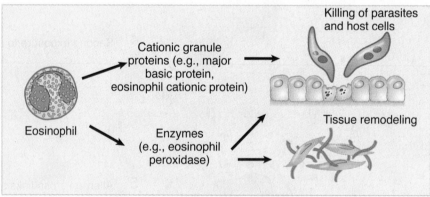

Figure I-12-2. Mediators of Type I Hypersensitivity

Table I-12-2. Mast Cell Mediators

Mediators Stored and Released	Effect
Histamine	Smooth muscle contraction; increased vascular permeability
Heparin	Anticoagulant
Eosinophil chemotactic factor A (multiple chemokines)	Chemotactic
Mediators Newly Synthesized from Arachidonic Acid	**Effect**
Prostaglandin D_2, E_2, $F_{2\alpha}$	Increased smooth muscle contraction and vascular permeability
Leukotrienes C_4, D_4, E_4 (lipoxygenase pathway)	Increased smooth muscle contraction and vascular permeability
Leukotriene B_4	Chemotactic for neutrophils

Table I-12-3. Allergic Diseases Due to Specific Allergens and Their Clinical Manifestations

Allergic Disease	Allergens	Clinical Findings
Allergic rhinitis (hay fever)	Trees, grasses, dust, cats, dogs, mites	Edema, irritation, mucus in nasal mucosa
Systemic anaphylaxis	**Insect stings, drug reactions**	Bronchial and tracheal constriction, complete vasodilation and death
Food allergies	Milk, eggs, fish, cereals, grains	Hives and gastrointestinal problems
Wheal and flare	In vivo skin testing for allergies	Local skin edema, reddening, vasodilation of vessels
Asthma	Inhaled materials	Bronchial and tracheal constriction, edema, mucus production, massive inflammation

TYPE II (ANTIBODY-MEDIATED) HYPERSENSITIVITY

Antibodies against cell surface or extracellular matrix antigens cause diseases that are **specific to the tissues** where those antigens are present; they are not usually systemic. In most cases, these antibodies are **autoantibodies**, but they may be produced against a foreign antigen that is cross-reactive with self-components of tissues.

These antibodies can cause tissue damage by 3 main mechanisms:

- Opsonization of cells

- Activation of the complement system which recruit neutrophils and macrophages that cause tissue damage

- Possible binding to normal cellular receptors and interference with their function

In some types of type II hypersensitivity, complement is activated and/or ADCC is active (e.g., hemolytic disease of the newborn [HDNB]). In other types, cell function is altered in the absence of complement activation and ADCC (e.g., myasthenia gravis and Graves disease). Eventually, as these diseases progress, complexes of antigen and antibody may cause localized damage, but they **do not circulate** so the damage is localized to the specific tissue.

Table I-12-4. Type II Hypersensitivities

Disease	Target Antigen	Mechanism of Pathogenesis	Clinical Manifestations
Cytotoxic			
Autoimmune hemolytic anemia (HDNB)	RBC membrane proteins (Rh, I Ags)	Opsonization, phagocytosis, and complement-mediated destruction of RBCs	Hemolysis, anemia
Acute rheumatic fever	**Streptococcal cell-wall Ag;** Ab cross-reacts with myocardial Ag	Inflammation, macrophage activation	**Myocarditis, arthritis**
Goodpasture syndrome	**Type IV collagen** in basement membranes of kidney glomeruli and lung alveoli	Complement- and Fc-receptor–mediated inflammation	**Nephritis,** lung hemorrhage, **linear Ab deposits**
Transfusion reaction	ABO blood glycoproteins	IgM isohemagglutinins formed naturally in response to normal bacterial flora cause opsonization + complement activation	Hemolysis
Autoimmune thrombocytopenic purpura	Platelet membrane proteins	Ab-mediated platelet destruction through opsonization and complement activation	Bleeding
Non-cytotoxic			
Myasthenia gravis	**Acetylcholine receptor**	Ab inhibits acetylcholine binding, downmodulates receptors	**Muscle weakness, paralysis**
Graves disease	**TSH receptor**	Ab-mediated stimulation of TSH receptors	**Hyperthyroidism followed by hypothyroidism**
Type II (insulin-resistant) diabetes	Insulin receptor	Ab inhibits binding of insulin	Hyperglycemia
Pernicious anemia	Intrinsic factor of gastric parietal cells	Neutralization of intrinsic factor, decreased absorption of vitamin B12	Abnormal erythropoiesis, anemia

An important example of type II hypersensitivity is **HDNB**, also known as erythroblastosis fetalis. In the fetus, this disease is due to transport of IgG specific for one of the Rhesus (Rh) protein antigens (RhD) across the placenta.

About 85% of people are Rh+. If a pregnant woman is Rh– and the father is Rh+, there is a chance that the fetus will also be Rh+. This situation will pose no problem in the first pregnancy, as the mother's immune system will not usually encounter fetal blood cell antigens until placental separation at the time of birth. At that time, however, Rh+ fetal red blood cells will enter the maternal circulation and stimulate a T-dependent immune response, eventually resulting in the generation of memory B cells capable of producing IgG antibody against RhD.

In a subsequent pregnancy with another Rh+ fetus, this maternal IgG can be transported across the placenta, react with fetal Rh+ red cells, and activate complement, producing hemolytic disease. Hemolytic disease of the newborn can be prevented by treating the Rh– mother with RhoGAM™, a preparation of human anti-RhD antibody, at 28 weeks of gestation and again within 72 hours after birth. This antibody effectively eliminates the fetal Rh+ cells before they can generate RhD-specific memory B cells in the mother. Anti-RhD antibody should be given to any Rh– individual following any termination of pregnancy.

TYPE III (IMMUNE COMPLEX) HYPERSENSITIVITY

The immune complexes that cause disease may involve either self or foreign antigens bound to antibodies. These immune complexes are filtered out of the circulation in the small vasculature, so their sites of ultimate damage do not reflect their sites of origin. These diseases tend to be systemic, with little tissue or organ specificity.

Table I-12-5. Type III Hypersensitivities

Disease	Antigen Involved	Clinical Manifestations
Systemic lupus erythematosus⁺	**dsDNA,** Sm, other nucleoproteins	Nephritis, arthritis, vasculitis, **butterfly facial rash**
Poststreptococcal glomerulonephritis	Streptococcal cell wall Ags (may be "planted" in glomerular basement membrane)	Nephritis, **"lumpy-bumpy" deposits**
Arthus reaction	Any injected protein	Local pain and edema
Serum sickness	Various proteins	Arthritis, vasculitis, nephritis
Polyarteritis nodosa	Hepatitis B virus Ag	Systemic vasculitis

+Other autoimmune diseases correlated with production of antinuclear antibodies include diffuse systemic sclerosis (antibodies to DNA topoisomerase 1), limited scleroderma (CREST; antibodies to centromeric proteins) and Sjögren syndrome (antibodies to ribonucleoproteins).

TYPE IV (T-CELL–MEDIATED) HYPERSENSITIVITY

T lymphocytes may cause tissue injury by triggering delayed-type hypersensitivity (DTH) reactions or by directly killing target cells. These reactions are elicited by CD4+ Th1, Th17 cells, or CD8+ CTLs, which activate macrophages, recruit neutrophils, and induce inflammation. These T cells may be autoreactive or specific against foreign protein antigens bound to tissues. T-cell-mediated tissue injury is common during the protective immune response against persistent intracellular microbes.

Table I-12-6. Type IV Hypersensitivities

Disease	Specificity of Pathogenic T Cells	Clinical Manifestations
Tuberculin test	PPD (tuberculin & mycolic acid)	Indurated skin lesion (granuloma)
Contact dermatitis	**Nickel, poison ivy/oak catechols, hapten/carrier**	Vesicular skin lesions, pruritus, rash
Hashimoto thyroiditis*	Unknown Ag in thyroid	**Hypothyroidism**
Multiple sclerosis	Myelin Basic Protein	Progressive demyelination, blurred vision, paralysis
Rheumatoid arthritis*	Unknown Ag in joint synovium (type II collagen?)	Rheumatoid factor (IgM against Fc region of IgG), alpha-cyclic citrullinated peptide (α-CCP) antibodies, chronic arthritis, inflammation, destruction of articular cartilage and bone
Insulin-dependent diabetes mellitus (type I)*	Islet-cell antigens, insulin, glutamic acid decarboxylase, others	Chronic inflammation and destruction of β cells, polydipsia, polyuria, polyphagia, ketoacidosis
Guillain-Barré syndrome*	Peripheral nerve myelin or gangliosides	Ascending paralysis, peripheral nerve demyelination
Celiac disease	CD4+ cells—gliadin, CD8+ cells—HLA class I-like molecule expressed during stress	Gluten-sensitive enteropathy
Crohn disease	Unknown Ag, commensal bacteria?	Chronic intestinal inflammation due to Th1 and Th17 cells, obstruction

*Diseases classified at type IV pathologies in which autoantibodies are present and used as clinical markers

THE PATHOGENESIS OF AUTOIMMUNITY

The key factor in the development of autoimmunity is the recognition of self-antigens by autoreactive lymphocytes, which then become activated, proliferate, and differentiate to produce effector cells and cytokines that cause tissue injury. Autoimmunity must initially result from a failure of mechanisms of **central tolerance,** as cells are "educated" in the bone marrow and thymus (*see* chapter 3).

Self-reactive lymphocytes that escaped central tolerance are subject to the different mechanisms of peripheral tolerance. The 3 primary mechanisms that induce peripheral tolerance are anergy, deletion and supression.

B lymphocytes that recognize self-antigen in the absence of the T-cell signaling become anergic and express high levels of IgD on their surface, excluding them from secondary lymphoid tissues. Anergic B lymphocytes are then unable to receive the signals necessary for survival and undergo apoptosis. Additionally, B lymphocytes have inhibitory receptors that can be engaged when self-antigen is recognized suppressing their activity.

Similar to self-reactive B lymphocytes, T lymphocytes that recognize self-antigen in the absence of the appropriate costimulatory signals are subject to anergy or deletion. Anergy is the result of a breakdown in either TCR signaling or the binding of an inhibitory receptor, CTLA-4 or PD-1. Deletion of self-reactive T lymphocytes is due to apoptosis by activation of the caspase signaling pathway or the Fas signaling pathway.

Self-reactive T lymphocytes are also subject to suppression by Tregs. Although a majority of Tregs are generated during central tolerance, some arise in the periphery. Tregs secrete IL-10 and TGF-beta that inhibit the activation of lymphocytes, macrophage and dendritic cells. CTLA-4 is expressed at high levels on Tregs and is thought to bind to and sequester the costimulatory molecule B7 which would otherwise be used to activate T lymphocytes.

Development of autoimmune disease is due to a combination of genetic and environmental factors as well as hormonal triggers. Among the strongest genetic associations with the development of autoimmune disease are the **HLA genes**. Also known to contribute to autoimmunity are polymorphisms in non-HLA genes.

Table I-12-7. Examples of HLA-Linked Immunologic Diseases

Disease	HLA Allele
Rheumatoid arthritis	DR4
Insulin-dependent diabetes mellitus	DR3/DR4
Multiple sclerosis, Goodpasture's	DR2
Systemic lupus erythematosus	DR2/DR3
Ankylosing spondylitis, psoriasis, inflammatory bowel disease, reactive arthritis	B27
Celiac disease	DQ2 or DQ8
Graves disease	B8

Infections and tissue injury may alter the way that self-antigens are presented to lymphocytes and serve as an inciting factor in the development of disease. Because autoimmune reactions against one self-antigen may injure other tissues and expose other potential self-antigens for recognition, autoimmune diseases tend to be chronic and progressive.

Chapter Summary

- There are 4 types of hypersensitivity:
  - Immediate
  - Antibody-mediated (cytotoxic, blocking, enhancing)
  - Immune complex-mediated
  - T cell-mediated

- Hypersensitivity reactions require initial sensitization, and subsequent exposures to the same or cross-reactive antigens cause the damage.

- **Type I hypersensitivities** (immediate) involve IgE antibodies and mast cells, show symptoms in minutes, and are mounted against harmless environmental antigens in atopic or allergic individuals.
  - Initial tissue damage in immediate hypersensitivities is due to release of mast cell mediators, and late-phase reactions involve products of the arachidonic acid cascade.
  - Examples include hay fever, asthma, food allergies, and systemic anaphylaxis.

- **Type II (antibody-mediated) hypersensitivities** are tissue-specific and involve autoantibodies that opsonize or activate complement. Some noncytotoxic forms (myasthenia gravis, Graves disease, type II diabetes) cause interference with cellular function.
  - Examples (cytotoxic) include autoimmune hemolytic anemia, hemolytic disease of the newborn, autoimmune thrombocytopenic purpura, Goodpasture syndrome, rheumatic fever, and pernicious anemia.

- Type III (immune complex) hypersensitivities cause systemic damage by activating complement wherever immune complexes of antibodies against self or foreign antigens are filtered from the circulation.
  - Examples include systemic lupus erythematosus, polyarteritis nodosa, poststreptococcal glomerulonephritis, serum sickness, and the Arthus reaction.

- Type IV hypersensitivities are delayed-type (manifesting symptoms 48-72 hrs after reexposure); are caused by TH1 and TH17 cells, CD8+ cells, and macrophages; and are common results of infection with persistent intracellular microbes.
  - Examples include the tuberculin test, insulin-dependent diabetes mellitus, celiac disease, contact dermatitis, Guillain-Barré syndrome, RA, Crohn disease and Hashimoto thyroiditis.

- Autoimmune diseases may associate with specific class II MHC haplotypes, envi-ronmental factors, hormonal factors, or be triggered by infections.

Learning Objectives

❏ Solve problems concerning definitions

❏ Use knowledge of mechanisms of graft rejection

❏ Answer questions about graft versus host disease

OVERVIEW

Transplantation is the process of taking cells, tissues, or organs (a **graft**) from one individual (the **donor**) and implanting them into another individual or another site in the same individual (the **host** or **recipient**). **Transfusion** is a special case of transplantation and the most frequently practiced today, in which circulating blood cells or plasma are infused from one individual into another. As we have seen in previous chapters, the immune system is elaborately evolved to recognize minor differences in self antigens that reflect the invasion of harmful microbes or pathologic processes, such as cancer. Unfortunately, it is this same powerful mechanism of self-protection which thwarts tissue transplantation because tissues derived from other individuals are recognized as **"altered-self"** by the educated cells of the host's immune system.

Types of Graft Tissue

Several different types of grafts are used in medicine:

- Autologous grafts (or **autografts**) are those where tissue is moved from one location to another in the same individual (skin grafting in burns or coronary artery replacement with saphenous veins).

- **Isografts (or syngeneic grafts)** are those transplanted between genetically identical individuals (monozygotic twins).

- **Allogeneic** grafts are those transplanted between genetically different members of the same species (kidney transplant).

- **Xenogeneic** grafts are those transplanted between members of different species (pig heart valves into human).

MECHANISMS OF GRAFT REJECTION

The recognition of transplanted cells as self or foreign is determined by the extremely polymorphic genes of the major histocompatibility complex, which are expressed in a **codominant** fashion. This means that each individual inherits a complete set or **haplotype** from each parent and virtually assures that 2 genetically unrelated individuals will have distinctive differences in the antigens expressed on their cells.

Note

MHC alleles are expressed codominantly.

The net result is that all grafts except autografts are ultimately identified as foreign invading proteins and destroyed by the process of **graft rejection**. Even syngeneic grafts between identical twins can express recognizable antigenic differences due to somatic mutations that occur during the development of the individual. For this reason, all grafts except autografts must be followed by some degree of lifelong immunosuppression of the host to attempt to avoid rejection reactions.

The time sequence of allograft rejection differs depending on the tissue involved but always displays specificity and memory. As the graft becomes vascularized, CD4+ and CD8+ cells that migrate into the graft from the host become sensitized and proliferate in response to both major and minor histocompatibility differences. In the **effector phase** of the rejection, Th cytokines play a critical role in stimulating macrophage, cytotoxic T cell, and even antibody-mediated killing. Interferons and TNF-α and -β all increase the expression of class I MHC molecules in the graft, and IFN-γ increases the expression of class II MHC as well, increasing the susceptibility of cells in the graft to MHC-restricted killing.

Four different classes of allograft rejection phenomena are classified according to their time of activation and the type of effector mechanism that predominates.

Hyperacute Graft Rejection

- Occurs within minutes to hours
- Due to pre-formed antibodies due to transfusions, multi-parity, or previous organ transplants (type II cytotoxic hypersensitivity)
- Antibodies bind to the grafted tissue and activate complement and the clotting cascade resulting in thrombosis and ischemic necrosis
- Rare because of cross-matching blood, **but common vignette**

Acute Graft Rejection

- Occurs within days to weeks; the timing and mechanism are similar to a primary immune response
- Induced by alloantigens (predominantly MHC) in the graft
- Both CD4 and CD8 T cells play a role as well as antibodies (think normal immune response)
- Immunosuppressive therapy works to prevent this type of graft rejection mainly

Accelerated Acute Graft Rejection

- Occurs within days; the timing and mechanism are similar to a memory response.

Chronic Graft Rejection

- Occurs within months to years
- Predominantly T cell mediated
- Difficult to treat and usually results in graft rejection
- Etiology not well understood, possibly triggered by viral infections

Table I-13-1. Type and Tempo of Rejection Reactions

Type of Rejection	Time Taken	Mechanism & Pathogenesis
Hyperacute rejection	Minutes to hours	 Endothelial cell, Blood vessel, Alloantigen (e.g., blood group antigen), Circulating alloantigen specific antibody (pre-formed) Complement activation, endothelial damage, inflammation and thrombosis
Acute rejection	Days to weeks	 Parenchymal cells, Alloreactive antibody, Endothelial cell Parenchymal cell damage, interstitial inflammation Endothelialitis
Accelerated acute rejection	Days	As above, but mediated by memory cell responses
Chronic rejection	Months to years	 Macrophage, Vascular smooth muscle cell, Cytokines, Alloantigen-specific CD4+ T cell Causes unclear: chronic DTH reaction in vessel wall, intimal smooth muscle cell proliferation, vessel occlusion

GRAFT VERSUS HOST DISEASE

A special case of tissue transplantation occurs when the grafted tissue is bone marrow. Because the bone marrow is the source of pluripotent hematopoietic stem cells, it can be used to reconstitute myeloid, erythroid, and lymphoid cells in a recipient who has lost these cells as a result of malignancy or chemotherapeutic regimens. Because the bone marrow is a source of some mature T lymphocytes, it is necessary to remove these cells before transplantation to avoid the appearance of **graft-versus-host disease** in the recipient. In this special case of rejection, any mature T cells remaining in the bone marrow inoculum can attack allogeneic MHC-bearing cells of the recipient and cause widespread epithelial cell death accompanied by rash, jaundice, diarrhea, and gastrointestinal hemorrhage.

Clinical Correlate

Monoclonal antibodies are used in the treatment and prevention of graft rejection along with the classic therapies (corticosteroids, cyclosporine A, rapamycin, etc.).

Drug/Target	Mechanism of Action
Daclizumab, basiliximab (anti-IL-2 receptor antibody)	Blocks T cell proliferation via blocking the binding of IL-2, opsonization of IL-2R bearing cells
Muromonab (anti-CD3)	Blocks T cell activation by causing apoptosis
Belatacept (CTLA-4-Ig)	Inhibits T cell activation by blocking the B7 costimulatory molecule binding to CD28
Alemtuzumab (anti-CD52)*	Depletes pool of T cells by binding to them and causing complement mediated lysis

*CD52 is a marker found on all lymphocytes.

Chapter Summary

- In transplantation, tissues are taken from a donor and given to a host or recipient.

- During graft rejection, MHC allele products are recognized as foreign by CTLs, macrophages, and antibodies, and the graft is destroyed.
  - Graft rejection is hyperacute when preformed antidonor antibodies and complement destroy the graft in minutes to hours.
  - Graft rejection is acute when T cells are activated for the first time and destroy the graft in days to weeks.
  - Graft rejection is accelerated when sensitized T cells are reactivated to destroy the graft in days
  - Graft rejection is chronic when antibodies, immune complexes, or cytotoxic cells destroy the graft in months to years.

- Graft-versus-host disease occurs when mature T cells inside bone marrow transplants become activated against the MHC products of the graft recipient.

CD Markers

CD Designation	Cellular Expression	Known Functions
CD2 (LFA-2)	T cells, thymocytes, NK cells	Adhesion molecule
CD3	T cells, thymocytes	Signal transduction by the TCR
CD4	Th cells, thymocytes, monocytes, and macrophages	Coreceptor for TCR-MHC II interaction, receptor for HIV
CD8	CTLs, some thymocytes	Coreceptor for MHC class I–restricted T cells
CD14 (LPS receptor)	Monocytes, macrophages, granulocytes	Binds LPS
CD16 (Fc receptor)	NK cells, macrophages, neutrophils	Opsonization ADCC
CD18	Leukocytes	Cell adhesion molecule (missing in leukocyte adhesion deficiency)
CD19	B cells	Coreceptor with CD21 for B-cell activation (signal transduction)
CD20	Most or all B cells	Unknown role in B-cell activation
CD21 (CR2, C3d receptor)	Mature B cells	Receptor for complement fragment C3d, forms coreceptor complex with CD19, Epstein-Barr virus receptor
CD25	Activated Th cells and T_{Reg}	Alpha chain of IL-2 receptor
CD28	T cells	T-cell receptor for costimulatory molecule B7
CD34	Precursors of hematopoietic cells, endothelial cells in HEV	Cell–cell adhesion, binds L-selectin
CD40	B cells, macrophages, dendritic cells, endothelial cells	Binds CD40L, role in T-cell–dependent B cell, macrophage, dendritic cell and endothelial cell activation
CD56	NK cells	Cell adhesion
CD152 (CTLA-4)	Activated T cells	Negative regulation: competes with CD28 for B7 binding

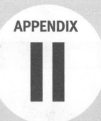
Cytokine	Secreted by	Target Cell/Tissue	Activity
Interleukin (IL)-1	Monocytes, macrophages, B cells, dendritic cells, endothelial cells, others	Th cells	Costimulates activation
		B cells	Promotes maturation and clonal expansion
		NK cells	Enhances activity
		Endothelial cells	Increases expression of ICAMs
		Macrophages and neutrophils	Chemotactically attracts
		Hepatocytes	Induces synthesis of acute-phase proteins
		Hypothalamus	Induces fever
IL-2	Th cells	Antigen-primed Th and CTLs	Induces proliferation, enhances activity
IL-3	Th cells, NK cells	Hematopoietic cells (myeloid)	Supports growth and differentiation
IL-4	Th2 cells	Antigen-primed B cells	Costimulates activation
		Activated B cells	Stimulates proliferation and differentiation, induces class switch to IgE
IL-5	Th2 cells and mast cells	Bone marrow cells	Induces eosinophil differentiation
IL-6	Monocytes, macrophages, Th2 cells, bone marrow stromal cells	Proliferating B cells	Promotes terminal differentiation into plasma cells
		Plasma cells	Stimulates Ab secretion
		Myeloid stem cells	Helps promote differentiation
		Hepatocytes	Induces synthesis of acute-phase proteins
IL-7	Bone marrow, thymic stromal cells	Lymphoid stem cells	Induces differentiation into progenitor B and T cells

(Continued)

Cytokine	Secreted by	Target Cell/Tissue	Activity
IL-8	Macrophages, endothelial cells	Neutrophils	Chemokine, induces adherence to endothelium and extravasation into tissues
IL-10	Th2 cells T$_{Reg}$ cells	Macrophages	Suppresses cytokine production by Th1 cells
IL-11	Bone marrow stroma	Bone marrow	↑ platelet count
IL-12	Macrophages, B cells	Activated CD8+ cells	Acts synergistically with IL-2 to induce differentiation into CTLs
		NK and LAK cells and activated Th1 cells	Stimulates proliferation
IL-13	Th2 cell	B cells	Induces isotype switch to IgE
IL-17	Th17 cells	Fibroblasts, endothelial cells, macrophages	Increases inflammation. Attracts PMNs, induces IL-6, IL-1, TGFβ, TNFα, IL-8
IL-18	Macrophages	IFN-γ synthesis	NK cells, Th cells, IFN-γ synthesis
Interferon-α (type I)	Leukocytes	Uninfected cells	Inhibits viral replication
IL-22	Th17	Endothelium	Stabilizes endothelial barrier, induces secretion of microbials
Interferon-β (type I)	Fibroblasts	Uninfected cells	Inhibits viral replication
Interferon-γ (type II)	Th1, CTLs, NK cells	Macrophages	Enhances activity
		Many cell types	Increases expression of classes I and II MHC
		Proliferating B cells	Induces class switch to IgG2a, blocks IL-4–induced class switch to IgE and IgG1
		Th2 cells	Inhibits proliferation
		Phagocytic cells	Mediates effects important in DTH, treatment for CGD
Transforming growth factor-β	Platelets, macrophages, lymphocytes, mast cells	Proliferating B cells	Induces class switch to IgA
Tumor necrosis factor-α	Macrophages, NK cells	Tumor cells	Has cytotoxic effect
		Inflammatory cells	Induces cytokine secretion, causes cachexia of chronic inflammation

(Continued)

Cytokine	Secreted by	Target Cell/Tissue	Activity
Tumor necrosis factor-β	Th1 and CTL	Tumor cells	Has cytotoxic and other effects, like TNF-α
		Macrophages and neutrophils	Enhances phagocytic activity
Granulocyte colony-stimulating factor (G-CSF)	Macrophages and Th cells	Bone marrow granulocyte precursors	Induce proliferation, used clinically to counteract neutropenia following ablative chemotherapy
Granulocyte– macrophage colony-stimulating factor (GM-CSF)	Macrophages and Th cells	Bone marrow granulocyte and macrophage precursors	Induces proliferation; used clinically to counteract neutropenia following ablative chemotherapy

CYTOKINES AVAILABLE IN RECOMBINANT FORM

Cytokine	Clinical Uses
Aldesleukin (IL-2)	$\uparrow$ lymphocyte differentiation and $\uparrow$ NKs—used in renal cell cancer and metastatic melanoma
Interleukin-11	$\uparrow$ platelet formation—used in thrombocytopenia
Filgrastim (G-CSF)	$\uparrow$ granulocytes—used for marrow recovery
Sargramostim (GM-CSF)	$\uparrow$ granulocytes and macrophages—used for marrow recovery
Erythropoietin	Anemias, especially associated with renal failure
Thrombopoietin	Thrombocytopenia
Interferon-α	Hepatitis B and C, leukemias, melanoma
Interferon-β	Multiple sclerosis
Interferon-γ	Chronic granulomatous disease $\rightarrow \uparrow$ TNF

Immunology Practice Questions

CELLS OF THE IMMUNE SYSTEM

1. Isotype switching during B-cell ontogeny dedicates mature B cells to production of a single heavy chain isotype, except in the case of IgM and IgD, which can be expressed concomitantly. How is this expression of both isotypes simultaneously possible?

   (A) Allelic exclusion

   (B) Allelic codominance

   (C) Affinity maturation

   (D) Alternative RNA splicing

   (E) Somatic hypermutation

2. A 4-year-old Caucasian boy is brought to his pediatrician with complaints of abnormal bruising and repeated bacterial infections. A blood workup reveals thrombocytopenia and neutropenia and the presence of numerous small, dense lymphoblasts with scant cytoplasm. Immunophenotyping of the abnormal cells determines them to be extremely primitive B cells, which are CD19+, HLA-DR+, and Tdt+. Which of the following best describes the status of immunoglobulin chain synthesis most likely in these cells?

   (A) IgM monomers inserted in the membrane

   (B) IgM monomers present in the cytoplasm

   (C) Mu (μ) chains inserted in the membrane

   (D) Mu (μ) chains present in the cytoplasm

   (E) No immunoglobulin chain synthesis present

3. A young woman with acute myeloblastic leukemia is treated with intensive chemotherapy and achieves remission of her symptoms. Because the prognosis for relapse is relatively high, a bone marrow transplant is undertaken in her first remission. Which of the following cytokines administered with the bone marrow cells would have the beneficial result of stimulating lymphoid-cell development from the grafted stem cells?

   (A) Interleukin (IL)-1

   (B) IL-2

   (C) IL-3

   (D) IL-6

   (E) IL-7

4. A 2-year-old boy is evaluated for a severe combined immunodeficiency disease. His bone marrow has normal cellularity. Radioactive tracer studies demonstrate a normal number of T-cell precursors entering the thymus, but no mature T lymphocytes are found in the blood or peripheral organs. Cells populating the thymus are found to lack CD3. Which of the following capabilities would his cells lack?

(A) Ability to bind cell-bound peptides

(B) Ability to express CD4/CD8 coreceptors

(C) Ability to produce terminal deoxyribonucleotidyl transferase

(D) Ability to proliferate in response to specific antigen

(E) Ability to rearrange T-cell receptor gene segments

5. A patient with advanced metastatic melanoma decides to join an experimental treatment protocol in the hope that it will cause regression of his tumor masses. Malignant cells are aspirated from several of his lesions and transfected in vitro with the gene encoding IL-3 production. The transfected tumor cells are then reinfused into the patient. Mobilization of which of the following cells from the bone marrow would be likely to result from this treatment?

(A) Antigen-presenting cells

(B) B lymphocytes

(C) NK cells

(D) Plasma cells

(E) T lymphocytes

THE SELECTION OF LYMPHOCYTES

6. An 8-year-old boy is diagnosed with acute lymphoblastic leukemia. Flow cytometry is used to determine the immunophenotype of the malignant cells. The patient's cells are evaluated with monoclonal antibodies for MHC class II, CD19, and CD34, and are found to have high levels of fluorescence with all of these markers. They also possess cytoplasmic μ heavy chains. What is the developmental stage of these cells?

(A) Immature B cell

(B) Lymphoid progenitor cell

(C) Mature B cell

(D) Pre-B cell

(E) Pro-B cell

7. The blood from an 8-year-old boy was analyzed by flow cytometry. The cells were treated with fluorescent-labeled antibodies to various cell surface markers before they were evaluated by flow cytometry. Which of the following markers would identify the B lymphocytes in the sample?

   (A) CD3
   (B) CD4
   (C) CD8
   (D) CD19
   (E) CD56

8. An 18-year-old member of a college soccer team is seen by a physician because of chest tightness and dyspnea on exertion. A 15-cm mediastinal mass is detected radiographically. Eighty percent of the white blood cells in the peripheral blood are small, abnormal lymphocytes with lobulated nuclei and scant cytoplasm. Immunophenotyping of the abnormal cells shows them to be CD4+ and CD8+. Where would such cells normally be found in the body?

   (A) Bone marrow
   (B) Peripheral blood
   (C) Thymic cortex
   (D) Thymic medulla
   (E) Splenic periarteriolar lymphoid sheaths

9. A 12-year-old child is diagnosed with a T-cell lymphoma. The phenotype of the malignant cell matches that of normal progenitor cells that leave the bone marrow to enter the thymus. What cell surface markers would you expect to find on the malignant cells?

   (A) CD4–, CD8–, TCR–
   (B) CD4–, CD8–, TCR+
   (C) CD4–, CD8+, TCR+
   (D) CD4+, CD8–, TCR+
   (E) CD4+, CD8+, TCR+

10. Herpes simplex viruses are extremely successful pathogens because they have a variety of immunologic evasion mechanisms. For example, both HSV 1 and 2 depress the expression of MHC class I molecules on the surface of infected cells. Which coreceptor's binding would be inhibited by this technique?

    (A) CD2
    (B) CD4
    (C) CD8
    (D) CD16
    (E) CD56

11. A patient with a B-cell lymphoma is referred to an oncology clinic for the analysis of his condition. The malignant cells are found to be producing IgM monomers. Which of the following therapeutic regimens is most likely to destroy the malignant cells and no others?

    (A) Anti-CD3 antibodies plus complement

    (B) Anti-CD19 antibodies plus complement

    (C) Anti-CD20 antibodies plus complement

    (D) Anti-idiotype antibodies plus complement

    (E) Anti-μ chain antibodies plus complement

LYMPHOCYTE RECIRCULATION AND HOMING

12. A lymph node biopsy of a 6-year-old boy shows markedly decreased numbers of lymphocytes in the paracortical areas. Analysis of his peripheral blood leukocytes is likely to show normal to elevated numbers of cells expressing surface

    (A) CD2

    (B) CD3

    (C) CD4

    (D) CD8

    (E) CD19

13. A 65-year-old woman was involved in an automobile accident that necessitated the removal of her spleen. To which of the following pathogens would she have the most increased susceptibility?

    (A) *Babesia microti*

    (B) *Bordetella pertussis*

    (C) *Corynebacterium diphtheriae*

    (D) Enteroaggregative *Escherichia coli*

    (E) Human papilloma virus

14. A 6-year-old child is taken to his pediatrician because the parents are alarmed about an indurated fluctuant mass on the posterior aspect of his neck. The mass is nontender and shows no signs of inflammation. The child is examined carefully, and no other masses are found. The pediatrician decides to submit a biopsy of this area to a pathologist. The pathologist reports back that the mass is a lymph node with markedly increased numbers of cells in the cortical area. Fluorescent antisera to which of the cell surface markers is most likely to bind to cells in this area?

    (A) CD2

    (B) CD3

    (C) CD4

    (D) CD16

    (E) CD19

15. A radioactive tracer dye is injected subcutaneously into the forearm of an experimental subject. What is the first area of the first draining lymph node that would develop significant radioactivity?

    (A) Cortex

    (B) Medulla

    (C) Paracortex

    (D) Primary follicle

    (E) Subcapsular sinus

THE FIRST RESPONSE TO ANTIGEN

16. A rabbit hunter in Arkansas is diagnosed with ulceroglandular tularemia and treated with streptomycin. Within a week, he returns to the hospital. The tularemic papule, lymphadenopathy, and bacteremia have resolved, but he has now developed a raised, itching skin rash and a fever. The drug was discontinued, and the symptoms subsided. What was the role of streptomycin in this case?

    (A) It acted as a B-cell mitogen

    (B) It acted as a hapten

    (C) It acted as a provider of costimulatory signals

    (D) It acted as a superantigen

    (E) It acted as an immunogen

17. A 2-year-old child who has suffered recurrent bacterial infections is evaluated for immunologic deficiency. The child has age-normal numbers of CD19+ and CD3+ cells in the peripheral blood and an extreme neutrophilia. The nitroblue tetrazolium dye reduction test is normal. What is the most likely defect in this child?

    (A) Absence of CCR4

    (B) Absence of CD18

    (C) Absence of interleukin-1

    (D) Absence of interleukin-4

    (E) Absence of tumor necrosis factor-α

18. A 2-year-old boy is admitted to the hospital for workup of a possible immunologic disorder. His history is remarkable for the occurrence of multiple skin infections involving *Staphylococcus*, *Pseudomonas*, and *Candida*. On examination the child has cervical lymphadenopathy and mild hepatosplenomegaly. Blood tests reveal an elevated erythrocyte sedimentation rate and neutrophilia. The nitroblue tetrazolium dye reduction test and neutrophil oxidative index are negative. What is the most likely defect in this child?

    (A) C3 deficiency

    (B) Deficiency of CD18

    (C) Deficiency of myeloperoxidase

    (D) NADPH oxidase deficiency

    (E) Phagocyte granule structural defect

19. It has been learned in animal experiments that there are advantages to eliciting nonspecific inflammation at the site of inoculation of antigen toward the ultimate development of a protective immune response to that immunogen. Which of the following substances, if introduced with a vaccine, would serve the purpose of attracting a neutrophilic infiltrate into the area?

    (A) Complement component 3b

    (B) Immunoglobulin G

    (C) Interleukin-8

    (D) Myeloperoxidase

    (E) Tumor necrosis factor-α

THE PROCESSING AND PRESENTATION OF ANTIGEN

20. Human infections with *Mycobacterium leprae* express a spectrum of clinical presentations depending on the extent and expression of their immune response to the intracellular organism. On one end of the spectrum, patients with tuberculoid leprosy produce an effective cell-mediated immune response, which is successful at killing the intracellular organisms and, unfortunately, produces tissue damage. Patients with tuberculoid leprosy have granulomas that have elevated amounts of IL-2, IFN-γ, and TNF-β. The immune cell responsible for this pattern of cytokine production is the

    (A) Cytotoxic T lymphocyte

    (B) Epithelioid cell

    (C) Macrophage

    (D) Th1 cell

    (E) Th2 cell

21. There is evidence that the immunologic pathway that distinguishes the selection between the two polar forms of leprosy depends on the initial means of antigen presentation, as well as individual human differences in response. If early events of antigen recognition elicit production of IL-4, IL-5, IL-6, and IL-10, lepromatous leprosy is more likely to result, with the outcome of failure to mount a protective delayed-type hypersensitivity response. What differential characteristic of the lepromatous form is predicted based on the fact of overproduction of IL-4, IL-5, IL-6, IL-10, IL-13 and TGFβ in lepromatous lesions?

    (A) Autoimmunity

    (B) Granuloma formation

    (C) Hypergammaglobulinemia

    (D) Immediate hypersensitivity

    (E) Inflammation

22. An elderly man with diabetes develops a blister on the heel of his foot, which becomes infected. Although nursing staff in the home where he is a resident clean and treat the wound with topical antibiotic ointment, he develops a fever and hypotension, and a desquamating rash spreads from the site of the original blister. How does the toxin responsible for his symptoms cause these signs?

    (A) It acts as an IL-1 homologue

    (B) It activates B lymphocytes polyclonally

    (C) It activates complement

    (D) It cross-links MHC class II molecules to TCRs polyclonally

    (E) It stimulates neutrophils

23. It has been learned in several experimental systems that proliferation and differentiation of T lymphocytes in response to tumor cells is low because tumor cells lack the necessary costimulatory molecules for lymphocyte activation. If melanoma cells from a patient were induced to express these costimulatory molecules by transfection, production of an effective antitumor response might occur. Which of the following molecules would be the best candidate for transfection of tumor cells to achieve this end?

    (A) B7

    (B) CD2

    (C) CD4

    (D) CD28

    (E) LFA-1

24. A 50-year-old woman with severe rheumatoid arthritis is started on infliximab (anti-tumor necrosis factor-alpha). This therapy has been shown to increase the production of CD25-positive T cells. Which of the following is likely, therefore, to become elevated in this patient?

    (A) Interferon-gamma

    (B) Interleukin-1

    (C) Interleukin-2

    (D) Interleukin-10

    (E) Transforming growth factor-beta

THE GENERATION OF HUMORAL EFFECTOR MECHANISMS

25. An antibody preparation is being used in a laboratory protocol to study B lymphocytes. The preparation does not activate the cells or cause capping. It does not cause precipitation of its purified ligand, and it does not cause agglutination of latex beads covalently coupled to its ligand. Which of the following is the most likely antibody preparation?

    (A) Monoclonal anti-CD19 IgG

    (B) Monoclonal anti-CD56 IgG

    (C) Papain-treated anti-CD19 IgG

    (D) Papain-treated anti-CD56 IgG

    (E) Pepsin-treated anti-CD19 IgG

    (F) Pepsin-treated anti-CD56 IgG

26. IgM isohemagglutinins from an individual of blood group A are treated with pepsin. When the product of this reaction is added to group B erythrocytes, they will be

    (A) agglutinated

    (B) lysed

    (C) phagocytized

    (D) precipitated

    (E) unaffected

27. A 26-year-old obstetric patient becomes ill during the first trimester of pregnancy with fever and lymphadenopathy. She is found to have a rising titer of anti-*Toxoplasma gondii* antibodies. She delivers a full-term baby with no apparent signs of in utero infection. The best test to diagnose acute infection in the neonate would be a parasite-specific ELISA for which isotype of immunoglobulin?

    (A) IgA

    (B) IgD

    (C) IgE

    (D) IgG

    (E) IgM

28. A 4-year-old boy is evaluated for a possible immunologic deficiency. He has suffered repeated infections of mucosal-surface pathogens and has shown delayed development of protective responses to the standard childhood vaccinations. Immunoelectrophoresis of his serum demonstrates absence of a macroglobulin peak, and his sputum is devoid of secretory IgA. Normal numbers of B lymphocytes bearing monomeric IgM are found by flow cytometry, and serum levels of monomeric IgA, IgE, and each of the 4 subisotypes of IgG are normal. Which of the following deficiencies could account for these findings?

    (A) Absence of CD40

    (B) Absence of J chains

    (C) Absence of IL-4

    (D) Absence of Tdt

    (E) Absence of Th2 cells

29. A 56-year-old homeless, alcoholic, and febrile man is brought to the emergency department after a difficult night during which his coughing kept everyone at the shelter awake. On arrival his pulse is rapid, and his breathing is labored with diffuse rales. Endotracheal aspirates produce a mucopurulent discharge containing numerous gram-positive cocci in chains. His serum contains high titers of IgM antibodies specific for the polysaccharide capsule of *Streptococcus pneumoniae*. The effector mechanism most likely to act in concert with this early IgM production to clear infection is

    (A) ADCC

    (B) complement-mediated opsonization

    (C) cytotoxic T lymphocytes

    (D) LAK cells

    (E) NK cells

30. A 3-year-old boy has had several bouts with pneumonia. *Streptococcus pneumoniae* was isolated and identified in each of the cases. The child was treated with penicillin each time, and the condition resolved. He is now being evaluated for a potential immunologic deficiency. Serum electrophoresis shows age-normal values for all isotypes of immunoglobulin, but serum levels of some components of complement are depressed. Which of the following deficiencies could explain his problem?

    (A) C1

    (B) C2

    (C) C3

    (D) C4

    (E) C5

31. Up until the 1970s, tonsillectomies were routinely performed on children with swollen tonsils. This procedure has lost its widespread appeal as we have learned the important role of mucosal-associated lymphoid tissue (MALT) in the protective immune response. What is the major immuno-globulin produced by the MALT?

    (A) A dimeric immunoglobulin with secretory component

    (B) A monomeric immunoglobulin that crosses the placenta

    (C) A monomeric immunoglobulin bound by mast cells

    (D) A monomeric immunoglobulin that opsonizes

    (E) A pentameric immunoglobulin that activates complement

32. A 64-year-old man undergoes surgery to excise 18 inches of bowel with adenocarcinoma. When the tissue and draining mesenteric lymph nodes are sent for pathologist's examination, the Peyer patches are noted to be hyperplastic with IgA-secreting plasma cells, but there is no secretory IgA found in the lumen of the colon. Which of the following changes in the bowel epithelium could explain this finding?

    (A) Failure of isotype switching

    (B) Failure of variable domain gene-segment rearrangement

    (C) Loss of J chain synthesis

    (D) Loss of the polyimmunoglobulin receptor

    (E) Loss of Th2 cells

THE GENERATION OF CELL-MEDIATED EFFECTOR MECHANISMS

33. A 62-year-old accountant develops a solid tumor that is unresponsive to chemotherapy. He elects to participate in an experimental treatment pro-tocol to stimulate his own immune effector cells to recognize and kill the malignant cells. The tumor cells are found to have no expression of MHC class I antigens. Which of the following in vitro treatments of his tumor cells is likely to stimulate the most effective immune response when rein-fused into the patient?

    (A) IFN-γ

    (B) IL-2

    (C) IL-8

    (D) IL-10

    (E) TNF-β

34. *Toxoplasma gondii* is an intracellular parasite that lives inside phagocytic and nonphagocytic cells by generating its own intracellular vesicle. This may allow it to avoid recognition and killing by CD8+ lymphocytes, which require the presentation of foreign peptides transported into the endoplasmic reticulum and loaded onto MHC molecules that have

    (A) a β_2 domain instead of a β_2 microglobulin
    (B) invariant chains
    (C) a peptide-binding groove
    (D) a single transmembrane domain
    (E) two similar chains

35. Before 1960, children with enlarged thymus glands were frequently irradiated to functionally ablate this organ, whose role was not yet known. Over the lifetime of such individuals, which of the following conditions was likely to develop?

    (A) Depressed immune surveillance of tumors
    (B) Depressed oxygen-dependent killing by neutrophils
    (C) Depressed primary response to soluble antigens
    (D) Increased cellularity of lymph node paracortical areas
    (E) Increased tendency toward atopy

36. A 42-year-old Nigerian man who is in the United States visiting with his brother comes into the hospital clinic. He complains of several months of weight loss, night sweats, mild sputum production, and the spitting up of blood. You run a PPD skin test and the results are positive. What can you conclude from this result?

    (A) A cell-mediated immune response has occurred
    (B) A humoral immune response has occurred
    (C) The B-cell system is functional
    (D) The B- and T-cell systems are functional
    (E) The neutrophilic phagocyte system is functional

37. A woman with advanced metastatic breast cancer undergoes a radical mastectomy, followed by irradiation and chemotherapy. After a 2-year remission, a metastatic focus appears, and she enrolls in an experimental treatment protocol. In it, a sample of her aspirated bone marrow is treated with GM-CSF, TNF-α, and IL-2, then pulsed with membrane fragments of her tumor cells and reinfused. Which of the following cell subpopulations is the most directly targeted by this treatment?

    (A) B lymphocytes
    (B) Cytotoxic T lymphocytes
    (C) NK cells
    (D) Th1 cells
    (E) Th2 cells

THE GENERATION OF IMMUNOLOGIC MEMORY

38. In a lifetime, a person may receive a dozen or more tetanus toxoid inoculations. When boosters are administered at 10-year intervals, which of the following would be true of the B lymphocytes that respond?

    (A) Their receptors would have high avidity

    (B) They would be large and highly metabolic

    (C) They would have low levels of adhesion molecules

    (D) They would have surface IgG, IgA, or IgE

    (E) They would have surface IgM

VACCINATION AND IMMUNOTHERAPY

39. A 10-year-old child was bitten by a stray dog. The child is started on a course of anti-rabies post-exposure prophylaxis, beginning with inoculation of pooled human antirabies immunoglobulin. What would repeated inoculation of this antirabies immunoglobulin preparation be likely to induce?

    (A) Anti-allotype antibodies

    (B) Anti-epitope antibodies

    (C) Anti-idiotype antibodies

    (D) Anti-isotype antibodies

    (E) Anti-rabies antibodies

40. All residents of a Chicago nursing home are inoculated intramuscularly with an H3N2 influenza A preparation. The goal of this protocol is to stimulate which of the following types of immunity?

    (A) Adaptive

    (B) Artificial active

    (C) Artificial passive

    (D) Natural active

    (E) Natural passive

41. A city sanitation worker is struck by a car and his leg is crushed against his sanitation truck. The extreme trauma to the leg necessitates amputation above the knee. Although the patient's health records reflect a tetanus booster 6 years ago, the man is revaccinated and human, pooled antitetanus immunoglobulin is injected around the macerated tissue. Administration of immunoglobulin is an example of which of the following forms of immunization?

    (A) Adaptive

    (B) Artificial active

    (C) Artificial passive

    (D) Natural active

    (E) Natural passive

42. A 28-year-old man was brought into court for nonpayment of child support. A 20-year-old woman insists that he is the father of her child. The court suggests before hearing the paternity case that various genetic tests be performed on the man, woman, and child. One of the sets of tests was for genetic immunoglobulin identification. Which immunoglobulin marker would be useful in this case?

    (A) Allotype
    (B) Idiotype
    (C) IgA2
    (D) IgM
    (E) Isotype

43. In 1988 a new childhood vaccine was developed to protect against epidemic meningitis by mixing *Haemophilus influenzae* type B capsular polysaccharide with whole, killed *Bordetella pertussis* bacteria. The function of the whole, killed bacteria in this vaccine was as a(n)

    (A) carrier
    (B) hapten
    (A) mitogen
    (D) adjuvant
    (E) immunogen

IMMUNODEFICIENCY DISEASES

44. A newborn is evaluated for immunologic function. He has a distortion of the shape of his mouth, low-set and malformed ears, and widely spaced eyes. Radiographically, there is evidence of cardiac malformation and absence of a thymic shadow. Which of the following parameters would be normal in this child?

    (A) Antibody-dependent cell-mediated cytotoxicity of parasite targets
    (B) Cellularity of splenic periarteriolar lymphoid sheaths
    (C) Cytotoxic killing of virus-infected targets
    (D) Generation of oxygen metabolites in phagocytic cells
    (E) Proliferative response to concanavalin A

45. A 14-month-old male infant is referred to a specialist for diagnosis of a potential immunologic deficiency. For the past 4 months, the child has suffered repeated episodes of bacterial infections and attempts to induce immunity using the pneumococcal vaccine have failed. Studies of peripheral blood indicate an absence of cells responsive to pokeweed mitogen. Bone marrow aspirates are remarkable for hypercellularity of pre-B cells. What is the most likely diagnosis?

    (A) Bruton agammaglobulinemia

    (B) Common variable hypogammaglobulinemia

    (C) DiGeorge syndrome

    (D) Selective immunoglobulin deficiency

    (E) Wiskott-Aldrich syndrome

46. A 31-year-old man is treated for a fourth episode of disseminated *Neisseria gonorrhoeae* infection in the last 5 years. He had no previous history of unusual or recurrent infections. If he has an immunologic defect, which of the following is most likely?

    (A) Common variable immunodeficiency

    (B) C8 deficiency

    (C) DiGeorge syndrome

    (D) Selective IgA deficiency

    (E) Severe combined immunodeficiency

47. A patient has been hospitalized 3 times for painful abdominal edema and is complaining now of swollen lips. What will laboratory findings in this patient most likely include?

    (A) Abnormal superoxide anion production by neutrophils

    (B) Abnormal T-cell function

    (C) Abnormal T-cell numbers

    (D) Defective neutrophil chemotaxis

    (E) Reduced C4 levels

48. A 4-year-old girl presents with a severe *Staphylococcus aureus* abscess. Her history is significant for a previous infection with *Serratia marcescens*. If she has an enzyme deficiency, which of the following is most likely?

    (A) Adenosine deaminase

    (B) C1 inhibitor

    (C) Myeloperoxidase

    (D) NADPH oxidase

    (E) Superoxide dismutase

49. An acutely ill, 2-year-old boy is hospitalized with *Staphylococcus aureus* pneumonia, which is treated appropriately. The patient's history indicates similar bouts of bacterial infections in the past. He had recovered uneventfully from measles 6 months ago. Physical examination discloses scant tonsillar tissue and no palpable lymphadenopathy. Immunoelectrophoresis reveals subnormal levels of gammaglobulins. The nitroblue tetrazolium and chemiluminescence assays indicate normal phagocytic killing. Which of the following disorders is most likely responsible for this child's condition?

    (A) Adenosine deaminase deficiency

    (B) Defect of the *Btk* gene

    (C) Defect of the *SAP* gene

    (D) Defect of the *WAS* gene

    (E) ICAM-1 deficiency

50. A 2-year-old boy suffering from repeated painful bouts of inflammation of mucosal surfaces, especially affecting the lips, is brought to the pediatrician's office. The mother remembers similar symptoms in previous generations of her family and fears a heritable tendency toward food allergy. What laboratory finding would best support the physician's suspicion?

    (A) Depressed C3

    (B) Depressed C4

    (C) Depressed C5

    (D) Elevated C1

    (E) Elevated C1, C4, and C2

51. A 10-month-old infant girl is admitted to the hospital with signs of *Pneumocystis jirovecii* pneumonia. Studies of her peripheral blood demonstrate age-normal counts of CD19+ cells, but CD3+ and CD4+ cell numbers are depressed. Immunoelectrophoresis of her serum reveals a moderate hypogammaglobulinemia. Her peripheral blood lymphocytes proliferate normally in response to phytohemagglutinin and MHC class I mismatched allogeneic cells. In a one-way mixed lymphocyte reaction using her cells as the stimulator cells, allogeneic T lymphocytes did not proliferate. Which of the following best describes the molecule most likely lacking from her lymphocytes?

    (A) It is designed to bind endogenously produced peptides

    (B) It is designed to bind exogenously processed peptides

    (C) It possesses β_2 microglobulin

    (D) It possesses two chains of unequal length

    (E) It should be present on all nucleated cells in the body

DISEASES CAUSED BY IMMUNE RESPONSES: HYPERSENSITIVITY AND AUTOIMMUNITY

52. A 36-year-old farmer has been exposed to poison ivy on several different occasions, and he usually gets very severe skin lesions. A pharmaceutical company is developing cytokines by recombinant DNA technology and formulating them in a fashion that they are readily absorbed through the skin. Which of the following cytokines administered topically could inhibit the severity of this reaction?

(A) γ-Interferon

(B) IL-2

(C) IL-3

(D) IL-8

(E) IL-10

53. In the 1960s, it was quickly ascertained that Peace Corps workers sent to schistosome-endemic areas were exposed to massive initial doses of cercariae before any protective immunity existed. In these individuals, IgG antibodies developed in response to the developing worms, and when the adults began their prodigious release of eggs into the circulation, the patients suffered acute and potentially life-threatening symptoms of fever, edema, arthralgia, and rash. Which of the following is another condition that arises by a similar immunologic mechanism?

(A) Arthus reaction

(B) Atopic allergy

(C) Goodpasture syndrome

(D) Tuberculin reaction

(E) Transfusion reaction

54. In native Egyptian populations, children are exposed to the cercariae of the fluke *Schistosoma mansoni* in early childhood when they wade in irrigation ditches throughout the Nile Delta. On first exposure, the cercariae penetrate the skin and become schistosomula, which enter the circulation and eventually mature in the mesenteric veins. On subsequent exposures, schistosomula are frequently killed within minutes by an immune response in the skin manifested by intense itching, stinging, and urticaria. What is this protective immune response a manifestation of?

(A) Arthus reaction

(B) Contact dermatitis

(C) Passive cutaneous anaphylaxis

(D) Serum sickness

(E) Type I hypersensitivity

TRANSPLANTATION IMMUNOLOGY

55. A 42-year-old auto mechanic has been diagnosed with end-stage renal disease. His twin brother is HLA identical at all MHC loci and volunteers to donate a kidney to his brother. What type of graft transplant terminology is correct in this situation?

   (A) Allograft

   (B) Autograft

   (C) Heterograft

   (D) Isograft

   (E) Xenograft

56. A patient with acute myelogenous leukemia (AML) undergoes irradiation and chemotherapy for his malignancy while awaiting bone marrow transplantation from a closely matched sibling. Six months after the transplant, the immune response appears to be reconstituting itself well—until 9 months postinfusion, when symptoms of generalized rash with desquamation, jaundice, and bloody diarrhea begin to appear. A second, more closely matched bone marrow donor is sought unsuccessfully, and 10 months after the transfer, the patient dies. What is the immunologic effector mechanism most closely associated with this rejection reaction?

   (A) Activated macrophages

   (B) Antibodies and complement

   (C) CD8+ lymphocytes

   (D) LAK cells

   (E) NK cells

57. A child who requires a kidney transplant has been offered a kidney by both parents and 3 siblings. A one-way mixed lymphocyte reaction between prospective donors and recipient is performed, and the stimulation indices are shown. The stimulation index is the ratio of proliferation (measured by [^{3}H]-thymidine incorporation) of the experimental group versus the negative control group. Which of the prospective donors would be the best choice?

Responder Cells	Irradiated Stimulator Cells					
	Recipient	Father	Mother	Sibling 1	Sibling 2	Sibling 3
Recipient	1.0	4.1	2.3	1.1	8.3	8.5
Father	5.3	1.0	12.3	5.6	4.9	5.9
Mother	3.2	12.6	1.0	4.5	3.9	4.8
Sibling 1	1.6	6.5	5.5	1.0	4.4	6.0
Sibling 2	7.6	5.9	4.9	4.4	1.0	7.8
Sibling 3	9.0	5.7	4.4	7.0	8.9	1.0

(A) Father

(B) Mother

(C) Sibling 1

(D) Sibling 2

(E) Sibling 3

58. A 6-year-old child from Zimbabwe is admitted to a U.S. oncology center for treatment of an advanced case of Burkitt lymphoma. Analysis of the malignant cells reveals that they are lacking MHC class I antigens on their surface. Which of the following cytokines produced by recombinant DNA technology could be injected into his solid tumor to increase this tumor cell's susceptibility to CD8+-mediated killing?

(A) IFN-γ

(B) IL-1

(C) IL-2

(D) IL-10

(E) TNF-α

LABORATORY TECHNIQUES IN IMMUNOLOGY

59. A 16-year-old runaway heroin user visits a family planning/STD clinic irregularly to receive birth control pills. In April 2004, the standard HIV screen performed by this clinic reports back that her test was positive. What does the primary test for HIV infection use?

    (A) Electrophoresis of HIV antigens in polyacrylamide gel

    (B) HIV antigen covalently coupled to RBC, patient serum, and anti-immunoglobulin

    (C) HIV antigen covalently coupled to RBC, patient serum, and complement

    (D) HIV antigen, patient serum, anti-immunoglobulin serum, and enzyme-substrate ligand

    (E) HIV antigen, patient serum, anti-immunoglobulin serum, and radioactive ligand

60. A direct Coombs test was performed on a baby in its seventh month of gestation. The mother has had trouble with two earlier pregnancies, and she has never received RhoGAM™. The physician is concerned about the possibility of erythroblastosis fetalis. What ingredients would be necessary to perform this procedure?

    (A) Mother's serum plus RhoGAM plus Coombs reagent

    (B) Mother's serum plus Rh– RBCs plus Coombs reagent

    (C) RhoGAM plus Rh+ RBCs from the baby

    (D) Rh+ RBCs from the baby plus Coombs reagent

    (E) Rh+ RBCs plus mother's serum plus Coombs reagent

61. A patient with Chediak-Higashi syndrome is analyzed for ability to mobilize NK cells into the peripheral blood. His peripheral blood leukocytes are treated with fluorescent-labeled antibodies to CD3, CD56, and CD20 before they are passed through a fluorescence-activated cell sorter. The computer-generated results of this process are shown. In which quadrant of which panel would the natural killer cells be found?

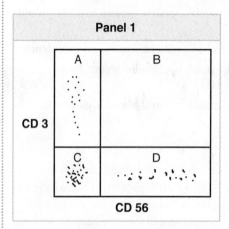
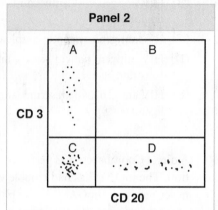

(A) Panel 1, quadrant A

(B) Panel 1, quadrant B

(C) Panel 1, quadrant C

(D) Panel 1, quadrant D

(E) Panel 2, quadrant A

(F) Panel 2, quadrant B

(G) Panel 2, quadrant C

(H) Panel 2, quadrant D

62. In both ABO blood typing and the Coombs test for detection of hemolytic disease of the newborn, agglutination of coated erythrocytes is a positive test result. Why is addition of Coombs reagent not a necessary step in ABO blood typing?

(A) All antibodies made in response to blood glycoproteins are IgG

(B) Complement-mediated lysis is not important in ABO incompatibilities

(C) Coombs serum identifies only anti-Rh antibodies

(D) IgM pentamers are large enough to agglutinate erythrocytes directly

(E) The high titer of natural isohemagglutinins makes Coombs reagent unnecessary

63. A young woman is in the care of an infertility specialist for evaluation of her inability to conceive since her marriage 5 years ago. As a first step in her examination, cervical scrapings are tested for the possibility of undiagnosed infection with *Chlamydia trachomatis*, which could cause fallopian tube scarring. Which of the following diagnostic tests could be used to identify chlamydial antigens in this specimen?

    (A) Direct fluorescent antibody test

    (B) Enzyme-linked immunosorbent assay (ELISA)

    (C) Indirect fluorescent antibody test

    (D) Radioimmunoassay

    (E) Western blot

64. An experimental treatment for melanoma involves in vitro stimulation of tumor-specific killer cells with tumor cells transfected with a gene for production of altered-self MHC class I molecules. As a first step, peripheral blood leukocytes from the patient are incubated with fluorescent-labeled antibodies against CD4, CD8, and CD20. The cells are then subjected to flow cytometry and separated into different populations based on their expression of these cell surface markers. In which quadrant would you find the cell subpopulation most likely to produce a beneficial anti-tumor response in this protocol?

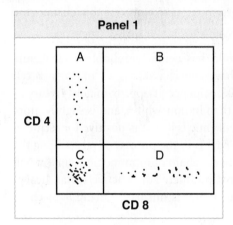
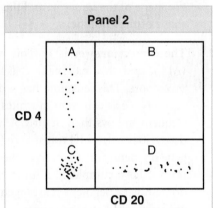

    (A) Panel 1, quadrant A

    (B) Panel 1, quadrant B

    (C) Panel 1, quadrant C

    (D) Panel 1, quadrant D

    (E) Panel 2, quadrant A

    (F) Panel 2, quadrant B

    (G) Panel 2, quadrant C

    (H) Panel 2, quadrant D

ANSWERS AND EXPLANATIONS

1. **The correct answer is D.** Alternative RNA splicing allows a mature B cell to attach either δ or μ constant domains on a single idiotype that has been generated by germ-line DNA rearrangements.

    Allelic exclusion (**choice A**) refers to the expression of products of either parental chromosome type, but not both. This allows lymphoid cells to express only one type of antigen receptor (one idiotype) per cell and is essential to cellular specificity of action.

    Allelic codominance (**choice B**) refers to the expression of products of both parental chromosomes simultaneously. It is found in the expression of MHC class I and II products, but not in the expression of antigen receptors.

    Affinity maturation (**choice C**) refers to the increase of affinity (binding strength) of a population of antibodies over time during the development of an immune response. Because the affinity of an antibody is dependent on the goodness-of-fit of its idiotype for its antigen, isotype switching does not affect the shape of the idiotype and does not change the affinity of the molecule.

    Somatic hypermutation (**choice E**) is the phenomenon that allows affinity maturation to occur. It is the accelerated mutation of DNA coding within the hypervariable region that occurs during B-cell proliferation in response to antigenic stimulation. Again, the isotype of the antibody does not affect the shape of the idiotype, and this term refers to a process that changes the shape of the idiotype.

2. **The correct answer is E.** This child has acute lymphoblastic leukemia (ALL), and the malignant cells have the characteristics of early B-cell precursors. This leukemia has peak incidence at approximately 4 years of age, is twice as common in whites than in non-whites, and is slightly more frequent in boys than in girls. A leukemic cell that is positive for terminal deoxyribonucleotidyl transferase (Tdt) is in the process of rearranging the gene segments for synthesis of the heavy chain of immunoglobulin but will not yet have completed a functional product. Tdt is active for all heavy-domain gene segment rearrangements but is not used during light-chain gene segment rearrangements.

    IgM monomers inserted in the membrane (**choice A**) would be found in leukemic cells that are at the mature B-cell stage. Such cells would have completed the rearrangements for both heavy and light chains and would lack Tdt as a marker. They would express surface MHC class II, CD19, and CD20 in addition to surface immunoglobulin.

    IgM monomers present in the cytoplasm (**choice B**) would be found in cells that have completed the rearrangement of their variable domain gene segments. They would no longer express Tdt.

    Mu (μ) chains inserted in the membrane (**choice C**) would be found in cells that have completed the rearrangement of their heavy chain variable domain gene segments, and these may transiently be expressed on the surface of a cell in association with a surrogate light chain before light chain rearrangement is complete. These cells would not be using their Tdt any more.

    Mu (μ) chains in the cytoplasm (**choice D**) would be found in leukemic cells that are more highly differentiated than those described. Once the variable domain gene segments for the heavy chain have been successfully rearranged in a cell, μ chains can be found in the cytoplasm. In ALL, this is usually associated with a decreased expression of Tdt and appearance of CD10 (the common acute lymphoblastic leukemia antigen; CALLA) and CD20.

3. **The correct answer is E.** The cytokine most strongly associated with stimulation of production of lymphoid cells from the bone marrow is interleukin (IL)-7.

IL-1 (**choice A**) is the endogenous pyrogen. It is produced by macrophages and acts on the hypothalamus to raise the temperature set point. It is associated with systemic inflammatory processes, but is not known to have an effect on lymphopoiesis.

IL-2 (**choice B**) is a product of T cells that stimulates proliferation of T cells in the periphery. It is not known to have an effect on lymphopoiesis.

IL-3 (**choice C**) is the cytokine that is most strongly associated with stimulation of myeloid cell precursors in the bone marrow.

IL-6 (**choice D**) is a second endogenous pyrogen. It causes production of acute-phase proteins from hepatocytes and acts on myeloid stem cells in the bone marrow to induce differentiation.

4. **The correct answer is D.** CD3 is the signal transduction complex in T lymphocytes. When specific antigen binding has occurred on the surface of the cell, this complex is responsible for transferring the message to the cytoplasm of the cell. This culminates in intracytoplasmic phosphorylation events, which activate the cell and induce its proliferation (cloning). A cell lacking CD3 would be capable of binding specific antigen, but incapable of activation and proliferation in response to that first signal.

Ability to bind cell-bound peptides (**choice A**) would not be affected by the absence of CD3. Binding to peptides presented by antigen-presenting cells is through interaction of the T-cell receptor with major histocompatibility antigens on the surface of other cells.

Ability to express coreceptors (**choice B**) would not be affected by the absence of CD3, although cells would not be able to complete their differentiation in the thymus and become fully committed T cells.

Ability to produce terminal deoxyribonucleotidyl transferase (**choice C**) would not be affected by the absence of the T-cell signal transduction complex. T-cell precursors rearrange their receptor gene segments (and use terminal deoxyribonucleotidyl transferase) in the absence of antigenic stimulation and before signal transduction through CD3 becomes critical.

Ability to rearrange T-cell receptor gene segments (**choice E**) would not be affected by the absence of the T-cell signal transduction complex. T-cell precursors rearrange their receptor gene segments in the absence of antigenic stimulation and before signal transduction through CD3 becomes critical.

5. **The correct answer is A.** Tumor cells transfected with the gene encoding IL-3 would produce IL-3. This is a cytokine that acts on the bone marrow to cause production and mobilization of myeloid cells. The goal of such therapy would be to induce the production of antigen-presenting cells, which might increase the presentation of tumor-cell antigens to cells important in cell-mediated cytotoxicity.

B lymphocytes (**choice B**) would not be mobilized by such a treatment. The cytokine that favors development of lymphoid precursors in the bone marrow is IL-7.

NK cells (**choice C**) would not be mobilized by such a treatment. Although NK cells are granular, they are derived from lymphoid, not granulocyte/monocyte, precursors. The cytokine that favors development of lymphoid precursors in the bone marrow is IL-7.

Plasma cells (**choice D**) are produced in the secondary lymphoid organs and submucosa. IL-7, which stimulates lymphoid precursors in the bone marrow, would have an indirect effect on plasma cell production, but they are not mobilized from the bone marrow.

T lymphocytes (**choice E**) would not be mobilized by such a treatment. The cytokine that favors development of lymphoid precursors in the bone marrow is IL-7.

6. **The correct answer is D.** The leukemic cells are pre-B cells. They have rearranged their immunoglobulin genes to encode a μ heavy chain. MHC class II antigens are expressed beginning at the pro-B cell stage, as are CD19 and CD20. CD34 is a marker for early lymphohematopoietic stem and progenitor cells, and it functions as a cell–cell adhesion molecule. These cells would also have expressed CD10, the common acute lymphoblastic leukemia antigen (CALLA), which functions as a metalloendopeptidase.

    Immature B cells (**choice A**) have accomplished both and heavy and light immunoglobulin chain rearrangements and therefore express IgM molecules on their cell surface. They would be Tdt-negative, CD19- and CD20-positive, MHC class II-positive, and CD34-negative.

    Lymphoid progenitor cells (**choice B**) would not have completed any of the gene rearrangements necessary to create an immunoglobulin molecule. They would be Tdt-negative, MHC class II–negative, CD19- and CD20-negative, and CD34-positive.

    Mature B cells (**choice C**) possess surface IgM and IgD molecules and are capable of responding to foreign antigen. They are Tdt-negative, MHC class II-positive, CD19- and CD20-positive, CD34-negative, and may express CD40.

    Pro-B cells (**choice E**) are rearranging their immunoglobulin heavy chain gene segments but have not yet completed the process. Therefore, they have no completed chains either cytoplasmically or on their cell surfaces. They would be positive for Tdt, MHC class II, CD19, and CD20.

7. **The correct answer is D.** The best markers for identification of B lymphocytes are CD19, CD20, and CD21. CD19 and CD21 form a coreceptor complex during B-cell activation. The role of CD20 in B-cell activation is unclear, although it forms a calcium-ion channel. CD21 is also a receptor for the C3d component of complement and the Epstein-Barr virus.

    CD3 (**choice A**) is the signal transduction complex of T cells. It is found on all T cells in association with the T-cell antigen receptor.

    CD4 (**choice B**) is found on all helper T lymphocytes.

    CD8 (**choice C**) is found on all cytotoxic T lymphocytes.

    CD56 (**choice E**) is a marker for human natural killer cells.

8. **The correct answer is C.** This patient has a T-cell lymphoblastic lymphoma. In his case, the malignant cell is "double-positive": it possesses both CD4 and CD8. In a normal individual, these would only be found as an early developmental stage in the cortex of the thymus. Once cells have rearranged their receptor genes and been subjected to positive and negative selection, the cells leaving the thymus will express one coreceptor or the other but never both.

    Bone marrow (**choice A**) would contain T lymphocyte precursors that are double negative: They will lack both CD4 and CD8.

    Peripheral blood (**choice B**) would have mature T cells that have differentiated into either helper (CD4+) or cytotoxic (CD8+) cells. There should be no double-positive T cells in the peripheral blood.

    Thymic medulla (**choice D**) is the location of maturing T cells ready to circulate into the bloodstream and peripheral lymphoid organs. It would have only single-positive cells.

    Splenic periarteriolar lymphoid sheaths (**choice E**) are the T-cell–dependent areas of the spleen. They would have fully committed helper (CD4+) or cytotoxic (CD8+) cells.

9. **The correct answer is A.** T-lymphocyte precursors that leave the bone marrow and move to the thymus have neither CD4 nor CD8 coreceptors, and they have not rearranged the DNA of the variable domains of their antigen receptor, the TCR.

    CD4–, CD8–, and TCR+ (**choice B**) is not a possible T-cell phenotype. Once the TCR gene segments are rearranged and the TCR is expressed, the cells will bear both CD4 and CD8 coreceptors.

    CD4–, CD8+, and TCR+ (**choice C**) is the phenotype of cytotoxic T cells that would be in the circulation, not in the thymus, unless it were immediately prior to their release into the circulation following the thymic selection process.

    CD4+, CD8–, and TCR+ (**choice D**) is the phenotype of helper T cells that would be in the circulation, not in the thymus, unless it were immediately prior to their release into the circulation following thymic selection processes.

    CD4+, CD8+, and TCR+ (**choice E**) is the phenotype of cells in the thymic cortex. These are the cells that have rearranged their receptor genes and bear both CD4 and CD8 coreceptors. As the specificity of their TCR is tested, they will be directed to express either CD4 (and become a helper T cell) or CD8 (and become a cytotoxic T cell).

10. **The correct answer is C.** The interaction between the TCR and MHC class I/peptide conjugates is stabilized by the CD8 coreceptor. By downregulating the expression of MHC class I antigens on the surface of infected cells, the virus protects the infected host cell from killing by cytotoxic T lymphocytes.

    CD2 (**choice A**), also known as LFA-2, is an adhesion molecule within the immunoglobulin superfamily of genes. Its ligand is the integrin LFA-3. It is found on T cells and mediates attachment to other lymphocytes and antigen-presenting cells. It does not have a coreceptor role that would impact MHC class I–restricted killing.

CD4 (**choice B**) is the coreceptor that stabilizes the interaction between MHC class II antigens and the TCR. It is thus important for helper T cells, not cytotoxic T cells.

CD16 (**choice D**) is the Fc receptor involved in binding to immune complexes and promoting antibody-dependent cell-mediated cytotoxicity. It is not involved in the MHC class I–restricted killing by cytotoxic T cells.

CD56 (**choice E**) is a cell surface marker found on NK cells. Its function is unknown. However, since NK activity is enhanced in the absence of MHC class I antigen expression, the downregulation of these molecules by herpes simplex 1 and 2 actually makes infected cells more susceptible to the NK cell form of lysis.

11. **The correct answer is D**. Because malignant cells are clonal in origin, all the cells in this patient's lymphoma should be producing IgM monomers of a single idiotype. Treatment with anti-idiotype antibodies plus complement, therefore, would specifically kill only malignant cells, and leave all other B lymphocytes unharmed.

Anti-CD3 antibodies plus complement (**choice A**) would kill all T lymphocytes in the body. This lymphoma is clearly of B-cell origin because it is bearing IgM monomers.

Anti-CD19 antibodies plus complement (**choice B**) would kill all B lymphocytes in the body. It would not specifically target malignant cells.

Anti-CD20 antibodies plus complement (**choice C**) would kill all B lymphocytes in the body. It would not specifically target malignant cells.

Anti-μ chain antibodies plus complement (**choice E**) would kill all mature and naive B cells and immature B cells that had completed VDJ rearrangement of their heavy chain genes. It would not be specific for malignant cells.

12. **The correct answer is E.** The paracortex of a lymph node is a T-cell–dependent area. If this area is lacking cellularity, then the patient has a deficiency of T lymphocytes. B-lymphocyte numbers could be normal or even elevated. The only B-cell marker on this list is CD19, the marker which is used clinically to enumerate B cells in the body.

CD2 (**choice A**), also known as LFA-2, is an adhesion molecule found on T cells, thymocytes, and NK cells. In a person with a T-cell deficiency, there would be decreased numbers of cells bearing this marker.

CD3 (**choice B**) is found on all T cells. It is also called the "pan-T" cell marker. In a person with a T-cell deficiency, there would be decreased numbers of cells bearing this marker.

CD4 (**choice C**) is found on all helper T lymphocytes. In a person with a T-cell deficiency, there would be decreased numbers of cells bearing this marker.

CD8 (**choice D**) is found on all cytotoxic T lymphocytes. In a person with a T-cell deficiency, there would be decreased numbers of cells bearing this marker.

13. **The correct answer is A.** The spleen is the secondary lymphoid organ that is responsible for primary surveillance against blood-borne antigens. *Babesia microti* is an intraerythrocytic parasite of humans, transmitted by

the same vector tick as Lyme disease. Red blood cells (and their parasites) are filtered by the spleen, so splenectomy is a predisposing factor in development of serious disease with this parasite.

Bordetella pertussis (**choice B**) is a mucosal surface pathogen that attaches to the upper airways. Although its toxin becomes blood-borne, the organism itself is confined to the respiratory tree.

Corynebacterium diphtheriae (**choice C**) is a mucosal surface pathogen that attaches to the upper airways. Although its toxin becomes blood-borne, the organism itself is confined to the respiratory tree.

Enteroaggregative *Escherichia coli* (**choice D**) is an organism that causes diarrhea by producing a biofilm-like aggregation of organisms on the surface of the colonic mucosa, which impedes absorption. It is not likely to be a blood-borne pathogen.

Human papilloma virus (**choice E**) produces localized infections in epithelial cells where it is transferred by human-to-human or human-to-fomite contact. It is not likely to be a blood-borne pathogen.

14. **The correct answer is E.** The cortex of lymph nodes is a B-lymphocyte area. Thus, cells in this area would stain with fluorescent antibodies against CD19, the molecule that serves as a portion of the B-cell signal transduction complex. This molecule would be found on all B cells, but would be absent from T cells, macrophages, and NK cells.

    CD2 (**choice A**) is a T-cell marker. T cells will be found in the paracortical areas of lymph nodes.

    CD3 (**choice B**) is a T-cell marker. It is the signal transduction complex of the T cell and will be found on all T cells. T cells will be found in the paracortical areas of lymph nodes.

    CD4 (**choice C**) is a marker for helper T cells. These cells would be found in the paracortical areas of lymph nodes.

    CD16 (**choice D**) is the Fc receptor for IgG antibodies. It would be found on natural killer and phagocytic cells, which would not be numerous in the cortex of the lymph nodes. Phagocytic cells typically are found in the medullary cords.

15. **The correct answer is E.** Lymph nodes are designed to filter tissue fluids. Fluids entering the lymph nodes do so through the afferent lymphatics and are released into the subcapsular sinus. From there, fluids percolate through the cortex, into the medulla, through the medullary cords, and finally exit through the efferent lymphatics in the hilum.

    The cortex (**choice A**) of the lymph node is directly beneath the subcapsular sinus. It would be the second region of the lymph node to be exposed to the radioactive tracer. The cortex is a B-lymphocyte–rich area.

    The medulla (**choice B**) of the lymph node is rich in macrophages. It would not receive the radioactive fluid until it had passed through the cortex and paracortex.

    The paracortex (**choice C**) of the lymph node is a T-cell area. It lies between the cortex and the medulla and thus would receive the radioactive fluid after the cortical areas.

Primary follicles (**choice D**) are found in the cortex of the lymph node. These are areas of active B-lymphocyte proliferation and cloning. They would receive the radioactivity after it left the subcapsular sinus.

16. **The correct answer is B.** Many drug allergies, such as the one described here, are hapten-carrier immune responses. The drug is not large enough by itself to elicit an immune response (it is a hapten), but when it becomes covalently coupled to the body's own proteins (which act as carriers), the combined molecule becomes immunogenic, and a response against one's own tissues is elicited.

    Acting as a B-cell mitogen (**choice A**) is not correct. B-cell mitogens, such as pokeweed mitogen and lipopolysaccharide, cause polyclonal proliferation of B cells and elaboration of IgM antibodies. The drug allergy described here is not a polyclonal response, but a specific anti–altered-self response generated by T and B lymphocytes and production of antibodies.

    Acting as a provider of costimulatory signals (**choice C**) is not correct. The costimulatory signals required to activate B and T lymphocytes include CD28/B7 and CD40/CD40L interactions. These are additional interactions (beyond the specific recognition of antigen) required for the activation of B and T lymphocytes. Although these costimulatory signals would be involved in the evolution of this allergic response, the streptomycin does not serve as a costimulatory signal.

    Acting as a superantigen (**choice D**) is not correct. Superantigens are materials that crosslink the variable β domain of the T-cell receptor and the α-chain of class II MHC molecules. They induce activation of all T cells that express receptors with a particular Vβ domain. The resulting T-cell mitogenesis causes overproduction of T-cell and macrophage cytokines and system-wide pathology. Toxic shock syndrome toxin-1 and *Streptococcus pyogenes* erythrogenic exotoxins act as superantigens.

    Acting as an immunogen (**choice E**) is not correct because streptomycin is not large enough to be immunogenic. Immunogens must be large enough to have at least two epitopes. It is only through binding to a larger carrier protein (the patient's own tissue proteins) that a hapten such as a drug can become immunogenic.

17. **The correct answer is B.** This child has leukocyte adhesion deficiency (LAD), which is a genetic deficiency of CD18. CD18 is an essential component of a number of integrins, and absence of these molecules causes the inability of WBCs to migrate into sites of inflammation. Thus in this patient, the blood contained abnormally high numbers of neutrophils, but they were unable to extravasate. CD18 is a component of LFA-1, CR3, and CR4.

    Absence of CCR4 (**choice A**) would cause difficulties in extravasation and migration of activated T cells and monocytes. This chemokine receptor is not found on neutrophils and therefore would have no effect on neutrophil migration.

    Absence of interleukin-1 (**choice C**) might cause difficulties in producing the acute and chronic inflammatory responses. This cytokine, frequently referred to as the endogenous pyrogen, produces fever, acute phase protein production, and many other results critical to inflammation. However, the actions of IL-1 are extremely redundant with those of IL-6 and tumor necrosis factor-α, so such a condition might have no clinically observable effects.

Absence of interleukin-4 (**choice D**) would result in defects in the ability to mount a normal IgE antibody response. This cytokine also serves as the major stimulus for the development of Th2 cells from naive helper T cells, so its absence would be likely to have profound effects on all aspects of the secondary antibody response.

Absence of tumor necrosis factor-α (**choice E**) might cause difficulties in producing the acute and chronic inflammatory responses. This cytokine has many functions that are redundant with those of IL-1 and IL-6, so such a condition might have no clinically observable effects.

18. **The correct answer is D.** This child has chronic granulomatous disease (CGD). The history indicates he has had recurrent infections with catalase-positive organisms and has a defect in generating oxygen radicals intracellularly in his phagocytic cells (the negative nitroblue tetrazolium test and neutrophil oxidative index). This genetic defect arises from a failure to produce one of the subunits of NADPH oxidase, which makes the individual incapable of producing intracellular oxygen radicals. Redundant intracellular killing mechanisms (myeloperoxidase and lysosomal contents) are still functional in these patients, but when they are infected with catalase-positive organisms, the substrate for myeloperoxidase (hydrogen peroxide) is destroyed, and the only remaining intracellular killing mechanism (lysosomes) is insufficient to protect from infection.

C3 deficiency (**choice A**) would cause increased susceptibility to pyogenic infections because C3b is an important opsonin that enhances phagocytosis of extracellular organisms. All extracellular bacteria would be included in this list, not simply catalase-positive ones, as mentioned here. The NBT and NOI would not be negative in this case.

Deficiency of CD18 (**choice B**) is the cause of leukocyte adhesion deficiency (LAD). Because CD18 is the common β chain of the β_2 integrins, its absence compromises leukocyte function antigen (LFA)-1, as well as complement receptors 3 and 4. Patients with LAD suffer recurrent infections with extracellular pathogens (not just catalase-positive ones) because of defective opsonization, mobilization, adhesion, and chemotaxis. The NBT and NOI would be positive.

Deficiency of myeloperoxidase (**choice C**) results from a deficiency of an important granule enzyme in phagocytic cells. However, because there are so many redundant mechanisms of intracellular killing, these patients generally have mild symptoms or none at all.

A phagocyte granule structural defect (**choice E**) is responsible for the Chediak-Higashi syndrome. These patients have chemotactic and degranulation defects, lack NK activity, and have partial albinism.

19. **The correct answer is C.** The only substance on the list that is chemotactic for neutrophils is IL-8. Other neutrophil chemotactic factors that might have been mentioned would include C5a, leukotriene B4, and formyl methionyl peptides.

Complement component 3b (**choice A**) is not chemotactic for neutrophils. It acts as an opsonin, enhancing the phagocytosis of coated particles.

Immunoglobulin G (**choice B**) is not chemotactic for neutrophils. It acts as an opsonin, enhancing the phagocytosis of coated particles.

Myeloperoxidase (**choice D**) is not chemotactic for neutrophils. It is an enzyme in the lysosomes of phagocytic cells that generates toxic halide radicals intracellularly when exposed to its substrate, hydrogen peroxide.

Tumor necrosis factor-α (**choice E**) is not chemotactic for neutrophils. It is produced by macrophages and is involved with the production of chronic inflammation and cytotoxicity.

20. **The correct answer is D**. IL-2, IFN-γ, and TNF-β are all elaborated by the Th1 cell. TNF-β can also be made by NK cells. In tuberculoid leprosy, the Th1 arm of the immune response is most active, resulting in a protective (but also damaging) cell-mediated response and a dampening of the antibody response. In lepromatous leprosy, the patient has an overabundance of Th2 responses, causing the production of a nonprotective antibody response.

Cytotoxic T lymphocytes (**choice A**) are an effector cell in the cell-mediated immune response. They do not elaborate many cytokines but produce cytotoxic molecules, which cause the destruction of specific target cells.

Epithelioid cells (**choice B**) are modified macrophages. They are extremely secretory and may produce IL-1, IL-6, TNF-α, IFN-γ, and GM-CSF. They are prominent in granulomas, and their cytokines would be elevated in a patient with tuberculoid leprosy, but that was not the question.

Macrophages (**choice C**), once activated, may produce IL-1, IL-6, TNF-α, IFN-γ, and GM-CSF. They are prominent in granulomas, and their cytokines would be elevated in a patient with tuberculoid leprosy, but again, that was not the question.

Th2 cells (**choice E**) would be elevated during lepromatous leprosy. The cytokines they secrete include IL-4, IL-5, IL-6, IL-10, IL-13 and TGFβ. These cells are stimulators of the humoral immune response.

21. **The correct answer is C.** In lepromatous leprosy, the activation of the Th2 arm of the immune response results in elicitation of those cytokines that stimulate production of antibody (IL-4, IL-5, IL-6, IL-10, IL-13 and TGFβ) and those that inhibit the development of the protective cell-mediated immune response (IL-4 and IL-10). Therefore, hypergammaglobulinemia is a frequent finding in lepromatous leprosy.

Autoimmunity (**choice A**) may develop after infectious processes, but there is no evidence that stimulation of Th2 cells, by itself, causes autoimmune disease.

Granuloma formation (**choice B**) would be decreased after exposure to these cytokines. Granulomas are an expression of the delayed-type hypersensitivity response, which is a function of Th1 cells. IL-10 and IL-4 would depress the Th1 response.

Immediate hypersensitivity (**choice D**) requires sensitized mast cells and IgE antibodies. Although this result could occur in persons predisposed to atopic allergy, it is not the most likely result of stimulation with Th2 cytokines.

Inflammation (**choice E**) is primarily mediated by substances released during tissue injury (leukotrienes, histamine, etc.) and the cytokines of activated macrophages (IL-1, IL-6, and TNF-α). It is not enhanced by Th2 cytokines.

22. **The correct answer is D**. This patient is showing signs of toxic shock syndrome, caused by infection of the blister with *Staphylococcus aureus* and the resultant elaboration of the exotoxin TSST-1. This toxin acts as a superantigen, cross-linking the variable β region of the TCR to the α chain of the class II MHC molecule. This binds Th cells and APC together without the specificity of antigen recognition, and so clonal proliferation of T cells and production of IFN-γ leads to activation of macrophages. As a result, the macrophages overproduce the cytokines IL-1, IL-6, and TNF-α, which are toxic at high levels.

It acts as an IL-1 homologue (**choice A**) is not true. IL-1 is produced by macrophages as a result of T-cell activation, but TSST-1 does not itself act as an IL-1 homologue.

It activates B lymphocytes polyclonally (**choice B**) is not true. TSST-1 acts on Th cells to stimulate macrophage cytokines. It does not have a direct effect on B-cell proliferation.

It activates complement (**choice C**) is not correct. TSST-1 does not have an effect on complement.

It stimulates neutrophils (**choice E**) is not correct. Although neutrophils are stimulated during *Staphylococcus aureus* infection and produce IL-1, which causes fever, the mechanism of action of TSST-1 and other superantigens is not through neutrophil activation.

23. **The correct answer is A.** The B7 molecule on antigen-presenting cells binds to the CD28 molecule on T lymphocytes and serves as a costimulatory signal for their activation. If the tumor cells could be induced to express this costimulatory molecule, they would provide the important activating signal to the T cells.

CD2 (**choice B**) is the molecule on T lymphocytes that binds to LFA-3 on antigen-presenting cells. If the tumor cell were induced to express CD2, it would bind to the complementary structure on macrophages and not activate the T cells.

CD4 (**choice C**) is the molecule on T lymphocytes that stabilizes the interaction of MHC class II and the TCR. If the tumor cell were induced to express CD4, it would not increase the tumor-specific response.

CD28 (**choice D**) is the molecule on T cells that binds to B7. If the tumor cell were induced to express CD28, it would bind to the complementary structure on macrophages and not activate the T cells.

LFA-1 (**choice E**) is the molecule on T cells that binds ICAM-1 on the antigen-presenting cells. If the tumor cells were induced to express LFA-1, it would bind to the complementary structure on macrophages and not activate the T cells.

24. **The correct answer is D.** CD25-positive T_{Reg} cells have been shown to have a role in maintenance of self-tolerance, and therefore, defects in these cells are being blamed in many cases of autoimmune disease. T_{Reg} cells secrete interleukin-10 which is an anti-inflammatory cytokine.

Interferon-gamma (**choice A**) is a product of Th1 which activates macrophages and amplifies pro-inflammatory pathways in the body. It is not a product of T_{Reg} cells and would cause additional damage in a case of rheumatoid arthritis, so it would not be a logical goal of therapy.

Interleukin-1 (**choice B**) is endogenous pyrogen which is responsible for the setting of the hypothalamic temperature point. It is a product of macrophages which activates Th1 cells, and therefore would be considered a pro-inflammatory cytokine rather than an anti-inflammatory one.

Interleukin-2 (**choice C**) is a product of Th0 and Th1 cells which causes the proliferation of T cells and the effector cells of cell-mediated immunity. Although IL-2 is required for natural T_{Reg} development, it would not be expected to be increased with the therapy mentioned here.

Transforming growth factor-beta (**choice E**) is a product of T cells and macrophages which is required for natural T_{Reg} development, but with this artificial therapy to increase T_{Reg} numbers, it would not be expected to be elevated.

25. **The correct answer is C.** The cell surface marker which is typically used to identify B lymphocytes is CD19. This is a component of the B-cell/signal transduction complex and thus will be found on all B cells. Treatment of IgG with papain yields two monovalent antigen binding (Fab) fragments and destroys the function of the Fc portion of the molecule. Immunoglobulin molecules that are disrupted this way lose their ability to cross-link the receptors on cells, to promote precipitation or agglutination, and to activate cells by providing a first stimulatory signal.

   Monoclonal anti-CD19 IgG (**choice A**) is a divalent antibody molecule that recognizes the signal transduction complex on B cells. Monoclonal antibodies can cross-link cell-surface receptors and cause capping, cell activation, and precipitation. Agglutination is usually accomplished using IgM because a very large molecule is needed to overcome the zeta potential (repulsive charge) of erythrocytes. If IgG is used, a second developing antibody must be added.

   Monoclonal anti-CD56 IgG (**choice B**) is a divalent antibody molecule that recognizes a molecule found on NK cells. Because both arms of the molecule are intact, it is capable of causing capping, cell activation, precipitation, and agglutination if a developing antiserum is added.

   Papain-treated anti-CD56 IgG (**choice D**) would not be used for the study of B lymphocytes because CD56 is a marker for NK cells.

   Pepsin-treated anti-CD19 IgG (**choice E**) is a divalent molecule possessing two Fab fragments joined together ($F[ab']_2$), and a fragmented Fc region. The $F(ab')_2$ portion of the antibody is capable of causing capping, cell activation, precipitation, and, with a developing antiserum, agglutination.

   Pepsin-treated anti-CD56 IgG (**choice F**) is a divalent molecule possessing two Fab fragments joined together ($F[ab']_2$) and a fragmented Fc region. Its specificity is for NK cells. Additionally, the $F(ab')_2$ portion of the antibody is capable of causing capping, cell activation, precipitation, and, with a developing antiserum, agglutination.

26. **The correct answer is A.** Isohemagglutinins are IgM antibodies that will agglutinate the RBCs of individuals with another blood type. They are believed to be made due to exposure to cross-reactive antigens found on the surface of normal gut flora organisms. Thus, a person of blood group A will produce isohemagglutinins that will agglutinate type B cells. If these antibodies are pretreated with pepsin, a divalent $F(ab')_2$ fragment and

destruction of the Fc will result. A divalent fragment is capable of causing agglutination.

Lysed (**choice B**) is not correct because it would require the integrity of the complement-binding regions of the IgM, which are found in the Fc, and the question stem does not provide complement in the mix.

Phagocytized (**choice C**) is not correct because it would require an intact cell-binding region in the Fc, and the question stem does not provide phagocytic cells in the mix.

Precipitated (**choice D**) would be the correct answer if the antigen in question were a soluble protein. Proteins precipitate when treated with specific antibodies, particles agglutinate. The two particles used in laboratory medicine are latex beads and erythrocytes. If neither of these is mentioned, then the student can assume that treatment would result in precipitation, not agglutination. Precipitation has exactly the same requirements as agglutination: a divalent antigen-binding molecule.

Unaffected (**choice E**) would be the correct answer if papain had been used to treat the isohemagglutinins. Because papain produces two monovalent Fab fragments, these are incapable of cross-linking antigen (whether soluble protein or particle), so neither agglutination nor precipitation would be possible.

27. **The correct answer is E.** The only way to identify a neonatal infection serologically is by detection of pathogen-specific IgM antibodies. This is because the fetus receives IgG antibodies from the mother by active transport across the placenta. Because you cannot identify the source of the antibodies, IgG detection in the child can simply reflect this natural passive type of protection. Because IgM does not cross the placenta, any IgM detected in the neonate is being produced in the child and is reflective of a response to infection. In this way, all children born to HIV-infected mothers will be seropositive by both ELISA and Western blot, but only 20% will actually be infected in utero, even in the absence of antiviral therapy.

IgA (**choice A**) does not usually begin to be produced by a child until one to two years after birth. At the end of the first year, most children have no more than 20% of adult values, so it would not be a useful diagnostic in the neonate. Additionally, because *Toxoplasma gondii* is an intracellular parasite, IgA would not be the most effective immune response in any individual.

IgD (**choice B**) will be produced by an infected neonate along with IgM because of alternative RNA splicing, but this is not a useful diagnostic. IgD rarely reaches levels easily detected by serology, and the immunoglobulin has the shortest half-life of all the immunoglobulins. The function of secreted IgD, if any, is not clear, so it is not a useful serologic test.

IgE (**choice C**) does not usually begin to be produced by a child until well into the second year after birth. Additionally, because *Toxoplasma gondii* is an intracellular parasite, IgE would not be the most effective immune response in any individual.

IgG (**choice D**) is not a useful serologic test in a neonate because it is impossible to determine the origin of such molecules. Children infected in utero will begin to produce IgG due to isotype switching late in gestation, but because the placenta is actively transporting all maternal IgG into the fetus, it is not possible to distinguish whether the child is actually infected or simply passively protected using this technique.

28. **The correct answer is B.** IgM and secretory IgA are similar in that they are held together by a J chain synthesized by the B cell or plasma cell. Without the presence of the J chain, IgM would exist only in monomeric form, and the macroglobulin peak would be absent on electrophoresis. Because pentameric IgM is important for capturing newly introduced foreign antigen and thus beginning the immune response, the child is delayed in his development of protective responses to vaccination. Because secretory IgA is a dimer that protects the mucosal surfaces, such a child would be especially susceptible to infectious agents crossing the mucosal surfaces.

Absence of CD40 (**choice A**) would affect the production of IgG, IgA, and IgE, but would not prevent macroglobulin synthesis. Indeed, most patients with this defect have hyper-macroglobulinemia because the CD40/CD40L interaction is necessary for isotype switching.

Absence of IL-4 (**choice C**) would cause problems with the ability to produce IgG, IgA, and IgE. This cytokine, produced by Th2 cells, is necessary for the differentiation and development of most antibody responses other than IgM. Thus, IgM levels either would not be affected or would be increased in a compensatory fashion.

Absence of Tdt (**choice D**) would cause problems with the patient's ability to perform the genetic rearrangements necessary to form the idiotype of the antibody molecule. They would not affect the isotype of antibody produced.

Absence of Th2 cells (**choice E**) would affect the production of IgG, IgA, and IgE, but would not affect IgM production.

29. **The correct answer is B.** One of the most effective protective responses to infections with extracellular, encapsulated bacteria, such as *Streptococcus pneumoniae*, is complement-mediated opsonization. Because IgM is the most effective antibody at activating complement, generation of C3b fragments during this process coats the bacteria and makes them more susceptible to ingestion and intracellular killing by cells of the phagocytic system.

ADCC (**choice A**), or antibody-dependent cell-mediated cytotoxicity, is a mechanism by which NK cells, neutrophils, macrophages, and eosinophils can use their Fc receptor to bind specific antibody and target an agent for lysis. No cells have Fc receptors for IgM, so this is not a mechanism that could act in concert with early IgM production.

Cytotoxic T lymphocytes (**choice C**) identify altered-self/MHC class I molecule conjugates on the surfaces of cells that are malignantly transformed or infected with intracellular pathogens. They are not a protective mechanism that acts in concert with any antibody molecule.

LAK cells (**choice D**), or lymphokine-activated killer cells, are NK cells that have been stimulated in vitro with cytokines that enhance their killing activity. These cells have a function in early surveillance against altered-self cells, but are not believed to play a role in protection against extracellular pathogens, such as this one.

NK cells (**choice E**) are members of the innate immune system and are believed to play a role in surveillance against tumor cells and other altered-self cells that fail to express MHC class I antigens on their surfaces. They would not act in concert with IgM production, and they would not be effective against an extracellular pathogen, such as this one.

30. **The correct answer is C.** The component of complement that is most important in clearance of extracellular pathogens such as *Streptococcus pneumoniae* is C3b. This fragment acts as an opsonin and enhances the ingestion and intracellular killing of the bacteria by phagocytic cells.

    C1 (**choice A**) is the first component of the complement cascade activated in the classic pathway. Although it is critical to initiating those events that can culminate in the production of the membrane attack complex, it is not the most important component for the clearance of infections such as this one.

    C2 (**choice B**) is the third component of the complement cascade activated in the classic pathway. Although it is critical to initiating those events that can culminate in the production of the membrane attack complex, it is not the most important component for the clearance of infections such as this one.

    C4 (**choice D**) is the second component of the complement cascade activated during the classic pathway. Although it is critical to initiating those events that can culminate in the production of the membrane attack complex, it is not the most important component for the clearance of infections such as this one.

    C5 (**choice E**) is the fifth component of the complement cascade activated during the classic pathway and the first step in the formation of the membrane attack complex (C5b–9). It is not the most important component for the clearance of infections such as this one.

31. **The correct answer is A.** The mucosal-associated lymphoid tissues (MALT) are the major sites of synthesis of IgA. IgA is a dimeric molecule held together by a J chain similar to that used in IgM. As IgA is transported across the epithelial surface, it acquires the secretory component, which functions both in transepithelial transport and protection from proteolytic cleavage.

    A monomeric immunoglobulin that crosses the placenta (**choice B**) describes IgG. IgG is the major immunoglobulin of the blood and is produced in lymph nodes and spleen, but less commonly in the MALT.

    A monomeric immunoglobulin bound by mast cells (**choice C**) describes IgE. IgE is the immunoglobulin that causes immediate hypersensitivity by virtue of its attraction to the Fc receptors of mast cells. It is not the major immunoglobulin produced in the MALT, although it may be produced there.

    A monomeric immunoglobulin that opsonizes (**choice D**) describes IgG. IgG is the major immunoglobulin of the blood and is produced in lymph nodes and spleen, but less commonly in the MALT.

    A pentameric immunoglobulin that activates complement (**choice E**) describes IgM. IgM is the major immunoglobulin of the primary immune response and is produced in lymph nodes and spleen, but less commonly in the MALT.

32. **The correct answer is D**. The transport of IgA dimers from the abluminal side of the mucosa to the lumen is mediated via attachment to polyimmunoglobulin receptors on mucosal cells. This allows endocytosis of IgA into the mucosal cell and secretion onto the other side. Secretory IgA found in the lumen of the bowel retains a residue of this receptor, secretory component, which further protects it from proteolytic cleavage inside the intestine. If this receptor were lacking, transport of IgA across the mucosa would not be possible, and the IgA dimers would be trapped on the abluminal side of the mucosa.

Failure of isotype switching (**choice A**) is not a potential cause of such a condition because isotype switching occurs in secondary lymphoid organs and not in epithelial cells. Because the IgA dimers were present, isotype switching had been successful, but transepithelial transport was not occurring.

Failure of variable domain gene segment rearrangement (**choice B**) is not a potential cause of such a condition because variable domain gene-segment rearrangement occurs in the primary lymphoid organs and not in epithelial cells. Because immunoglobulin was being produced, these gene segment rearrangements had occurred successfully, but transepithelial transport was not occurring.

Loss of J chain synthesis (**choice C**) would result in the inability of an individual to join dimers of IgA and pentamers of IgM. Because the question states that the individual was making IgA dimers, J chain is clearly being made successfully by the B cell.

Loss of Th2 cells (**choice E**) would cause the patient to be unable to switch isotypes. These persons could make only IgM, and this patient clearly has successfully produced IgA.

33. **The correct answer is A**. The killer cells cytotoxic to targets lacking MHC class I antigens are NK cells. These cells are members of the innate immune response, and as such their response is not enhanced over time. The most specific, inducible cytotoxic cells in the body are cytotoxic T lymphocytes (CTLs), which depend on MHC class I recognition of their target. Because this question asks how the tumor cells can be altered to make them better stimulators of an immune response, one approach would be to increase their expression of MHC class I molecules. This can be accomplished by treatment of the tumor cells with interferon (IFN)-γ. IFN-γ increases expression of both class I and II MHC products on cells.

IL-2 (**choice B**) is a product of Th1 lymphocytes and induces proliferation of antigen-primed Th and cytotoxic T cells. It also supports their long-term growth. It would not have an effect on this patient's tumor cells.

IL-8 (**choice C**) is a product of macrophages and endothelial cells and acts on neutrophils to cause their chemotaxis and extravasation into tissues. It would not have an effect on this patient's tumor cells.

IL-10 (**choice D**) is a product of Th2 cells and acts on macrophages to suppress their cytokine production. It therefore indirectly reduces cytokine production by Th1 cells and dampens the activation of the cell-mediated arm of the immune response. It would not have an effect on this patient's tumor cells.

TNF-β (**choice E**) is a product of macrophages and NK cells and acts on tumor cells to cause direct cytotoxicity. It acts on inflammatory cells to induce cytokine secretion and causes the cachexia associated with chronic inflammation. It would not cause the patient's tumor cells to stimulate better immunity.

34. **The correct answer is D.** CD8+ lymphocytes, or cytotoxic T lymphocytes recognize their target cells by binding to MHC class I molecules containing altered-self peptides. The class I molecule is a two-chain structure, with one long α chain that passes through the cellular membrane and a shorter chain called β_2 microglobulin that becomes associated with the α chain.

A β_2 domain instead of a β_2 microglobulin (**choice A**) describes the class II MHC molecule. It is loaded with peptides by the endosomal (exogenous) pathway and is recognized by CD4+ T cells.

Invariant chains (**choice B**) are found blocking the peptide-binding groove of the class II MHC molecule immediately after synthesis. These chains are digested away when the class II MHC is exposed to the contents of the phagocytic vesicles of macrophages, and the groove is loaded with peptides from the ingested particle.

A peptide-binding groove (**choice C**) would be found in both class I and II MHC molecules and is therefore not the best answer.

Two similar chains (**choice E**) would be found in the class II MHC molecule. It is composed of an α and a β chain of similar lengths, both of which have transmembrane domains. The class II MHC molecule is loaded with peptides by the endosomal (exogenous) pathway and is recognized by CD4+ T cells.

35. **The correct answer is A.** Although the ablation of the thymus in early childhood will ultimately have far-reaching consequences in the development of many immune responses, the immune surveillance of tumors is performed only by cytotoxic T cells and NK cells, and thus would be profoundly affected by this treatment. Although NK cell numbers would not be affected by loss of the thymus, in the absence of Th1 cell cytokines, they would not be able to increase in number in response to challenge. Other parameters that could be depressed include immune responses to intracellular pathogens and secondary antibody responses.

Depressed oxygen-dependent killing by neutrophils (**choice B**) would not be expected in this case because neutrophils are components of the innate immune response and function in the absence of T-cell help.

Depressed primary response to soluble antigens (**choice C**) would not be expected in this case because the IgM response to many antigens is T-cell independent. It is class switching that would be impossible without T-cell help.

Increased cellularity of lymph node paracortical areas (**choice D**) would not be expected in this case because the paracortex of lymph nodes is a T-cell area. Therefore, following thymic irradiation, decreased cellularity of these regions would occur.

Increased tendency toward atopy (**choice E**) would not be expected in this case because atopic allergies are those that involve IgE antibodies and mast cells. IgE cannot be produced without T-cell help, so athymic individuals will have decreased tendency toward atopy.

36. **The correct answer is A.** The Mantoux test, or tuberculin test (or simply the TB skin test), is the classic clinical demonstration of the function of the delayed-type hypersensitivity response. This is a cell-mediated reaction caused by sensitization of Th1 cells and demonstrated by the influx and activation of macrophages in response to the cytokines that they elaborate.

That a humoral immune response has occurred (**choice B**) is not true. Antibodies are not involved in the production of a DTH response, and they are not important products during infections with most intracellular pathogens.

That the B-cell system is functional (**choice C**) is not true. B cells do not play a role in the DTH response, and they do not play a major role in defense during infections with most intracellular pathogens.

That the B- and T-cell systems are functional (**choice D**) is not true. The DTH response certainly demonstrates that the Th1 response is functional, but it says nothing about the function of B cells.

That the neutrophilic phagocyte system is functional (**choice E**) is not true. Neutrophils do not play a role in the elicitation of the DTH response. Neutrophils are the important cells in abscess formation, not granuloma formation.

37. **The correct answer is D.** The goal of this therapy is to provide an increased population of activated antigen-presenting cells primed with tumor cell antigens so that these can be presented to the Th cells involved in stimulation of cell-mediated immunity. The Th1 cell is the first cell listed which would be activated by such a treatment.

B lymphocytes (**choice A**) would not be stimulated by such treatment. B lymphocytes bind to and are activated by unprocessed (not cell-bound) antigens.

Cytotoxic T lymphocytes (**choice B**) would be indirectly stimulated by this treatment. Cytokines secreted by the activated Th1 cells would have the effect of increasing the number and cytotoxic activity of killer cells.

NK cells (**choice C**) would be indirectly stimulated by this treatment. Cytokines secreted by the activated Th1 cells would have the effect of increasing the number and cytotoxic activity of killer cells.

Th2 cells (**choice E**) would be stimulated by this treatment, but this is not the major goal of such therapy. Th2 cells stimulate humoral immunity, which is not the most important protective mechanism against tumor cells.

38. **The correct answer is D.** The protective response to the tetanus toxoid depends on production of antibodies that prevent the binding of the toxin. After repeated immunizations, the population of memory B cells is stimulated, which is the goal of such prophylaxis. Memory B cells may have IgG, IgA, or occasionally IgE on their surfaces serving as antigen receptors.

That their receptors would have high avidity (**choice A**) is not true because avidity decreases with repeated booster inoculations. This is because IgM, which is the immunoglobulin of the primary immune response and is the receptor on mature naive B lymphocytes, is replaced in secondary and subsequent responses by isotype switching to other isotypes such as IgG or IgA or IgE. All of these molecules have less avidity than IgM because they have fewer combining sites than IgM. The secondary and subsequent responses should have increased affinity (goodness-of-fit of idiotype for epitope), but decreased avidity.

That they would be large and highly metabolic (**choice B**) is not true because memory lymphocytes are usually small and in a resting phase of the cell cycle. Activated lymphocytes are large and highly metabolic.

That they would have low levels of adhesion molecules (**choice C**) is not true because memory lymphocytes express high levels of adhesion molecules. This allows them to migrate to areas of active inflammation where they can have maximum benefit in protection of the host.

That they would have surface IgM (**choice E**) is not true because this would describe mature, naive B lymphocytes that have not met their antigen before. As soon as the primary response begins, isotype switching to other classes of immunoglobulin is directed by Th cells.

39. **The correct answer is A.** Because rabies antitoxin is a pooled, human immunoglobulin product, repeated inoculation will cause a patient to produce anti-allotype antibodies. Allotypes are minor amino-acid sequence variations in the constant domains of heavy and light immunoglobulin chains. Their expression is genetically determined, and repeated exposure to molecules of foreign allotype can cause antibodies to be produced which recognize these sequence variations.

Anti-epitope antibodies (**choice B**) would be produced by repeated inoculation of an immunogen. The epitope of the antigen has a three-dimensional complementarity with the idiotype of the antibody molecule. In this case, anti-epitope antibodies would be generated by rabies vaccination, but the question asks what the result of repeated exposure to immunoglobulins would be.

Anti-idiotype antibodies (**choice C**) would be generated in a human if a monoclonal antibody preparation were repeatedly inoculated. The idiotype of an antibody is the three-dimensional shape of its antigen-combining site. It is unique to the antibodies produced by a clone of cells. Because the material mentioned in this case is a pooled human immunoglobulin, it would contain many different idiotypes and would be unlikely to elicit any one specific anti-idiotype antibody.

Anti-isotype antibodies (**choice D**) are usually raised across species barriers. For example, to produce anti-human IgG, IgG pooled from many humans is repeatedly injected into rabbits, goats, or sheep. These animals will recognize the human determinants in the constant domains of the heavy and light chains (the isotypes) and will produce antibodies that specifically recognize those determinants.

Anti-rabies antibodies (**choice E**) are generated during vaccination. When the killed virus is administered, the patient makes an active, artificial response to the immunogen and produces immunoglobulins, which will protect against virus attachment. In this case, anti-rabies antibodies were inoculated, so there is no possibility that more of the same will be generated.

40. **The correct answer is B.** In this case, high-risk individuals are vaccinated with the serotype of influenza virus that is predicted to be most common in this flu season. This elicits an active immunologic response in the patient

and is artificial by definition because it is being administered in a medical setting. This sort of immunization causes the development of memory in the patient that will protect for the whole season, but it requires approximately two weeks for development of protection.

Adaptive (**choice A**) immunity describes all immune responses that have specificity and memory. These immune responses are produced by specific B and T lymphocytes. Although adaptive immunity will be elicited in these patients, this is not the best answer because it is imprecise.

Artificial passive (**choice C**) immunity is achieved when preformed immunologic products (immune cells or antibodies) are given to a patient. These procedures provide passive protection that is rapid but lacks immunologic memory. Because it is administered in a medical setting, it is, by definition, artificial.

Natural active (**choice D**) immunity would result following recovery from an infection.

Natural passive (**choice E**) immunity is acquired across the placenta and in the colostrum and breast milk, from mother to child. The child receives preformed antibodies (IgG across the placenta and IgA in milk) that protect the child until a natural active immune response can be mounted.

41. **The correct answer is C.** In this case, an attempt at postexposure prophylaxis against tetanus is made by inoculating antitetanus immunoglobulin into the patient. When preformed immunologic products (immune cells or antibodies) are given to a patient, the procedure provides passive protection that is rapid but lacks immunologic memory. Because it is being administered in a medical setting, it is by definition artificial.

Adaptive (**choice A**) immunity describes all immune responses that have specificity and memory. These immune responses are produced by specific B and T lymphocytes. Because this patient is being given a product of the adaptive immune response (antibodies), there will be no elicitation of an adaptive immune response in this individual.

Artificial active (**choice B**) immunity is produced during the process of vaccination. The patient is exposed to a modified pathogen or product. As a result, an active immune response to that inoculation is made. This sort of immunization causes the development of memory in the patient.

Natural active (**choice D**) immunity would result after a recovery from an infection.

Natural passive (**choice E**) immunity is acquired across the placenta and in the colostrum and breast milk, from mother to child. The child receives preformed antibodies (IgG across the placenta and IgA in milk), which serve to protect the child until a natural active immune response can be mounted.

42. **The correct answer is A.** Allotypes are minor amino-acid sequence variations in the constant domains of heavy and light immunoglobulin chains. Their expression is genetically determined, and variations can be used as evidence in favor of paternity in some cases. Allotypic markers are most frequently used in studies of population genetics, as certain ethnic groups are likely to have similar allotypic markers on their immunoglobulins.

Allotypic markers do not affect the biologic function of the immunoglobulin molecule.

The term "idiotype" (**choice B**) describes the 3-dimensional shape of the antigen-combining site of an antibody or T-cell receptor molecule. Because each human is capable of producing many millions of different idiotypic sequences, these would not be useful in paternity cases.

IgA2 (**choice C**) is an isotype of immunoglobulin. Because all normal human beings produce some amount of this immunoglobulin, it would not be useful in paternity cases.

IgM (**choice D**) is an isotype of immunoglobulin. Because all normal human beings produce some amount of this immunoglobulin, it would not be useful in paternity cases.

An isotype (**choice E**) is found in the heavy- or light-chain constant domains of an immunoglobulin. Thus, there are 5 heavy-chain isotypes (A, E, G, M, and D) and two light-chain isotypes (κ and λ). Because all human beings produce heavy- and light-chain isotypes, this would not be useful in paternity testing.

43. **The correct answer is D.** Although this vaccine is no longer in use because of the possible side effects of *Bordetella pertussis* inoculation, in this case the whole, killed bacteria served as an adjuvant. They increased local inflammation, thus calling inflammatory cells to the site and prolonging exposure to the immunogen, the capsular polysaccharide of *Haemophilus*.

A carrier (**choice A**) is not correct because a carrier is a protein covalently coupled to a hapten to elicit a response. There is no mention in the question stem here that the polysaccharide is chemically coupled to the bacteria; it is stated that they are only mixed together.

A hapten (**choice B**) is not correct because a hapten is a single antigenic epitope, and a whole, killed bacterium such as *Bordetella* has many epitopes.

A mitogen (**choice C**) is not correct because mitogens are substances that cause the polyclonal activation of immune cells. The mitogens most commonly used in clinical laboratory medicine are lipopolysaccharide, concanavalin A, and pokeweed mitogen.

An immunogen (**choice E**) is not correct because the immunogen in a vaccine is the substance to which the immune response is being made. Because the object of the Hib vaccine is to immunize against *Haemophilus influenzae*, *Bordetella pertussis* bacteria cannot be the immunogen.

44. **The correct answer is D.** This is a case of DiGeorge syndrome, which is a congenital failure in the formation of the third and fourth pharyngeal pouches. As a result, individuals with this defect have aplastic thymus and parathyroids and facial, esophageal, and cardiac malformations. Immunologically, the absence of the thymus will ultimately have global effects on the development of all T-cell–mediated immune responses. At birth, the child will have IgG antibodies that have been transplacentally transferred from the mother, but by 9 months or so after birth, these will be gone and IgM will be the only isotype of immunoglobulin present. Phagocytic killing will be normal until that point, although after all the maternal IgG is gone, opsonization of bacteria will no longer be possible.

Antibody-dependent cell-mediated cytotoxicity of parasite targets (**choice A**) will be depressed in this child because eosinophil-mediated ADCC requires IgE antibodies, and these cannot be produced without T-cell help.

Cellularity of splenic periarteriolar lymphoid sheaths (**choice B**) will be decreased in this child because these are T-cell–dependent areas of the spleen.

Cytotoxic killing of virus-infected targets (**choice C**) will be depressed in this child because cytotoxic T cells will be absent, and only NK cells will be available for antiviral protection.

The proliferative response to concanavalin A (**choice E**) will be depressed in this child because concanavalin A is a T-cell mitogen. If there are no T cells, there will be no proliferation in response to this mitogen.

45. **The correct answer is A.** This is a case of X-linked agammaglobulinemia, or Bruton agammaglobulinemia. It is caused by a mutation in a tyrosine kinase gene, which is important in B-cell maturation. The bone marrow becomes hypercellular with cells that cannot progress beyond the pre-B stage, while the peripheral blood lacks mature B lymphocytes. There will be no proliferative response to B-cell mitogens (pokeweed mitogen), and CD19+ cells will be absent from the blood. Persons with this condition are unable to mount a normal antibody response; therefore, symptoms appear after the disappearance of maternal antibodies. Susceptibility to extracellular, encapsulated pathogens is profound.

Common variable hypogammaglobulinemia (**choice B**) is a condition that usually appears in the late teens or early twenties. It is believed to be an autoimmune disease and is associated with the disappearance of immunoglobulin isotypes over time.

DiGeorge syndrome (**choice C**), or congenital thymic aplasia, is a condition in which there is failure of formation of the third and fourth pharyngeal pouches. These infants have facial abnormalities, failure of formation of the parathyroids, and cardiac defects, as well as absence of T-lymphocyte development.

Selective immunoglobulin deficiency (**choice D**) would not be manifested by a failure of B-cell development in the bone marrow. Selective IgA deficiency is most common of these and would manifest as increased susceptibility to mucosal-surface pathogens.

Wiskott-Aldrich syndrome (**choice E**) is a complex immune deficiency with a triad of symptoms: eczema, thrombocytopenia, and immunodeficiency. It is inherited in an X-linked recessive fashion. These patients are prone to development of malignant lymphomas and have inability to respond to polysaccharide antigens.

46. **The correct answer is B.** Unusual frequency or severity of *Neisseria* infections should always lead to a suspicion of a terminal complement component deficiency (C5, C6, C7, or C8). *Neisseria* seem to be highly susceptible to complement-mediated lysis, so any failure of production of the membrane attack complex predisposes the patient to recurrent bacteremias with these organisms.

Common variable immunodeficiency (**choice A**) is a condition that usually appears in the late teens or early twenties. It is believed to be an autoimmune disease and is associated with the disappearance of immunoglobulin isotypes over time.

DiGeorge syndrome (**choice C**) is a condition in which there is failure of formation of the third and fourth pharyngeal pouches. Diagnosed in infancy, these individuals have facial abnormalities, failure of formation of the parathyroids, and cardiac defects, as well as an absence of T-lymphocyte development. This condition predisposes to early viral and fungal infections.

Selective IgA deficiency (**choice D**) would be expected to result in respiratory and gastrointestinal tract infections, autoimmune disease, and allergies.

Severe combined immunodeficiency (**choice E**) typically presents with early susceptibility to viral and fungal agents. It is most frequently diagnosed in infancy, after the disappearance of maternally derived IgG antibodies.

47. **The correct answer is E.** The description of painful abdominal edema and edema in the oral mucosa are typical of hereditary angioedema. This is a genetic deficiency of complement C1 inhibitor. When this important control protein is missing, there is excessive use of the classic complement pathway components, especially C4. This causes abnormal inflammation along the mucosal surfaces.

    Abnormal superoxide anion production by neutrophils (**choice A**) would result in predisposition to infections with extracellular pathogens.

    Abnormal T-cell function (**choice B**) would result in predisposition to infections with viral and fungal pathogens, not edema of the mucosal surfaces.

    Abnormal T-cell numbers (**choice C**) would result in predisposition to infections with viral and fungal pathogens, not edema of the mucosal surfaces.

    Defective neutrophil chemotaxis (**choice D**) would result in neutrophilia and failure to produce pus and abscesses in response to extracellular bacterial invasion.

48. **The correct answer is D.** The infections of this child with catalase-positive bacteria are characteristic of chronic granulomatous disease (CGD). While two thirds of CGD patients are male, one third has the autosomal recessive form of NADPH oxidase deficiency and can be female.

    Adenosine deaminase deficiency (**choice A**) produces a severe combined immunodeficiency. The infections seen are likely to be the result of T-cell deficiency (viral and fungal agents). In the absence of adenosine deaminase, deoxyadenosine phosphate builds up in T cells and is toxic to them.

    C1 inhibitor (**choice B**) is not an enzyme, and its absence does not predispose to infections. It is absent in the condition known as hereditary angioedema, represented by recurrent, painful bouts of mucosal edema.

    Myeloperoxidase (**choice C**) deficiency is normally without clinical symptoms. This is an enzyme that is important in intracellular killing in phagocytes because it causes formation of toxic halide radicals. However, because oxygen radicals are more important in intracellular killing, MPO deficiency will present without symptoms.

    Superoxide dismutase (**choice E**) deficiency has not been described in leukocytes, and its absence would not be likely to predispose to infection.

49. **The correct answer is B.** This is a case of X-linked agammaglobulinemia, or Bruton agammaglobulinemia. During the early 1990s, the gene responsible for this condition was cloned. The normal counterpart of the mutant gene encodes a protein tyrosine kinase (Bruton tyrosine kinase, *Btk*), which is important in B-cell signaling. When it is absent or altered, B lymphocytes are unable to progress beyond the pre-B cell stage in the bone marrow. Thus, the bone marrow becomes hypercellular, while the peripheral blood is lacking mature B lymphocytes. Persons with this condition are unable to mount a normal antibody response; therefore, symptoms appear after the disappearance of maternal antibodies, and susceptibility to extracellular, encapsulated pathogens such as *Streptococcus pneumoniae* and *Haemophilus influenzae* is profound.

Adenosine deaminase deficiency (**choice A**) is an example of a severe combined immunodeficiency disease (SCID). When this enzyme is absent, toxic metabolites build up in B and T lymphocytes and cause a general failure of the immune response. It would have clinical manifestations of both B- and T-lymphocyte defects, and not exclusively B lymphocytes, as described in this case history.

A defect of the *SAP* gene (**choice C**) is believed to cause X-linked proliferative disease, in which uncontrolled T-cell proliferation follows infection with Epstein-Barr virus. *SAP* stands for SLAM-associated protein, and SLAM (signaling lymphocytic activation molecule) is a potent T-cell coactivator.

Defect of the *WAS* gene (**choice D**) causes Wiskott-Aldrich syndrome, in which a defect in CD43 (a cytoskeletal protein) causes defects in T cells and platelets. Patients with Wiskott-Aldrich syndrome display a triad of signs: thrombocytopenia, eczema, and immunodeficiency.

ICAM-1 deficiency (**choice E**) would cause defects of antigen recognition and activation of lymphocytes. ICAM-1 is an adhesion molecule in the immunoglobulin superfamily of genes and is bound by LFA-1 integrin.

50. **The correct answer is B.** This is a case of hereditary angioedema, caused by a deficiency in an important complement regulatory protein, C1-INH. When it is absent, the early components of the classical complement cascade are overused. It is normally diagnosed by the finding of depressed levels of complement component C4 in the blood.

Depressed C3 (**choice A**) would not be a correlate of C1-INH deficiency. There are separate regulatory controls on abnormal complement activation that operate at the C3 level, so this condition is rarely found.

Depressed C5 (**choice C**) would not be a correlate of C1-INH deficiency. There are separate regulatory controls on abnormal complement activation that operate at the C5 level, so this condition is rarely found.

Elevated C1 (**choice D**) would not be found in this case because the condition results in the overuse of early components of the classical complement cascade. Therefore, serum levels of C1, C4, and C2 would be decreased from normal values.

Elevated C1, C4, and C2 (**choice E**) would not be found in this case because the condition results in the overuse of early components of the classical complement cascade. Therefore, serum levels of C1, C4, and C2 would be decreased from normal values.

51. **The correct answer is B.** This child has bare lymphocyte syndrome, a rare autosomal-recessive disease in which there is absence of MHC class II molecules on cells. Thus, her cells can recognize other cells as foreign and proliferate to T-cell mitogens, but they cannot be recognized by allogeneic lymphocytes because they do not express class II MHC antigens on their surface. The phrase which best describes the MHC class II molecule on this list is that it is designed to bind exogenously processed peptides. Other descriptions that could apply would be that it has two chains of similar length, is produced with an invariant chain, and is designed to present foreign peptides to Th cells.

It is designed to bind endogenously produced peptides (**choice A**) is a description that fits the class I MHC molecule. If this were a case of class I MHC deficiency, she would not have made a normal proliferative response to mismatched allogeneic cells.

It possesses β_2 microglobulin (**choice C**) is a description that fits the class I MHC molecule.

It possesses two chains of unequal length (**choice D**) is a description of the class I MHC molecule. It has an α chain with 3 domains, and a smaller chain, β_2 microglobulin, becomes associated with the α chain.

It should be present on all nucleated cells in the body (**choice E**) describes the class I MHC molecule. Class II MHC will be found on all antigen-presenting cells in the body.

52. **The correct answer is E.** IL-10 is produced by Th2 cells and inhibits Th1 cells. Because the response to poison ivy is a delayed-type hypersensitivity response and therefore is mediated by Th1 cells and macrophages, inhibiting their activity would minimize the severity of the reaction.

γ-Interferon (**choice A**) is a product of Th1 cells, CTLs, and NK cells. It inhibits the proliferation of Th2 cells and therefore would skew the immune response toward a more potent cell-mediated arm. This is not a cytokine that would help this patient: It would make his condition worse.

IL-2 (**choice B**) is a product of Th cells that induces the proliferation and enhances the activity of antigen-primed Th cells and CTLs. It would tend to increase the symptoms of this patient, not ameliorate them.

IL-3 (**choice C**) is a product of Th cells and NK cells. It acts on hematopoietic cells to encourage myeloid cell development. It would neither hinder nor help this man's condition.

IL-8 (**choice D**) is a product of macrophages and endothelial cells and acts on neutrophils to attract them to areas of inflammation. It would increase inflammation in the area.

53. **The correct answer is A.** The condition described here is an immune complex–mediated pathology. When large amounts of antigen are added into a situation where there is pre-existence of a large amount of antibody, the precipitation of those complexes in the small vasculature causes a type III hypersensitivity response. The only syndrome on this list that also has a type III etiology is the Arthus reaction.

Atopic allergy (**choice B**) is a type I hypersensitivity, mediated by IgE antibodies and mast cells. Although many parasitic diseases elicit IgE and

ADCC by eosinophils, the question stem clearly stipulates the presence of IgG antibodies, so a type I hypersensitivity reaction is ruled out.

Goodpasture syndrome (**choice C**) and transfusion reaction (**choice E**) are examples of a type II, cytotoxic antibody hypersensitivity response. In these cases, antibody binds to cells or tissues of the body and elicits complement activation in those locations. The result is a tissue- or organ-specific pathology, and not a systemic problem as described here.

The tuberculin reaction (**choice D**) is a type IV hypersensitivity response. Delayed-type hypersensitivities are mediated by Th1 and Th17 cells and their mediators and have no contribution whatsoever from antibodies.

54. **The correct answer is E.** The description in the vignette is a type I hypersensitivity reaction—the only type of hypersensitivity that can be manifested in minutes. These are IgE-mediated responses and are an important protective response against helminth parasites that migrate through the tissues.

    The Arthus reaction (**choice A**) is an example of a type III (immune complex–mediated) pathology. These hypersensitivities develop when antigen is added to pre-existing antibody and immune complexes are filtered out of the circulation in the small vasculature. Complement is activated in these locations, and the underlying tissue is damaged. In this vignette, the killing is occurring in the skin and is associated within minutes with stinging, itching, and urticaria.

    Contact dermatitis (**choice B**) is an example of a type IV (delayed-type) hypersensitivity response. After the sensitizing exposure, symptoms of this type of hypersensitivity will occur in 48 to 72 hours (not minutes, as described here).

    Passive cutaneous anaphylaxis (**choice C**) is an example of a type I hypersensitivity reaction, but it is used to diagnose these conditions using passive transfer of serum. It is not a mechanism of protection, but a diagnostic technique.

    Serum sickness (**choice D**) is an example of a type III (immune complex-mediated) pathology. These hypersensitivities develop when antigen is added to pre-existing antibody and immune complexes are filtered out of the circulation in the small vasculature. Complement is activated in these locations, and the underlying tissue is damaged. In this vignette, the killing is occurring in the skin and is associated within minutes with stinging, itching, and urticaria.

55. **The correct answer is D.** An isograft is performed between genetically identical individuals. In human medicine, these are performed between monozygotic twins. In reality, even these "identical" individuals are not identical because minor mutations can occur during development. These sorts of grafts still require immunosuppression for success. They are, however, the best chance for success other than autografts.

    An allograft (**choice A**) is a transplant between two members of the same species who are not genetically identical. These are the most common types of transplants used in medicine, but in this vignette, the twins are described as having identical MHC haplotypes.

An autograft (**choice B**) is a transplant from one location in the body to another. This is the only form of transplantation that will succeed without immunosuppression.

"Heterograft" (**choice C**) is not a word that is used in transplantation immunology.

A xenograft (**choice E**) is a transplant that is performed across species barriers.

56. **The correct answer is C.** Graft-versus-host disease (GVHD) is primarily a manifestation of sensitization of transplanted T cells against recipient tissues. The killing of mucosal and other epithelial cells is largely mediated through recognition of MHC class I incompatibility by transferred cytotoxic cells or their precursors. However, eventually, continuous priming by the host's own tissues will elicit immune responses at the level of all the cells of the immune system.

    Activated macrophages (**choice A**) are involved in the delayed-type hypersensitivity response, but are not stimulated by MHC incompatibility, so if they become involved in pathology, it has to be secondary to Th stimulation.

    Antibodies and complement (**choice B**) are not involved in GVHD. Because bone marrow is a cellular transplant, it is the cells inside it that start the problem, not accidentally transferred antibodies or complement.

    LAK (lymphokine-activated killer) cells (**choice D**) are believed to be involved in the rejection of bone marrow transplants by the recipient (host-versus-graft), but not in GVHD.

    NK cells (**choice E**) are believed to be involved in the rejection of bone marrow transplants by the recipient (host-versus-graft), but not in GVHD.

57. **The correct answer is C.** The lowest stimulation index (and the lowest amount of proliferation) is shown between sibling 1 and the prospective recipient, both when the donor cells are used as stimulators and as responders. This means (most importantly) that the recipient will make little response to the graft and (less importantly, except in graft-versus-host disease) that the donor will make little response against the recipient.

    The father (**choice A**) is not the best choice of donors because the recipient makes 4 times the proliferative response to his cells as to those of sibling 1.

    The mother (**choice B**) is not the best choice of donors because the recipient makes twice the proliferative response to her cells as to those of sibling 1. She would be the second-best choice, unless sibling 1 had an incompatible ABO blood group.

    Sibling 2 (**choice D**) is not the best choice of donors because the recipient makes 8 times the proliferative response to his cells as to those of sibling 1.

    Sibling 3 (**choice E**) is not the best choice of donors because the recipient makes 8 times the proliferative response to his cells as to those of sibling 1.

58. **The correct answer is A.** IFNs of all types increase cellular expression of MHC class I and II products. Because CD8+ cells recognize their targets by MHC class I–dependent mechanisms, increases in the amount of these antigens on tumor-cell targets would increase susceptibility to cytotoxic killing.

IL-1 (**choice B**) does not increase MHC class I molecule expression. The endogenous pyrogen is responsible for alteration of the hypothalamic temperature set point during acute inflammatory events.

IL-2 (**choice C**) does not increase MHC class I molecule expression. It is produced by Th cells and causes proliferation of many classes of lymphocytes.

IL-10 (**choice D**) does not increase MHC class I molecule expression. It is a product of Th2 cells and inhibits Th1 cells; thus, it inhibits the cell-mediated arm of the immune response.

TNF-α (**choice E**) does not increase MHC class I molecule expression. It may act directly on tumor cells to cause their necrosis and decrease angiogenesis. It is a product of Th1 cells that stimulates the effector cells of cell-mediated immunity.

59. **The correct answer is D.** The standard screening test for HIV infection is the enzyme-linked immunosorbent assay, or ELISA. In this test, the virus p24 antigen is coated onto microtiter plates. Serum from the test subjects is added, followed by antihuman-immunoglobulin, which is labeled with an enzyme. When the substrate for the enzyme is added, if the antibodies listed have bound in sequence, there will be a color change in that microtiter well.

Electrophoresis of HIV antigens in polyacrylamide gel (**choice A**) describes the Western blot, which is used as a confirmatory test of HIV infection.

HIV antigen covalently coupled to RBC, patient serum, and anti-immunoglobulin (**choice B**) describes an erythrocyte agglutination test. There is no such test in use for diagnosis of HIV. The indirect Coombs test, which is used to detect Rh– mothers who have become sensitized to the Rh antigens of their fetuses, operates on this principle, however.

HIV antigen covalently coupled to RBC, patient serum, and complement (**choice C**) describes either a complement-fixation or complement-mediated hemolysis assay. There is no such test in use for the diagnosis of HIV.

HIV antigen, patient serum, anti-immunoglobulin serum, and radioactive ligand (**choice E**) describes a radioimmunoassay. This is not used in the standard screening for HIV.

60. **The correct answer is D.** If the child is developing hemolytic disease of the newborn, then his erythrocytes will already be coated with maternal anti-Rh antibodies. Adding Coombs serum (antihuman gammaglobulin) to the baby's RBCs then will cause agglutination. This is the direct Coombs test.

Mother's serum plus RhoGAM plus Coombs reagent (**choice A**) is not a set of reagents that will accomplish any diagnosis. RhoGAM is anti-RhD immunoglobulin, which is given to Rh– mothers at the termination of any Rh+ pregnancy. If the mother is sensitized, she is making IgG antibodies of the same specificity. Adding these 3 reagents together would tell you nothing of the baby's condition.

Mother's serum plus Rh– RBCs plus Coombs reagent (**choice B**) is not a set of reagents that will accomplish any diagnosis. If the mother is Rh–, she will not make a response to Rh– RBCs, and addition of Coombs reagent will accomplish nothing.

RhoGAM plus Rh+ RBCs from the baby (**choice C**) is not a set of reagents that will accomplish any diagnosis. RhoGAM will bind to Rh+ RBCs from the baby by definition, but adding these reagents together would tell you nothing of the baby's condition.

Rh+ RBCs plus mother's serum plus Coombs (**choice E**) is the set of reagents necessary for the performance of the indirect Coombs test. This is a test used to determine if the mother is making IgG anti-Rh antibodies, which could cross the placenta and harm a fetus. The question asks about the direct Coombs test, not the indirect.

61. **The correct answer is D.** The cell surface marker that would be useful to identify NK cells is CD56. The cells that have the highest fluorescence with antibodies to CD56 are found in quadrant D of panel 1.

Panel 1, quadrant A (**choice A**) contains the cells with maximum fluorescence with antibodies to CD3. These would be T lymphocytes.

Panel 1, quadrant B (**choice B**) contains the cells double-labeled with CD3 and CD56. Because CD3 is the pan-T-cell marker and CD56 is an NK-cell marker, there are no double-labeled cells in this case.

Panel 1, quadrant C (**choice C**) contains the cells that have background fluorescence with both CD3 and CD56. These are non-T, non-NK cells, so they could be B lymphocytes or any other leukocyte.

Panel 2, quadrant A (**choice E**) contains the cells with maximum fluorescence with antibodies to CD3. These are T lymphocytes.

Panel 2, quadrant B (**choice F**) contains double-labeled cells, which fluoresce with both antibody to CD3 and antibody to CD20. Because CD3 is a T-cell marker and CD20 is a B-cell marker, there are no cells in this quadrant.

Panel 2, quadrant C (**choice G**) contains the cells with background fluorescence with both antibodies to CD3 and CD20. These would be non-B, non-T cells and would contain some NK cells, but other leukocytes would be included here, so this is not the best choice.

Panel 2, quadrant D (**choice H**) contains the cells with maximum fluorescence with antibody to CD20, which is a B-cell marker.

62. **The correct answer is D.** Coombs reagent is antihuman IgG. It is necessary in the direct and indirect Coombs tests because in those cases, one is looking for IgG antibodies that could be transported across the placenta to harm an unborn child. IgG is a much smaller molecule than IgM, and is not capable of agglutinating erythrocytes without the addition of a "developing" antibody. In the ABO blood typing test, the important isohemagglutinins are of the IgM variety, capable of agglutinating erythrocytes by themselves because of their sheer size.

The statement that all antibodies made in response to blood glycoproteins are IgG (**choice A**) is not true because isohemagglutinins against ABO blood group antigens are IgM.

The statement that complement-mediated lysis is not important in ABO incompatibilities (**choice B**) is not true because isohemagglutinins of the IgM variety are extremely powerful activators of complement-mediated lysis. The agglutination tests here, however, do not use complement-mediated lysis as the indicator system.

That Coombs serum identifies only anti-Rh antibodies (**choice C**) is not true. Coombs serum is antihuman IgG. It will bind to the Fc portion of any human IgG molecule, regardless of its antigenic specificity.

The statement that the high titer of natural isohemagglutinins makes Coombs reagent unnecessary (**choice E**) is not true. It is the isotype of these antibodies (IgM) and the size of that molecule that allows agglutination to proceed without a developing antibody.

63. **The correct answer is A.** The direct fluorescent antibody test is used to detect antigens in the tissues of a patient.

The enzyme-linked immunosorbent assay (**choice B**) is a test usually used to detect antibody production. It can be modified to detect antigen, but not from a tissue specimen such as this one.

The indirect fluorescent antibody test (**choice C**) is used to detect antibodies being produced in a patient. It is not used for detection of microbial antigens.

Radioimmunoassay (**choice D**) is generally used to detect antibodies in a patient.

Western blot (**choice E**) is used to detect antibodies in a patient, not antigen.

64. **The correct answer is D.** To generate tumor-specific killer cells in vitro that would kill tumor cells transfected with an altered-self MHC class I gene, one would need to start with potential killer cells that use MHC I as a stimulatory signal. The only cytotoxic cell in the body that meets these criteria is the cytotoxic T lymphocyte (CTL). In panel I, increasing levels of fluorescence with antibody to CD8 are plotted as one moves to the right, and increasing levels of fluorescence with antibody to CD4 are plotted as one moves upward. Thus, the cells most strongly positive with CD8 are found the farthest to the right in quadrant D of panel I.

Panel I, quadrant A (**choice A**) would contain cells that are CD4+ and CD8–. These would be helper cells, and they would not be cytotoxic to transfected tumor cells.

Panel I, quadrant B (**choice B**) would contain cells that are double-positive for CD4 and CD8. These cells would be found as immature thymocytes in the thymus and not in the blood; thus, there are no double-labeled cells shown in this quadrant.

Panel I, quadrant C (**choice C**) contains the cells that have only background levels of fluorescence with antibodies to CD4 and CD8. These would be nonhelper, noncytotoxic cells, so they could be B lymphocytes, NK cells, or any other peripheral blood leukocyte.

Panel II, quadrant A (**choice E**) would contain cells which are strongly CD4+ and CD20–. These are helper T lymphocytes.

Panel II, quadrant B (**choice F**) would contain cells positive for CD4 and CD20. Because CD4 is a Th cell marker, and CD20 is a B-cell marker, such cells do not exist and thus this quadrant is empty.

Panel II, quadrant C (**choice G**) contains the cells that have only background levels of fluorescence with antibodies to CD4 and CD20. These would be nonhelper, non-B cells, so they could be cytotoxic T lymphocytes, NK cells, or any other peripheral blood leukocyte. Although this quadrant clearly contains some of the cytotoxic cells that this question asks about, there are other cells present, so this is not the best answer.

Panel II, quadrant D (**choice H**) contains the cells strongly positive for CD20 and negative for CD4. These are B lymphocytes.

SECTION II

Microbiology

General Microbiology ①

Learning Objectives

❏ Answer questions about bacterial structure, and bacterial growth and death

❏ Demonstrate knowledge about bacterial toxins

BACTERIAL STRUCTURE

Both Gram-positive and Gram-negative cell envelopes have the following properties:.

- **Cytoplasmic membranes**, which contain transpeptidases and carboxypeptidases that help construct the cell wall or peptidoglycan; they are also known as penicillin-binding proteins because they are targets for the β-lactam antibiotics

- **Peptidoglycan**, of which Gram-positives have a thick layer to protect it from osmotic damage, while Gram-negatives have a very thin layer; Gram stain reflects this difference

Gram-positive bacteria may utilize teichoic acid for attachment or lipoteichoic acid. Cell surface proteins are variable among the different genera but may include proteins such as the M protein found within the genus *Streptococcus*.

Gram-negative bacteria have an outer membrane covering the peptidoglycan. The outer membrane contains the endotoxin lipopolysaccharide (LPS).

- LPS is comprised of **lipid A (the toxic portion)**, and polysaccharide.

- LPS is highly immunogenic and binds specifically to receptors (LPS receptor, or **TLR-4**, see Immunology chapter 3) to activate macrophages.

- LPS can also non-specifically activate B cells without the help of T cells.

- LPS can be serotyped to classify bacteria.

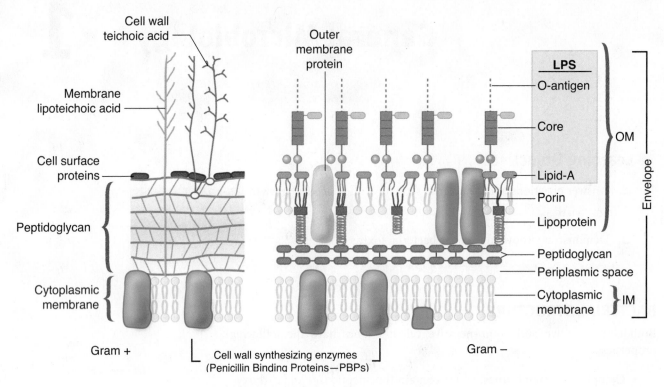

Figure II-1-1. Bacterial Cell Envelope

Peptidoglycan is comprised of polysaccharide chains N-acetylglucosamine (GlcNAc, NAG) and N-acetylmuramic acid (MurNAc, NAM) that are crosslinked by peptides. The peptide which crosslinks NAG and NAM is a tetrapeptide (begins as a pentapeptide but terminal D-alanine is released upon crosslinking to create the tetrapeptide) in which the first 2 amino acids may vary among different organisms.

The third amino acid in the peptide must include an amine group (e.g., L-lysine, diaminopimelic acid, diaminobutyric acid) which forms the cross link with the fourth peptide (D-alanine from another chain). The peptidoglycan is very thick in Gram positive cells and only 1 layer thick in gram negative cells.

Synthesis of the peptidoglycan is a several step process.

- The NAG and NAM precursors are synthesized inside of the cell and the pentapeptide is added.

- At the cytoplasmic membrane, the individual units are attached to a carrier called bactoprenol.

- The NAG is added and the unit (NAG-NAM-peptide) is translocated to the outside of the cell.

- The individual unit is then added to the peptidoglycan chain through transglycosylases which use a pyrophosphate link between the unit and the bactoprenol as energy to drive the reaction.

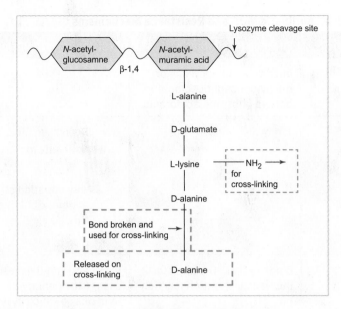

Figure II-1-2. Synthesis of Peptodoglycan

The cross-linking is catalyzed by transpeptidases and carboxypeptidases (remove the terminal D-alanines) that are also called penicillin-binding proteins (PBP's).

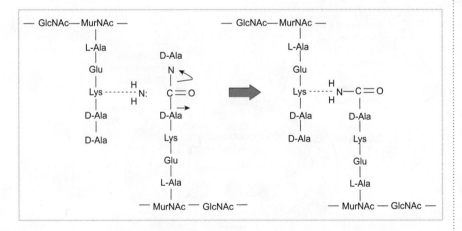

Figure II-1-3. Transpeptidation Reaction

Clinical Correlate

Peptidoglycan synthesis is a major target for antimicrobial chemotherapy for the following reasons:

- The process is utilized only in prokaryotes.

- Its inhibition has few side effects on eukaryotic cells (human cells).

As effective as antibiotics are, bacteria have become very clever at getting around them and becoming resistant to antibiotics.

Table II-1-1. Antibiotic MOA and Resistance Mechanisms

Antibiotic	Effect on PG synthesis	Resistance mechanisms
Bacitracin	Interferes with recycling of the pyrophosphobactoprenol back to phosphobactoprenol	
β-lactams	Target the PBPs	• Decreased binding of antibiotic to the PBP • Decreased concentration of antibiotic at target (Gram negative only) • β-lactamases
Vancomycin	Binds to D-ala-D-ala to block the transpeptidation reaction	Van-A and Van-B genes change the pentapeptide terminus so vancomycin will no longer bind

See Pharmacology Lecture Notes for more on the MOA of antibiotics.

The mechanism of action (MOA) of antibiotics is covered in the Pharmacology Lecture Notes but an overview can be seen below.

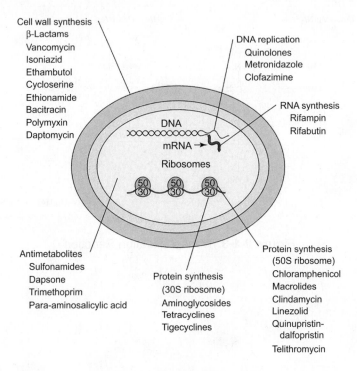

Figure II-1-4. Antibiotic MOA

ENDOSPORES

Organisms: *Bacillus* and *Clostridium*

Function: survival not reproductive (1 bacterium → 1 spore); resistance to chemicals, dessiccation, radiation, freezing, and heat

Mechanism of resistance

- New enzymes (i.e., dipicolinic acid synthetase, heat-resistant catalase)

- Increases or decreases in other enzymes

- Dehydration: calcium dipicolinate in core

- Keratin spore coat

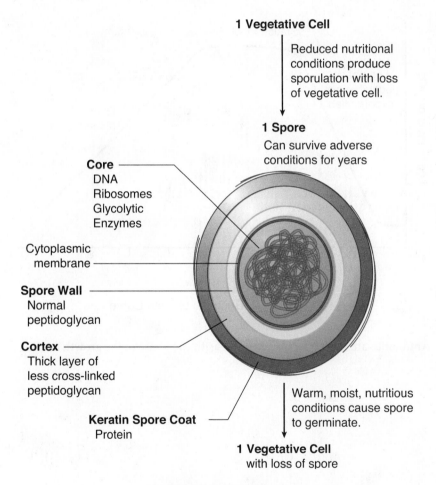

1 Vegetative Cell

Reduced nutritional conditions produce sporulation with loss of vegetative cell.

1 Spore

Can survive adverse conditions for years

Core
DNA
Ribosomes
Glycolytic
Enzymes

Cytoplasmic
membrane

Spore Wall
Normal
peptidoglycan

Cortex
Thick layer of
less cross-linked
peptidoglycan

Keratin Spore Coat
Protein

Warm, moist, nutritious conditions cause spore to germinate.

1 Vegetative Cell
with loss of spore

Figure II-1.5. Endospore

Note

Spores of fungi have a reproductive role.

BACTERIAL GROWTH AND DEATH

In a Nutshell

Lag Phase

- Initial Phase (only 1 lag phase)
- Detoxifying medium
- Turning on enzymes to utilize medium
- For exam, number of cells at beginning equals number of cells at end of lag phase.

Log Phase

- Rapid exponential growth
- Generation time = time it takes one cell to divide into two. This is determined during log phase.

Stationary Phase

- Nutrients used up
- Toxic products like acids and alkali begin to accumulate.
- Number of new cells equals the number of dying cells.

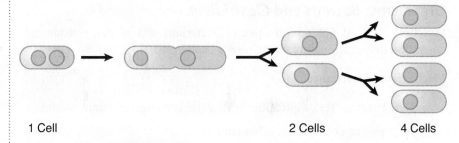

Figure II-1-6. Exponential Growth by Binary Fission

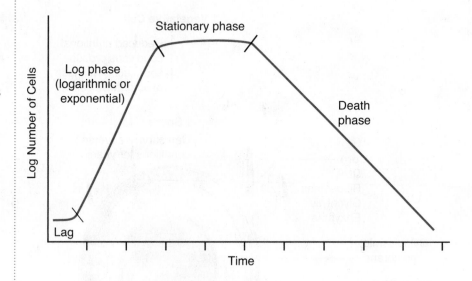

Figure II-1-7. Bacterial Growth Curve

Antibiotics are most effective at the logarithmic phase of the growth curve.

CULTURE OF MICROORGANISMS

Obligate intracellular pathogens (viruses, rickettsias, chlamydias, etc.) cannot be cultured in vitro on articial media. Therefore, tissue cultures (cell cultures), eggs, animals are utilized for growth. Some pathogens cannot be cultured at all (e.g., syphilis).

Facultative intracellular or extracellular organisms can be grown on inert lab media such as broth or agar. Selective media selects for certain bacteria by inclusion of special nutrients and/or antibiotics. Differential media differentiates bacteria by colony morphology or color.

Table II-1-2. Special Media for Selected Organisms

Organism	Medium
Anaerobes	Thioglycolate
Corynebacterium	Löffler's coagulated serum medium (S) Tellurite agar (D)
Enteric bacteria	Eosin methylene blue (D) MacConkeys (D and S)
Enteric pathogens	Hektoen enteric agar (D) Xylose-lysine-deoxycholate agar
Vibrio cholerae (likes alkaline growth medium)	TCBS (Thiosulfate Citrate Bile Salts Sucrose agar) (S)
Legionella	Charcoal-yeast extract agar (CYE agar) (S)
Mycobacterium	Löwenstein-Jensen medium (S)
Neisseria from normally sterile sites, *Haemophilus*	Chocolate agar
Neisseria from sites with normal flora	Thayer-Martin selective medium* (S)

*Thayer-Martin media is a chocolate agar supplemented with vancomycin, nystatin and colistin to inhibit the normal flora, including nonpathogenic Neisseria.

Table II-1-3. Miscellaneous Growth Requirements

Cholesterol and purines and pyrimidines	*Mycoplasma*
Cysteine*	*Francisella, Brucella, Legionella, Pasteurella*
X (protoporphyrin) and V (NAD)	*Haemophilus* (*influenzae* and *aegypticus* require both)

*The 4 Sisters Ella and the Cysteine Chapel

Note

Mnemonic

The 4 sisters "Ella" worship in the "Cysteine" chapel:

- *Francisella*
- *Brucella*
- *Legionella*
- *Pasteurella*

PATHOGENICITY (INFECTIVITY AND TOXICITY) MAJOR MECHANISMS

Colonization

(Important unless organism is traumatically implanted.)

Adherence to cell surfaces involves

- **Pili/fimbriae:** primary mechanism in most gram-negative cells.
- **Teichoic acids:** primary mechanism of gram-positive cells.
- **Adhesins:** colonizing factor adhesins, pertussis toxin, and hemagglutinins.
- **IgA proteases:** make it easier for pathogens to colonize.

Partial adherence to inert materials, **biofilms:** *Staph. epidermidis, Streptococcus mutans, Pseudomonas aeruginosa*

Avoiding Immediate Destruction by Host Defense System

- **Anti-phagocytic surface components** (inhibit phagocytic uptake):
  - **Capsules**/slime layers:

    ***Streptococcus pyogenes* M protein**

    ***Neisseria gonorrhoeae* pili**

    ***Staphylococcus aureus* A protein**
- **IgA proteases,** destruction of mucosal IgA: *Neisseria, Haemophilus, S. pneumoniae*

"Hunting and Gathering" Needed Nutrients

- **Siderophores** steal (chelate) and import iron.

Antigenic Variation

- Changing surface antigens to avoid immune destruction
- *N. gonorrhoeae*—pili and outer membrane proteins
- *Trypanosoma brucei rhodesiense* and *T. b. gambiense*—phase variation
- Enterobacteriaceae: capsular and flagellar antigens may or may not be expressed
- HIV, influenza—antigenic drift

Note

Mnemonic

*S*treptococcus pneumoniae

*K*lebsiella pneumoniae

*H*aemophilus influenzae

*P*seudomonas aeruginosa

*N*eisseria meningitidis

*C*ryptococcus neoformans

(**S**ome **K**illers **H**ave **P**retty **N**ice **C**apsules)

Note

Intracellular organisms

- Elicit different immune responses
- Different pathology
- Different antibiotics
- Different culture techniques

Ability to Survive Intracellularly

- **Evading intracellular killing by professional phagocytic cells** allows intracellular growth:

  - *M. tuberculosis* survives by inhibiting phagosome-lysosome fusion.

  - *Listeria* quickly escapes the phagosome into the cytoplasm **before** phagosome-lysosome fusion.

- **Invasins**: surface proteins that allow an organism to bind to and invade normally non-phagocytic human cells, escaping the immune system. Best studied invasin is on *Yersinia pseudotuberculosis* (an organism causing diarrhea).

- Damage from viruses is largely from intracellular replication, which either kills cells, transforms them or, in the case of latent viruses, may do no noticeable damage.

Type III Secretion Systems

- Tunnel from the bacteria to the host cell (macrophage) that delivers bacterial toxins directly to the host cell

- Have been demonstrated in many pathogens: *E. coli, Salmonella* species, *Yersinia* species, *P. aeruginosa*, and *Chlamydia*

Inflammation or Immune-Mediated Damage

Examples

- **Cross-reaction of bacteria-induced antibodies with tissue antigens** causes disease. Rheumatic fever is one example.

- **Delayed hypersensitivity and the granulomatous response** stimulated by the presence of intracellular bacteria is responsible for neurological damage in leprosy, cavitation in tuberculosis, and fallopian tube blockage resulting in infertility from *Chlamydia* PID (pelvic inflammatory disease).

- **Immune complexes** damage the kidney in post streptococcal acute glomerulonephritis.

- **Peptidoglycan-teichoic acid** (large fragments) of gram-positive cells:

  - Serves as a structural toxin released when cells die.

  - Chemotactic for neutrophils.

Physical Damage

- Swelling from infection in a fixed space damages tissues; examples: meningitis and cysticercosis.

- Large physical size of organism may cause problems; example: *Ascaris lumbricoides* blocking bile duct.

TOXINS

Toxins may aid in invasiveness, damage cells, inhibit cellular processes, or trigger immune response and damage.

Structural Toxins

- **Endotoxin** (lipopolysaccharide = LPS)

  - LPS is part of **gram-negative outer membrane**

  - **Toxic portion is lipid A**: generally not released (and toxic) until death of cell (exception: *N. meningitidis,* which over-produces outer membrane fragments)

  - **LPS is heat stable** and not strongly immunogenic, so **cannot be converted to a toxoid**

  - **LPS is primary virulence factor in Gram negative septic shock**

  - Mechanism: **LPS activates macrophages**, leading to release of TNF-alpha, IL-1, and IL-6. IL-1 is a major mediator of fever. Macrophage activation and products lead to tissue damage. Damage to the endothelium from **bradykinin-induced vasodilation leads to shock. Coagulation** (DIC) is mediated through the **activation of Hageman factor**.

- **Peptidoglycan, Teichoic Acids**

Exotoxins

- Are **protein toxins,** generally **quite toxic** and **secreted by** bacterial **cells** (some gram +, some gram −)

- **Can be modified** by chemicals or heat to produce a **toxoid** that still is **immunogenic, but no longer toxic** so can be used as a vaccine

- **A-B** (or "two") **component** protein toxins

  - **B** component **binds** to specific cell receptors to facilitate the internalization of A.

  - **A** component is the **active (toxic) component** (often an enzyme such as an ADP ribosyl transferase).

  - Exotoxins may be subclassed as enterotoxins, neurotoxins, or cytotoxins.

- **Cytolysins:** lyse cells from outside by damaging membrane.

  - *C. perfringens* **alpha toxin** is a **lecithinase.**

  - *Staphylococcus aureus* **alpha toxin** inserts itself to form **pores** in the membrane.

Table II-1-4. Major Exotoxins

	Organism (Gram)	Toxin	Mode of Action	Role in Disease
Inhibitors of Protein Synthesis	*Corynebacterium diphtheriae* (+)	Diphtheria toxin	ADP ribosyl transferase; inactivates eEF-2; 1´ targets: heart/nerves/epithelium	Inhibits eukaryotic cell protein synthesis
	Pseudomonas aeruginosa (−)	Exotoxin A	ADP ribosyl transferase; inactivates eEF-2; 1´ target: liver	Inhibits eukaryotic cell protein synthesis
	Shigella dysenteriae (−)	Shiga toxin	Interferes with 60S ribosomal subunit	Inhibits protein synthesis in eukaryotic cells. Enterotoxic, cytotoxic, and neurotoxic
	Enterohemorrhagic *E. coli* (EHEC) (−)	Verotoxin (a shiga-like toxin)	Interferes with 60S ribosomal subunit	Inhibits protein synthesis in eukaryotic cells
Neurotoxins	*Clostridium tetani* (+)	Tetanus toxin	Blocks release of the inhibitory transmitters glycine and GABA	Inhibits neurotransmission in inhibitory synapses
	Clostridium botulinum (+)	Botulinum toxin	Blocks release of acetylcholine	Inhibits cholinergic synapses
Super-antigens	*Staphylococcus aureus* (+)	TSST-1	Superantigen	Fever, increased susceptibility to LPS, rash, shock, capillary leakage
	Streptococcus pyogenes (+)	Exotoxin A, a.k.a.: erythrogenic or pyrogenic toxin	Similar to TSST-1	Fever, increased susceptibility to LPS, rash, shock, capillary leakage, cardiotoxicity
cAMP Inducers	Enterotoxigenic *Escherichia coli* (−)	Heat labile toxin (LT)	LT stimulates an adenylate cyclase by ADP ribosylation of GTP binding protein	Both LT and ST promote secretion of fluid and electrolytes from intestinal epithelium
	Vibrio cholerae (−)	Cholera toxin	Similar to *E. coli* LT	Profuse, watery diarrhea
	Bacillus anthracis (+)	Anthrax toxin (3 proteins make 2 toxins)	EF = edema factor = adenylate cyclase; LF = lethal factor; PA = protective antigen (B component for both)	Decreases phagocytosis; causes edema, kills cells
	Bordetella pertussis (−)	Pertussis toxin	ADP ribosylates G_i, the negative regulator of adenylate cyclase → increased cAMP	Histamine-sensitizing Lymphocytosis promoting Islet activating
Cytolysins	*Clostridium perfringens* (+)	Alpha toxin	Lecithinase	Damages cell membranes; myonecrosis
	Staphylococcus aureus (+)	Alpha toxin	Toxin intercalates forming pores	Cell membrane becomes leaky

Medically Important Bacteria 2

Learning Objectives

❏ Answer questions about normal flora and their function

❏ Demonstrate understanding of microorganism cultures, strains, and gram stain techniques

❏ Answer questions about distinguishing features, transmission, pathogenesis, diagnosis, treatment, and prevention of gram-positive cocci, gram-positive rods, gram-negative cocci, gram-negative bacilli, spirochetes, and unusual bacteria

❏ Differentiate organisms in the *Chlamydophila*, *Rickettsia*, and *Ehrlichia* genuses

❏ Differentiate organisms in the *Mycoplasmataceae* and *Chlamydiaceae* families

Note

Nomenclature

Latin bacterial **family** names have **"-aceae,"** e.g., Enterobacteriaceae.

Genus and species names are **italicized** and **abbreviated**, e.g., *Enterobacter aerogenes = E. aerogenes*.

NORMAL FLORA

Normal flora are found on body surfaces contiguous with the outside environment. They are semi-permanent, varying with major life changes.

- Can cause infection
  - If misplaced, e.g., fecal flora to urinary tract or abdominal cavity, or skin flora to catheter
  - If person becomes compromised, normal flora may overgrow (oral thrush)
- Contribute to health
  - Protective host defense by maintaining conditions such as pH so other organisms may not grow
  - Serve nutritional function by synthesizing: K and B vitamins
  - Competition for space

Note

Definitions

Carrier: person colonized by a potential pathogen without overt disease.

Bacteremia: bacteria in bloodstream without overt clinical signs.

Septicemia: bacteria in bloodstream (multiplying) with clinical symptoms.

Table II-2-1. Important Normal Flora

Site	Common or Medically Important Organisms	Less Common but Notable Organisms
Blood, internal organs	None, generally sterile	
Cutaneous surfaces including urethra and outer ear	*Staphylococcus epidermidis*	*Staphylococcus aureus*, Corynebacteria (diphtheroids), streptococci, anaerobes, e.g., peptostreptococci, yeasts (*Candida* spp.)
Nose	*Staphylococcus aureus*	*S. epidermidis*, diphtheroids, assorted streptococci
Oropharynx	**Viridans streptococci** including *Strep. mutans*[1]	Assorted streptococci, **nonpathogenic *Neisseria*, nontypeable[2] *Haemophilus influenzae*, *Candida albicans***
Gingival crevices	Anaerobes: *Bacteroides, Prevotella, Fusobacterium, Streptococcus, Actinomyces*	
Stomach	None	
Colon (microaerophilic/anaerobic)	Babies; breast-fed only: *Bifidobacterium*	*Lactobacillus*, streptococci
	Adult: ***Bacteroides**/Prevotella* (Predominant organism) *Escherichia* *Bifidobacterium*	*Eubacterium, Fusobacterium, Lactobacillus*, assorted Gram-negative anaerobic rods, *Enterococcus faecalis* and other streptococci
Vagina	***Lactobacillus***[3]	Assorted streptococci, gram-negative rods, diphtheroids, yeasts, *Veillonella*

[1] ***S. mutans*** secretes a biofilm that glues it and other oral flora to teeth, producing **dental plaque**.

[2] Nontypeable for *Haemophilus* means no capsule.

[3] Group B streptococci colonize vagina of 15–20% of women and may infect the infant during labor or delivery, causing septicemia and/or meningitis (as may *E. coli* from fecal flora).

Table II-2-2. Oxygen Requirements and Toxicity

Classification	Characteristics	Important Genera
Obligate aerobes	Require oxygen Have no fermentative pathways Generally produce superoxide dismutase	*Mycobacterium* *Pseudomonas* *(Bacillus)*
Microaerophilic	Require low but not full oxygen tension	*Campylobacter* *Helicobacter*
Facultative anaerobes	Will respire aerobically until oxygen is depleted and then ferment	Most bacteria, e.g., *Enterobacteriaceae*
Obligate anaerobes	• Lack superoxide dismutase • Generally lack catalase • Are fermenters • Cannot use O_2 as terminal electron acceptor	*Actinomyces** *Bacteroides* *Clostridium*

*ABCs of anaerobiosis = *Actinomyces*, *Bacteroides*, and *Clostridium*

STAINS

Table II-2-3. Gram Stain

Reagent	Gram-Positive	Gram-Negative
Crystal violet (a very intense purple, small dye molecule)	Purple/blue	Purple/blue
Gram's iodine	Purple/blue (a large dye complex)	Purple/blue (a large dye complex)
Acetone or alcohol	Purple/blue	Colorless
Safranin (a pale dye)	Purple/blue	Red/pink

All cocci are gram-positive except *Neisseria*, *Moraxella* and *Veillonella*.

All spore formers are gram-positive.

Background in stain modified for tissues will be pale red.

Table II-2-4. Ziehl-Neelsen Acid Fast Stain (or Kinyoun)

Reagent	Acid Fast	Non-Acid Fast*
Carbol fuchsin with heat**	Red (hot pink)	Red (hot pink)
Acid alcohol	Red	Colorless
Methylene blue***	Red	Blue

* *Mycobacterium* is acid fast. *Nocardia* is partially acid fast. All other bacteria are non-acid fast. Two protozoan parasites (*Cryptosporidium* and *Isospora*) have acid fast oocysts.

** Without the heat, the dye would not go in the mycobacterial cells.

*** Sputa and human cells will be blue.

GRAM-STAINING REACTIONS

Table II-2-5. Gram-Negative Bacteria

Cocci		
	Neisseria** Moraxella	
Rods		
	Pseudomonas** Burkholderia Acinetobacter Eikenella Kingella Haemophilus** Bartonella	Legionella* Brucella Bordetella* Francisella* Capnocytophaga Pasteurella*
Curved or helical		
	Campylobacter** Helicobacter** Vibrio**	
Enterobacteriaceae		
	Escherichia** Shigella** Salmonella** Klebsiella* Proteus*	Yersinia** Aeromonas Serratia Citrobacter Enterobacter
Anaerobic Rods		
	Bacteroides Prevotella	Porphyromonas Fusobacterium
Gram-variable Rods		
	Gardnerella	Mobiluncus
Spirochetes		
	Treponema** Borrelia** Leptospira	

Table II-2-6. Gram-Positive Bacteria

Cocci	
	*Staphylococcus***
	*Streptococcus***
	Enterococcus
Rods	
Aerobic or facultative anaerobic	
	*Bacillus***
	*Listeria**
	*Corynebacterium**
	Nocardia
	*Mycobacterium***
Anaerobic	
	*Clostridium***
	Actinomyces
	Propionibacterium
	Lactobacillus

Note: Spore formers are *Bacillus* and *Clostridium*.

Note

*Typically considered high yield

** Extremely high yield organisms

Table II-2-7. Non-Gram–staining Bacteria*

Mycoplasmataceae	
	*Mycoplasma*** *Ureaplasma*
Rickettsiaceae	
	*Rickettsia** *Ehrlichia* *Coxiella*
Chlamydiaceae	
	*Chlamydia*** *Chlamydophila*

*Note:

Poorly visible on traditional Gram stain: *Mycobacterium* does not stain well with the Gram stain due to its waxy cell wall. It is considered gram-positive.

Most **spirochetes, chlamydiae,** and **rickettsias** are so thin that the color of the Gram stain cannot be seen. All have gram-negative cell walls.

Legionella (gram-negative) also does not stain well with the traditional Gram stain unless counterstain time is increased.

GRAM-POSITIVE COCCI

- *Staphylococcus*
- *Streptococcus*

Table II-2-8. Major Species of *Staphylococcus* and *Streptococcus* and Identifying Features*

	Catalase	Coagulase	Hemolysis†	Distinguishing Features	Disease Presentations
Staphylococcus Species					
S. aureus	+	+	β	Ferments mannitol Salt tolerant	Infective endocarditis (acute) Abscesses Toxic shock syndrome Gastroenteritis Suppurative lesions, pyoderma, impetigo Osteomyelitis
S. epidermidis	+	−	γ	Novobiocin^S Biofilm producer	Endocarditis in IV drug users Catheter and prosthetic device infections
S. saprophyticus	+	−	γ	Novobiocin^R	UTIs in newly sexually active females
Streptococcus Species (Grouped by analysis of C carbohydrate)					
S. pyogenes (Group A)	−	−	β	Bacitracin^S PYR†	Pharyngitis Scarlet fever Pyoderma/impetigo Suppurative lesions Rheumatic fever Acute glomerulonephritis
S. agalactiae (Group B)	−	−	β	Bacitracin^R CAMP+	Neonatal septicemia and meningitis
S. pneumoniae (not groupable)	−	−	α	Optochin^S Bile-soluble	Pneumonia (community acquired) Adult meningitis Otitis media and sinusitis in children
Viridans group (not groupable)	−	−	α/γ	Optochin^R Bile-soluble	Infective endocarditis Dental caries
Enterococcus sp. (Group D)	−	−	α, β, or γ	PYR† Bile-soluble Esculin agar	Infective endocarditis Urinary and biliary infections

† β hemolysis = clear; α hemolysis = partial; γ hemolysis = no hemolysis

Definition of abbreviations: PYR, pyrrolidonyl arylamidase; ^S, sensitive; ^R, resistant

*Many of the diseases caused by *Staphylococcus* and *Streptococcus* are similar (i.e., skin infections, endocarditis). Therefore, laboratory tests are extremely important in differentiating between these organisms.

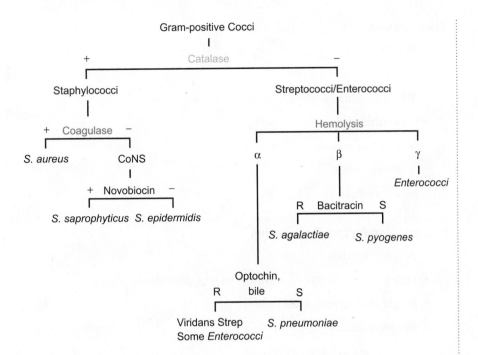

Figure II-2-1. Differentiation of Gram-Positive Cocci

GENUS: *STAPHYLOCOCCUS*

Genus Features
- Gram-positive cocci in clusters
- **Catalase positive (streptococci are catalase negative)**

Species of Medical Importance
- *S. aureus*
- *S. epidermidis*
- *S. saprophyticus*

Staphylococcus aureus

Distinguishing Features
- Small, yellow Staphylococcus aureuscolonies on blood agar
- **β-hemolytic**
- **Coagulase positive** (all other *Staphylococcus* species are negative)
- **Ferments mannitol** on mannitol salt agar

Reservoir
- Normal flora
  - Nasal mucosa (25% of population are carriers)
  - Skin

Key Vignette Clues
S. epidermidis
- Coagulase (–); gram (+) cocci
- Novobiocin sensitive
- Infections of catheters/shunts

S. saprophyticus
- Coagulase (–), gram (+) cocci
- Novobiocin resistant

Key Vignette Clues
Staphylococcus aureus
- Coagulase (+), gram (+) cocci in clusters
- Gastroenteritis: 2–6 h onset, salty foods, custards
- Endocarditis: acute
- Toxic shock syndrome: desquamating rash, fever, hypotension
- Impetigo: bullous
- Pneumonia: nosocomial, typical, acute
- Osteomyelitis: #1 cause unless HbS mentioned

Transmission

- Hands
- Sneezing
- Surgical wounds
- Contaminated food
  - Custard pastries
  - Potato salad
  - Canned meats

Predisposing Factors for Infection

- Surgery/wounds
- Foreign body (tampons, surgical packing, sutures)
- Severe neutropenia (<500/µL)
- Intravenous drug abuse
- Chronic granulomatous disease
- Cystic fibrosis

Pathogenesis

- Protein A binds Fc component of IgG, inhibits phagocytosis
- **Enterotoxins:** fast acting, heat stable
- **Toxic shock syndrome toxin-1 (TSST-1):** superantigen (see Chapter 6 of Immunology for further explanation of a superantigen)
- Coagulase: converts fibrinogen to fibrin clot
- Cytolytic toxin (α toxin): pore-forming toxin, Panton-Valentine leuko-cidin (PVL), forms pores in infected cells and is acquired by bacterio-phage; associated with increased virulence, MRSA strains
- Exfolatins: skin-exfoliating toxins (involved in scalded skin syndrome [SSS]) and bullous impetigo

Diseases

Table II-2-9. *Staphylococcus aureus*

Diseases	Clinical Symptoms	Pathogenicity Factors
Gastroenteritis (food poisoning)—toxin ingested preformed in food	**2–6 hours** after ingesting toxin: nausea, abdominal pain, vomiting, followed by diarrhea	Enterotoxins A–E preformed in food
Infective endocarditis (acute) (**most common cause**)	Fever, malaise, leukocytosis, heart murmur (may be absent initially)	Fibrin-platelet mesh, cytolytic toxins
Abscesses and mastitis	Subcutaneous tenderness, redness and swelling; hot	Coagulase, cytolysins
Toxic shock syndrome	Fever, hypotension, **scarlatiniform rash that desquamates (particularly on palms and soles)**, multiorgan failure	TSST-1
Impetigo	Erythematous papules to **bullae**	Coagulase, exfoliatins
Scalded skin syndrome	Diffuse epidermal peeling	Coagulase, exfoliatins
Pneumonia	Productive pneumonia with rapid onset, high rate of necrosis, and high fatality; nosocomial, ventilator, postinfluenza, IV drug abuse, cystic fibrosis, chronic granulomatous disease, etc. Salmon-colored sputum	Coagulase, cytolysins
Surgical infections	Fever with cellulitis and/or abscesses	Coagulase, exfoliatins, ± TSSTs
Osteomyelitis (most common cause)	Bone pain, fever, ± tissue swelling, redness; lytic bone lesions on imaging	Cytolysins, coagulase
Septic arthritis	Monoarticular joint pain; inflammation	Cytolysins, coagulase

Treatment

- Gastroenteritis is self-limiting.
- Nafcillin/oxacillin are drugs of choice because of widespread penicillinase-producing stains.
- Mupirocin for topical treatment.
- For methicillin-resistant *Staphylococcus aureus* (MRSA): vancomycin
- For vancomycin-resistant *Staphylococcus aureus* (VRSA) or vancomycin-intermediate *S. aureus* (VISA): quinupristin/dalfopristin

GENUS: *STREPTOCOCCUS*

Genus Features

- Gram-positive cocci in chains
- **Catalase negative**
- Serogrouped using known antibodies to the cell wall carbohydrates (Lancefield groups A–O): *S. pneumoniae* serotyped via capsule; *S. pyogenes* serotyped via M protein

Species of Medical Importance

- *S. pyogenes*
- *S. agalactiae* (group B streptococci; GBS)
- *S. pneumoniae*
- Viridans streptococci: *S. mutans*; *S. sanguinis*; *S. gallolyticus (bovis)*

Streptococcus pyogenes (Group Enterococcus Streptococcus; GAS)

Distinguishing Features

- **β hemolytic**
- **Bacitracin sensitive**
- **Pyrrolidonyl arylamidase (PYR) positive**

Reservoir: human throat; skin

Transmission: direct contact; respiratory droplets

Pathogenesis

- **Hyaluronic acid: is non-immunogenic**
- **M-protein: antiphagocytic**, associated with **acute glomerulonephritis**, rheumatic fever
- Streptolysin O: immunogenic, hemolysin/cytolysin
- Streptolysin S: not immunogenic, hemolysin/cytolysin

Spreading Factors

- Streptokinase: breaks down fibrin clot

- Streptococcal DNAse: liquefies pus, extension of lesion

- Hyaluronidase: hydrolyzes the ground substances of the connective tissues

- Exotoxins A–C (pyrogenic or erythrogenic exotoxins)

  – Phage-coded (i.e.,the cells are lysogenized by a phage.)

  – Cause **fever and rash** of scarlet fever: **superantigens**

Diseases

Table II-2-10. Acute Suppurative Group A Streptococcal Infections*

Diseases	Symptoms
Pharyngitis	Abrupt onset of sore throat, fever, malaise, and headache; tonsillar abscesses and tender anterior cervical lymph nodes
Scarlet fever	Above followed by a blanching **"sandpaper" rash** (palms and soles are usually spared), circumoral pallor, **strawberry tongue**, and nausea/vomiting
Pyoderma/impetigo	Pyogenic skin infection (honey-crusted lesions)

*Also, cellulitis/necrotizing fasciitis, puerperal fever, lymphangitis, erysipelas

Table II-2-11. Nonsuppurative Sequelae to Group A Streptococcal Infections

Disease	Sequelae of	Mechanisms/Symptoms
Rheumatic fever	Pharyngitis with group A strep	Antibodies to heart tissue/2 weeks post pharyngitis, fever, joint inflammation, carditis, erythema marginatum (chorea later)type II hypersensitivity
Acute glomerulonephritis (AGN)	Pharyngitis or skin infection	Immune complexes bound to glomeruli/pulmonary edema and hypertension, "smoky" urine (type III hypersensitivity)

Laboratory Diagnosis

- Rapid strep test (ELISA-based) misses approximately 25% of infections. Culture all negatives.

- Antibodies to streptolysin O (ASO) titer of >200 is significant for rheumatic fever.

- Anti-DNAse B and antihyaluronidase titers for AGN

Treatment: beta lactam drugs, macrolides in the case of penicillin allergy

Prevention: possible prophylactic antibiotics for at least 5 years post-acute rheumatic fever; beta lactams and macrolides

Streptococcus agalactiae (Group B Streptococci; GBS)

Key Vignette Clues

S. agalactiae

- Gram (+), catalase (–), β hemolytic, bacitracin resistant, CAMP test (+)

- Neonatal meningitis and septicemia: #1 cause, especially in prolonged labors

Distinguishing Features

- **β hemolytic**

- **Bacitracin resistant**

- **Hydrolyze hippurate**

- **CAMP test positive** (CAMP factor is a polypeptide which "complements" the sphingomyelinase of *S. aureus* to create an enhanced hemolytic pattern in shape of an arrowhead)

Reservoir: human vagina (15–20% of women); GI tract

Transmission: newborn infected during birth (increased risk with **prolonged labor after rupture of membranes**)

Pathogenesis: capsule; β hemolysin and CAMP factor

Diseases: neonatal septicemia and meningitis; most common causal agent

Treatment: ampicillin with an aminoglycoside or a cephalosporin

Prevention

- Prophylaxis during delivery in women with positive vaginal/rectal culture of GBS, history of recent infection with GBS, or prolonged labors after membrane rupture

- Ampicillin or penicillin drugs of choice

- Clindamycin or erythromycin for penicillin allergies

Streptococcus pneumoniae

Distinguishing Features

- α **hemolytic**
- **Optochin sensitive**
- **Lancet-shaped diplococci**
- **Lysed by bile** (bile soluble)

Reservoir: human upper respiratory tract

Transmission: respiratory droplets (not considered highly communicable; often colonize the nasopharynx without causing disease)

Predisposing Factors

- Antecedent influenza or measles infection
- Chronic obstructive pulmonary disease (COPD)
- Congestive heart failure (CHF)
- Alcoholism
- Asplenia predisposes to septicemia

Pathogenesis

- **Polysaccharide capsule** is the major virulence factor
- IgA protease
- Teichoic acid
- Pneumolysin O: hemolysin/cytolysin: damages respiratory epithelium; inhibits leukocyte respiratory burst and inhibits classical complement fixation

Diseases

- Typical pneumonia: **most common cause** (especially in decade 6 of life); shaking chills, high fever, lobar consolidation, **blood-tinged, "rusty" sputum**
- Adult meningitis: **most common cause**; peptidoglycan and teichoic acids are highly inflammatory in CNS; CSF reveals high WBCs (neutrophils) and low glucose, high protein
- Otitis media and sinusitis in children **most common cause**

Laboratory Diagnosis

- Gram stain and culture of CSF or sputum
- Quellung reaction: positive (swelling of the capsule with the addition of type-specific antiserum, no longer used but still tested!)
- Latex particle agglutination: test for capsular antigen in CSF
- Urinary antigen test

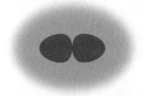

Streptococcus pneumoniae

Key Vignette Clues

Streptococcus pneumoniae

- Gram (+), catalase (–), α hemolytic, soluble in bile, optochin sensitive
- Pneumonia—typical, most common cause, rusty sputum
- Meningitis—many PMNs, ↓ glucose, ↑ protein in CSF, most common adult cause
- Otitis media and sinusitis—most common cause

In a Nutshell

Typical Pneumonia

Bacterial pneumonia such as *Streptococcus pneumoniae* elicits neutrophils; arachidonic acid metabolites (acute inflammatory mediators) cause pain and fever. *Pneumococcus* produces a lobar pneumonia with a productive cough, grows on blood agar, and usually responds well to penicillin treatment.

Treatment: beta lactams for bacterial pneumonia; ceftriaxone or cefotaxime for adult meningitis (add vancomycin if penicillin-resistant *S. pneumoniae* has been reported in community); amoxicillin for otitis media and sinusitis in children (erythromycin in cases of alltergy)

Prevention

- Antibody to capsule (>80 capsular serotypes) provides type-specific immunity
- Vaccine
  - Pediatric (PCV, pneumococcal conjugate vaccine): 13 of most common serotypes; conjugated to diphtheria toxoid; prevents invasive disease
  - Adult (PPV, pneumococcal polysaccharide vaccine): 23 of most common capsular serotypes; recommended for all adults age ≥65 plus at-risk individuals

Viridans Streptococci (*S. sanguis, S. mutans*)

Distinguishing Features

- α **hemolytic**
- **Optochin resistant**
- PYR-negative
- Bile insoluble

Reservoir: normal flora of human oropharynx (*S. mutans, S. sanguinis*), human colon (*S. gallolyticus*)

Transmission: endogenous

Pathogenesis: **dextran (biofilm)-mediated adherence** onto tooth enamel or damaged heart valve and to each other (vegetation); growth in vegetation protects organism from immune system

Diseases

- Dental caries: *S. mutans* dextran-mediated adherence glues oral flora onto teeth, forming plaque and causing dental caries
- Infective endocarditis (subacute): m
  - Malaise, fatigue, anorexia, night sweats, weight loss, splinter hemorrhages
  - Predisposing conditions: damaged (or prosthetic) heart valve *and* dental work without prophylactic antibiotics or extremely poor oral hygiene
  - *S. gallolyticus* associated with colon cancer

Treatment: penicillin G with aminoglycosides for endocarditis

Prevention: prophylactic antibiotics prior to dental work for individuals with damaged heart valve

Key Vignette Clues

Viridans Streptococci

- Gram (+), catalase (–), α hemolytic, optochin resistant, bile insoluble
- Plaque and dental caries
- Subacute bacterial endocarditis—preexisting damage to heart valves; follows dental work

GENUS: *ENTEROCOCCUS*

Genus Features

- Catalase negative
- PYR+

Species of Medical Importance

- *Enterococcus faecalis*
- *Enterococcus faecium*

Enterococcus faecalis/faecium

Distinguishing Features

- **Group D gram-positive cocci in chains**
- **PYR test positive**
- Catalase-negative, varied hemolysis
- **Hydrolyze esculin in 40% bile and 6.5% NaCl** (bile esculin agar turns black)

Reservoir: human colon, urethra ± and female genital tract

Transmission: endogenous

Pathogenesis

- Bile/salt tolerance allows survival in bowel and gall bladder.
- During medical procedures on GI or GU tract: *E. faecalis* → **blood-stream → previously damaged heart valves → endocarditis**

Diseases: urinary and biliary tract infection; infective (subacute) endocarditis in persons (often elderly) with damaged heart valves

Diagnosis

- Culture on blood agar
- Antibiotic sensitivities

Treatment: all strains carry some drug resistance

- Some **vancomycin-resistant strains of *Enterococcus faecium* or *E. faecalis*** have no reliably effective treatment; or low-level resistance use ampicillin, gentamicin, or streptomycin
- VanA strains have UDP-N-acetylmuramyl pentapeptide with terminal D-alanyl-D-alanine replaced with D-alanyl-D-lactate, which functions in cell wall synthesis but does not bind to vancomycin

Prevention: prophylactic use of penicillin and gentamicin for patients with damaged heart valves prior to intestinal or urinary tract manipulation

Key Vignette Clues

Enterococcus faecalis/faecium

- Gram (+), catalase (−), variable hemolysis, hydrolyzes esculin
- Urinary/biliary tract infections—elderly males
- Subacute bacterial endocarditis—elderly males, follows GI/GU surgery, preexisting heart valve damage

GRAM-POSITIVE RODS

Table II-2-12. Gram-Positive Rods

Genus	Spore	Aerobic Growth	Exotoxin	Facultative Intracellular	Acid Fast	Branching Rods
Bacillus	+	+	+	−	−	−
Clostridium	+	−	+	−	−	−
Listeria	−	+	−	+	−	−
Corynebacterium	−	+	+	−	−	−
Actinomyces	−	−	−	−	−	+
Nocardia	−	+	−	−	+†	+
Mycobacterium	−	+	−	+	+	−

†*Nocardia* is considered partially acid fast.

GENUS: *BACILLUS*

Bacillus anthracis

Distinguishing Features

- **Large,** boxcar-like, gram-positive, **spore-forming rods**
- **Capsule is polypeptide (poly-d-glutamate)**
- **Potential bioterrorism agent**

Reservoir: animals, skins, soils

Transmission: contact with infected animals or inhalation of spores (bioterrorism)

Pathogenesis

- Capsulepolypeptide, antiphagocytic, immunogenic
- **Anthrax toxin** includes 3 protein components:
  - **Protective antigen** (B component) mediates entry of LF or EF into eukaryotic cells
  - **Lethal factor** kills cells
  - **Edema factor** is an adenylate cyclase (calmodulin-activated like pertussis adenylate cyclase)

Key Vignette Clues

Bacillus anthracis

- Gram (+), spore forming, aerobic rods
- Contact with animal hides or bioterrorism; eschar or life-threatening pneumonia

Diseases

- Cutaneous anthrax: papule → papule with vesicles (malignant pustules) → central necrosis (eschar) with erythematous border often with painful regional lymphadenopathy; fever in 50%

- Pulmonary (wool sorter's disease): life-threatening **pneumonia**; cough, fever, malaise, and ultimately facial edema, dyspnea, diaphoresis, cyanosis, and shock with **mediastinal hemorrhagic lymphadenitis**

- GI anthrax (rare): edema and blockage of G tract can occur, vomiting and bloody diarrhea, high mortality

Diagnosis

- Mediastinal widening on chest x-ray

- Gram stain and culture of blood, respiratory secretions or lesions

- Serology

- PCR

Treatment: ciprofloxacin or doxycycline. (Genes encoding resistance to penicillin and doxycycline have been transferred to *B. anthracis*.)

Prevention: toxoid vaccine (AVA, acellular vaccine adsorbed) is given to those in high risk occupations such as military; raxibacumab for prophylaxis

Bacillus cereus

Distinguishing Feature: spores

Reservoir: ound in nature

Transmission

- Foodborne, intoxication

- Major association with fried rice from Chinese restaurants

- Associated with food kept warm, not hot (buffets)

Pathogenesis: 2 possible toxins:

- **Emetic toxin: preformed fast** (1–6 hours), similar to *S. aureus* with vomiting and diarrhea; associated with **fried rice**

- Diarrheal toxin produced in vivo (meats, sauces): 18 hours, similar to *E. coli*; LT: increasing cAMP → watery diarrhea

Diseases

- Gastroenteritis: nonbloody, ± vomiting

- Eye infection (rare)

Key Vignette Clues

Bacillus cereus

- Rapid-onset gastroenteritis

- Fried rice, Chinese restaurants

Diagnosis

- Clinical grounds
- Culture and Gram stain of implicated food

Treatment: self-limiting; vancomycin for eye infection

GENUS: *CLOSTRIDIUM*

Species of Medical Importance

- *Clostridium tetani*
- *botulinum*
- *Clostridium perfringens*
- *Clostridium septicum*
- *Clostridium difficile*

Clostridium tetani

Distinguishing Features: large gram-positive, spore-forming rods; anaerobes; produces tetanus toxin

Reservoir: soil

Transmission: puncture wounds/trauma (human bites); requires low tissue oxygenation (E_h)

Pathogenesis

- Spores germinate in tissues, producing **tetanus toxin** (an exotoxin also called **tetanospasmin**)
- Carried intra-axonally to CNS
- **Binds to ganglioside receptors**
- **Blocks release of inhibitory mediators (glycine and GABA) at spinal synapses**
- Excitatory neurons are unopposed → extreme muscle spasm
- **One of the most toxic substances known**

Disease: tetanus

- Risus sardonicus
- Opisthotonus
- Extreme muscle spasms
- Drooling, hydrophobia

Key Vignette Clues

Clostridium tetani

- Dirty puncture wound
- Rigid paralysis

Diagnosis: primarily a clinical diagnosis; organism rarely isolated

Treatment of Actual Tetanus

- **Hyperimmune human globulin (TIG) to neutralize toxin plus metronidazole or penicillin**

- **Spasmolytic drugs** (diazepam); debride; delay closure

Prevention: toxoid is formaldehyde-inactivated toxin (important because disinfectants have poor sporicidal action); care of wounds: proper wound cleansing and care plus treatment

Table II-2-13. Wound Management

Patient	Not Tetanus Prone	Tetanus Prone
	Linear, 1 cm deep cut, without devitalized tissue, without major contaminants, <6 hours old	Blunt/missile, burn, frostbite, 1 cm deep; devitalized tissue present + contaminants (e.g., dirt, saliva); any wound 6 hours old
Not completed primary or vaccination history unknown	Vaccine	Vaccine and tetanus immunoglobulin (human)
Completed primary series	Vaccine if >10 years since last booster	Vaccine if >5 years since last booster

Clostridium botulinum

Distinguishing Features
- **Anaerobic**
- **Gram-positive spore-forming rods**

Reservoir: soil/dust

Transmission: foodborne/traumatic implantation

Pathogenesis

- **Spores** survive in soil and dust; **germinate** in moist, warm, nutritious but **nonacidic and anaerobic conditions**

- **Botulinum toxin**

  - **A-B polypeptide neurotoxin** (actually a series of 7 antigenically different; type A and B most common)

  - **Coded for by a prophage** (lysogenized *Clostridium botulinum*).

  - Highly toxic

Key Vignette Clues

Clostridium botulinum

- Home-canned alkaline vegetables

- Floppy baby syndrome (infant with flaccid paralysis)

- Reversible flaccid paralysis

- **Heat labile** (unlike staph), 10 minutes 60.0°C
- **Mechanism of action: absorbed by gut** and carried by blood to peripheral nerve synapses; **blocks release of acetylcholine** at myoneuronal junction, resulting in a reversible **flaccid paralysis**

Disease(s)

Table II-2-14. Forms of Botulism

Disease	Adult	Infant
Acquisition	**Preformed toxin ingested (toxicosis)** Poorly canned alkaline vegetables (green beans)	**Spores ingested: household dust, honey** Toxin produced in gut (toxi-infection)
Symptoms	1–2 day onset of weakness, dizziness, blurred vision, flaccid paralysis (reversible), constipation	Constipation, limpness/flaccid paralysis (reversible): diplopia, dysphagia, weak feeding/crying; may lead to respiratory arrest
Toxin demonstrated in	Suspected food	Stool or serum
Treatment	Respiratory support Trivalent (A-B-E) antitoxin	Respiratory support in monitored intensive care; hyperimmune human serum Antibiotics generally not used as may worsen or prolong
Prevention	**Proper canning; heat all canned foods**	**No honey first 2 years**

Clostridium perfringens

Distinguishing Features

- Large **gram-positive, spore-forming** rods (spores rare in tissue), nonmotile
- **Anaerobic: "stormy fermentation" in milk media**
- **Double zone of hemolysis**

Reservoir: soil and human colon

Transmission: foodborne and traumatic implantation

Pathogenesis

- **Spores** germinate under anaerobic conditions in tissue.

- Vegetative cells produce **alpha toxin** (phospholipase C), a **lecithinase**, which disrupts membranes, damaging RBCs, platelets, WBCs, and endothelial cells. Can lead to massive hemolysis, tissue destruction, and hepatic toxicity.

- Identified by **Nagler reaction**: egg yolk agar plate: one side with anti-α-**toxin**; lecithinase activity is detected on side with no antitoxin

- Twelve other toxins damage tissues

- **Enterotoxin** produced in intestines in food poisoning: disrupts ion transport → watery diarrhea, cramps (similar to *E. coli*); resolution <24 hours.

Disease(s)

- Gas gangrene (myonecrosis)

  - Contamination of **wound with soil or feces**

  - **Acute** and **increasing pain** at wound site

  - **Tense tissue** (edema, gas) and exudate

  - Systemic symptoms include **fever** and **tachycardia** (disproportionate to fever), diaphoresis, pallor, etc.

  - **Rapid, high mortality**

- Food poisoning: **reheated meat dishes,** organism grows to high numbers; 8–24 hour incubation; **enterotoxin** production in gut; self-limiting noninflammatory, watery diarrhea

Diagnosis: clinical

Treatment: debridement, delayed closure, clindamycin and penicillin, hyperbaric chamber for gangrene; food poisoning is self-limiting

Prevention: extensive **debridement** of wound plus penicillin

Clostridium septicum

Distinguishing features: anaerobic, gram-positive rods

Transmission: endogenous

Disease: septic shock in colon cancer patients

Clostridium difficile

Reservoir: human colon/gastrointestinal tract

Transmission: endogenous

Key Vignette Clues

Clostridium difficile

- Hospitalized patient on antibiotics

- Develops colitis, diarrhea

Pathogenesis

- Toxin A: enterotoxin damaging mucosa leading to fluid increase; granulocyte attractant
- Toxin B: cytotoxin: cytopathic

Disease(s): antibiotic-associated (clindamycin, cephalosporins, amoxicillin, ampicillin) **diarrhea, colitis, or pseudomembranous colitis** (yellow plaques on colon)

Diagnosis: culture is not diagnostic because organism is part of normal flora; stool exam for toxin production

Treatment

- **Metronidazole** for severe disease; vancomycin only when no other drug is available to avoid selecting for vancomycin-resistant normal flora
- Fecal transplant for chronic infections
- Discontinuation of other antibiotic therapy for mild disease

Prevention: use caution in overprescribing broad-spectrum antibiotics (consider limited-spectrum drugs first); in nursing home setting, isolate patients who are symptomatic; use autoclave bed pans (treatment kills spores)

GENUS: *LISTERIA*

Listeria monocytogenes

Distinguishing Features

- Small gram-positive rods
- Beta hemolytic, nonspore-forming rod on blood agar, CAMP positive
- **Tumbling motility** in broth; actin jet motility in cells
- **Facultative intracellular parasite**
- **Cold growth**

Reservoir

- Widespread: animals (GI and genital tracts), **unpasteurized milk products**, plants, and soil
- Cold growth: contaminated food, soft cheese, deli meat, cabbage (coleslaw), hotdogs, fruit, ice cream

Transmission: foodborne or vertical

Pathogenesis

- **Listeriolysin O, a β-hemolysin**, facilitates rapid egress from phagosome into cytoplasm, thus evading killing when lysosomal contents are dumped into phagosome; "jets" directly (by actin filament formation) from cytoplasm to another cell
- **Immunocompromised status** predisposes to serious infection

Key Vignette Clues

Listeria monocytogenes

- Gram (+), β hemolytic bacilli, cold growth
- Facultative intracellular
- Foodborne (deli foods)
- Transplacental◻granulomatosis infantiseptica
- Neonatal septicemia and meningitis (third most common cause)
- Meningitis in renal transplant or cancer patients (most common cause)

Disease(s)

- Listeriosis (human, peaks in summer)

  - Healthy adults and children: generally asymptomatic or diarrhea with low % carriage

  - Pregnant women: symptomatic carriage, septicemia characterized by fever and chills; can cross the placenta in septicemia.

- Neonatal disease

  - **Early-onset:** (granulomatosis infantisepticum) in uterotransmission; sepsis with high mortality; disseminated granulomas with central necrosis

  - **Late-onset:** 2–3 weeks after birth from fecal exposure; meningitis with septicemia

- In immunocompromised patients

  - **Septicemia and meningitis** (most common clinical presentation)

  - *Listeria* meningitis most common cause of meningitis in **renal transplant patients and adults with cancer**

Diagnosis: blood or CSF culture at 4°C; CSF or Gram stain (>25% lymphocytes + PMNs)

Treatment: ampicillin with gentamicin added for immunocompromised patients

Prevention: pregnant and immunocompromised patients should avoid cold deli food

GENUS: CORYNEBACTERIUM

Corynebacterium diphtheriae

Distinguishing Features

- Gray-to-black colonies of **club-shaped** gram-positive rods arranged in V or L shapes on **Gram stain**

- **Granules (volutin)** produced on Loeffler coagulated serum medium stain metachromatically

- **Toxin-producing strains have β-prophage** carrying genes for the toxin (**lysogeny, β-corynephage**). The phage from one person with diphtheria can infect the normal nontoxigenic diphtheroid of another, and thus cause diphtheria.

Reservoir: throat and nasopharynx

Transmission: bacterium or phage via respiratory droplets

Key Vignette Clues

Corynebacterium diphtheriae

- Gram (+), aerobic, non–spore forming rods

- Bull neck, myocarditis, nerve palsies

- Gray pseudomembrane → airway obstruction

- Toxin produced by lysogeny

- Toxin ribosylates eEF-2; heart, nerve damage

Pathogenesis

- Organism **not invasive**; colonizes epithelium of oropharynx or skin in cutaneous diphtheria

- **Diphtheria toxin (A-B component)—inhibits protein synthesis by adding ADP-ribose to eEF-2**

- Effect on oropharynx: **Dirty gray pseudomembrane** (made up of dead cells and fibrin exudate, bacterial pigment)

- **Extension into larynx/trachea → obstruction**

- Effect of systemic circulation → **heart** and **nerve** damage

Disease: diphtheria (sore throat with **pseudomembrane, bull neck**, potential respiratory obstruction, **myocarditis**, cardiac dysfunction, **recurrent laryngeal nerve palsy**, and lower limb polyneuritis), renal failure

Diagnosis

- Elek test to document toxin production (ELISA for toxin is now gold standard)

- Toxin produced by Elek testtoxin-producing strains diffuses away from growth

- Antitoxin diffuses away from strip of filter paper

- Precipitin lines form at zone of equivalence

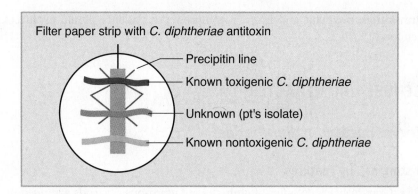

Filter paper strip with *C. diphtheriae* antitoxin

— Precipitin line

— Known toxigenic *C. diphtheriae*

— Unknown (pt's isolate)

— Known nontoxigenic *C. diphtheriae*

Figure II-2-2. Elek Test

Treatment

- Erythromycin and antitoxin

- For endocarditis, intravenous penicillin and aminoglycosides for 4–6 weeks

Prevention: toxoid vaccine (formaldehyde-modified toxin is still immunogenic but with reduced toxicity), part of DTaP, DTP, or Td, boosters 10-year intervals

GENUS: *ACTINOMYCES*

Actinomyces israelii

Distinguishing Features

- Anaerobic
- Branching rods
- Non–acid fast

Reservoir: human; normal flora of **gingival crevices** and **female genital tract**

Transmission: endogenous

Pathogenesis: invasive growth in tissues with compromised oxygen supply

Disease: actinomycosis

- Generally not painful but **very invasive**, penetrating all tissues including bone
- **Tissue swelling** can lead to **draining abscesses** (sinus tracts) with **"sulfur" granules** (hard yellow microcolonies) in exudate that can be used for microscopy or culture
- Only in tissues with low oxygenation (E_h)
    - **Cervicofacial (lumpy jaw): dental trauma or poor oral hygiene**
    - **Pelvic: from thoracic or sometimes IUDs**
    - Abdominal: surgery or bowel trauma
    - Thoracic: aspiration with contiguous spread
    - CNS: **solitary brain abscess** (*Nocardia* will produce multiple foci)

Diagnosis: identify gram-positive branching bacilli in "sulfur granules"; colonies resemble molar tooth

Treatment: penicillin V and surgical drainage; metronidazole not effective

GENUS: *NOCARDIA*

Nocardia asteroides and *Nocardia brasiliensis*

Distinguishing Features: aerobic; Gram-positive branching rods (some areas of smear will be blue and some red; **partially acid fast)**

Reservoir: soil and dust

Transmission: airborne or traumatic transplantation

Pathogenesis: no known toxins or virulence factors; **immunosuppression** and **cancer predispose** to pulmonary infection

Key Vignette Clues

- Patient with mycetoma on jaw line or spread from IUD
- Sulfur granules in pus grow anaerobic, gram (+), non-acid fast branching rods

Key Vignette Clues

Nocardia asteroides and *Nocardia brasiliensis*

- Gram (+) filamentous bacilli, aerobic, partially acid fast
- Cavitary bronchopulmonary disease, mycetomas

Disease(s)

- Nocardiosis

  - **Cavitary bronchopulmonary nocardiosis**

  - Mostly *N. asteroides*

  - Can be acute, subacute, chronic

  - Symptoms: cough, fever, dyspnea, localized or diffuse pneumonia with cavitation

  - May spread hematogenously to brain (**brain abscesses**)

- Cutaneous/subcutaneous nocardiosis

  - Mostly *N. brasiliensis*

  - Starts with traumatic implantation

  - Symptoms: **cellulitis** with swelling can lead to **draining subcutaneous abscesses** with **granules** (mycetoma)

Diagnosis: culture of sputum or pus from cutaneous lesion

Treatment: sulfonamides (high dose) or trimethoprim/sulfamethoxazole (TMP-SMX)

GENUS: *MYCOBACTERIUM*

Genus Features

- **Acid fast rods** with waxy cell wall

- **Obligate aerobe**

- Cell wall

  - Unique: **high concentration of lipids** containing long chain fatty acids called **mycolic acids**

  - Wall makes **mycobacteria highly resistant to desiccation** and **many chemicals** (including NaOH used to kill other bacteria in sputa before neutralizing and culturing)

- **Sensitive to UV**

Species of Medical Importance

- *M. tuberculosis*
- *M. leprae*
- *M. avium-intracellulare*
- *M. kansasii*
- *M. marinum*
- *M. ulcerans*

Mycobacterium tuberculosis

Distinguishing Features

- **Auramine-rhodamine staining bacilli** (fluorescent apple green); no antibody involved (sensitive but not specific)

- **Acid fast**

- **Aerobic, slow growing** on **Lowenstein-Jensen** medium; new culture systems (broths with palmitic acid) faster

- **Produces niacin**

- **Produces a heat-sensitive catalase**: catalase-negative at 68.0°C (standard catalase test); catalase active at body temperature

Reservoir: human lungs

Transmission: respiratory droplets

Pathogenesis

- **Facultative intracellular organism** (most important)

- **Sulfatides (sulfolipids** in cell envelope): **inhibit phagosome-lysosome fusion,** allowing intracellular survival (if fusion occurs, waxy nature of cell envelope reduces killing effect)

- **Cord factor (trehalose dimycolate)**: causes **serpentine growth** in vitro; **inhibits leukocyte migration; disrupts mitochondrial respiration and oxidative phosphorylation**

- **Tuberculin** (surface protein) along with mycolic acid → delayed hypersensitivity and **cell-mediated immunity** (CMI): granulomas and caseation mediated by CMI; no exotoxins or endotoxin; damage done by immune system

Disease(s)

- Primary pulmonary TB

  - Symptoms can include fever, dry cough

  - Organisms replicate in naive alveolar macrophages, killing the macrophages until CMI is set up (Ghon focus)

  - Macrophages transport the bacilli to the regional lymph node (**Ghon complex**) and most people heal without disease

  - Organisms that are walled off within the Ghon complex remain viable unless treated

- Reactivational TB

  - Symptoms can include fever, hemoptysis, night sweats, weight loss

  - Erosion of granulomas into airways (high oxygen) later in life under conditions of reduced T-cell immunity can lead to mycobacterial replication and disease symptoms

Key Vignette Clues

Mycobacterium tuberculosis

- High-risk patient (poverty, HIV+, IV drug user)

- Chronic cough, weight loss

- Ghon complex

- Auramine-rhodamine staining, acid fast bacilli in sputum

- Produce niacin, heat-sensitive catalase

- Positive PPD

- Facultative intracellular

Cord Factor

- Complex disease with the potential of infecting any organ system

- May disseminate (miliary TB): kidneys, GI tract, brain, spine (Pott disease)

Diagnosis

- Microscopy of sputum: screen with auramine-rhodamine stain (fluorescent apple-green); no antibody involved; very sensitive; if positive, confirm with

- acid fast stain

- **PPD skin test** (Mantoux): measure **zone of induration at 48–72 hours; positive if:**

  - ≥5 mm in HIV+ or anyone with recent TB exposure; AIDS patients have reduced ability to mount skin test.

  - ≥10 mm in high-risk population: IV drug abusers, people living in poverty, or immigrants from high TB area

  - ≥15 mm in low-risk population

- **Positive skin test indicates** only **exposure but not necessarily active disease.**

- Quantiferon-TB Gold Test: measures interferon-gamma production when leukocytes exposed to TB antigens

- Slow-growing (3–6 weeks) colonies on Lowenstein-Jensen medium (faster new systems)

- Organisms produce **niacin** and are **catalase-negative** (68°C).

- **No serodiagnosis**

Treatment

- **Multiple drugs critical** to treat infection

- Standard observed short-term therapy for uncomplicated pulmonary TB (rate where acquired resistance <4%):

  - First 2 months: rifampin + isoniazid + pyrazinamide + ethambutol (RIPE)

  - Next 4 months: rifampin and isoniazid

- Streptomycin added for possible drug-resistant cases until susceptibility tests are back (if area acquired has >4% drug-resistant mycobacteria)

- For MDR TB, use 3–5 previously unused drugs: aminoglycosides, fluoroquinolones, thioamide, cycloserine, bedaquiline

Prevention

- **Isoniazid** taken for 9 months can prevent TB in persons with infection but no clinical symptoms

- Bacille Calmette-Guérin (BCG) **vaccine** containing live, attenuated organisms may prevent disseminated disease; not used in U.S.

- UV light or HEPA filter used to treat potentially contaminated air

Mycobacteria Other than Tuberculosis (MOTTS)

Distinguishing Features

- Atypical mycobacteria
- **Noncontagious**
- Found in surface waters, soil, cigarettes

Note

- *M. tuberculosis* in HIV patient with normal count or low CD4 count (disseminated)
- MAI only in late HIV patient with low CD4 count

Table II-2-15. MOTTS

Organism	Disease	Transmission	Clinical Presentation	Treatment
M. avium-intracellulare	Pulmonary, GI, Disseminated	Respiratory, Ingestion	AIDS patients, cancer, chronic lung disease	AIDS patients prophylaxis <50 CD4+ cells/mm^3 Macrolide plus ethambutol
M. kansasii				
M. ulcerans	Buruli ulcer (Africa)	Wound contamination	Ulcer	Rifampin and streptomycin
M. marinum	Soft tissue infections "Fish tank granuloma"	Abrasions	Cutaneous granulomas in tropical fish enthusiasts	Isonazid Rifampin or ethambutol

Mycobacterium leprae

Distinguishing Features

- **Acid fast rods (seen in punch biopsy)**
- **Obligate intracellular parasite** (cannot be cultured in vitro)
- Optimal growth at less than body temperature

Reservoir: human mucosa, skin, and nerves are only significant reservoirs; some infected armadillos in Texas and Louisiana

Transmission: nasal discharge from untreated lepromatous leprosy patients

Pathogenesis: obligate intracellular parasite; cooler parts of body, e.g., skin, mucous membranes, and peripheral nerves

Disease(s): leprosy: a continuum of disease, which usually starts out with an indeterminate stage called "borderline"

Key Vignette Clues

Leprosy

- Acid fast bacilli in punch biopsy
- Immigrant patient with sensory loss in extremities

Table II-2-16. Extreme Forms of Leprosy

	Tuberculoid	B	Lepromatous
Cell-mediated immune system	Strong CMI (Th1)	o	Weak CMI (Th2)
Lepromin skin test	Lepromin test +	r / d	Lepromin test −
Number of organisms in tissue	Low	e / r	High (foam cells totally filled)
Damage from	• Immune response (CMI killing infected cells) • Granuloma formation → nerve enlargement/damage • Loss of sensation → burns and trauma	l / i / n / e	• Large number of intracellular organisms • Nerve damage from overgrowth of bacteria in cells • Loss of sensation → burns and trauma
Number of lesions and other symptoms	Fewer lesions: macular; nerve enlargement, paresthesia		• Numerous lesions becoming nodular; loss of eyebrows; destruction of nasal septum • Paresthesia • Leonine facies

Diagnosis

- **Punch biopsy or nasal scrapings; acid fast stain**
- **Lepromin skin test** is positive in the tuberculoid but not in the lepromatous form
- No cultures

Treatment: multiple-drug therapy with dapsone and rifampin, with clofazimine added for lepromatous

Prevention: dapsone for close family contacts

GRAM-NEGATIVE COCCI

GENUS: *NEISSERIA*

Table II-2-17. Medically Important *Neisseria* Species

Organism	Capsule	Vaccine	Portal of Entry	Glucose Fermentation	Maltose Fermentation	β-Lactamase Production
N. meningitidis	Yes	Yes	Respiratory	Yes	Yes	Rare
N. gonorrhoeae	No	No	Genital	Yes	No	Common

Neisseria meningitidis

Distinguishing Features

- **Gram-negative, kidney bean–shaped diplococci**
- **Oxidase-positive**
- **Large capsule; latex particle agglutination** (or CIE, counter immuno-electrophoresis) **to identify *N. meningitidis* capsular antigens in CSF**
- Grows on **chocolate (not blood) agar in 5% CO_2** atmosphere
- **Ferments maltose** in contrast to gonococci

Reservoir: human nasopharynx (5–10% carriers)

Transmission: respiratory droplets; oropharyngeal colonization, spreads to meninges via bloodstream; disease occurs in only small percentage of colonized individuals

Pathogenesis: important virulence factors

- Polysaccharide **capsule:** antiphagocytic, antigenic, 5 common serogroups: B is not strongly immunogenic (sialic acid); B strain is most common strain in U.S.; used for serogrouping, detection in CSF, and vaccine
- **IgA protease** allows oropharynx colonization.
- **Endotoxin** (lipo**oligo**saccharide): fever, septic shock in meningococcemia, **overproduction of outer membrane**
- Pili and outer membrane proteins important in ability to colonize and invade
- Deficiency in late complement components (C5–C9) predisposes to bacteremia

Note

Oxidase

- *Oxidase (cytochrome C oxidase) test:* flood colony with phenylenediamine; in presence of oxidase, phenylenediamine turns black. Rapid test.

- Major oxidase-negative gram-negative group is Enterobacteriaceae.

Key Vignette Clues

Meningococcal Meningitis

- Gram (–) diplococcus in CSF
- Young adults with meningitis
- Abrupt onset with signs of endotoxin toxicity

Disease(s): meningitis and meningococcemia

- **Abrupt onset with fever, chills, malaise, prostration, and rash that is generally petechial;** rapid decline

- Fulminant cases: ecchymoses, DIC, shock, coma, and death (Waterhouse-Friderichsen syndrome)

Diagnosis: Gram stain of CSF; PCR; latex agglutination

Treatment: ampicillin and cefotaxime (neonates/infants); cefotaxime or ceftriaxone with or without vancomycin (children and adults)

Prevention: vaccine: conjugate for strains **Y, W-135, C,** and **A,** recombinant for serotype **B,** prophylaxis of close contacts with **rifampin** (or ciprofloxacin)

Neisseria gonorrhoeae

Distinguishing Features

- **Gram-negative**, kidney bean–shaped **diplococci**
- Oxidase-positive

Reservoir: human genital tract

Transmission: sexual contact, birth; sensitive to drying and cold

Pathogenesis

- **Pili: attachment** to mucosal surfaces; **inhibit phagocytic uptake; antigenic variation:** >1 million variants

- **Outer membrane proteins:** OMP I structural, antigen used in serotyping; Opa proteins (opacity) **antigenic variation,** adherence; **IgA protease** aids in colonization and cellular uptake

- **Organism invades mucosal surfaces and causes inflammation.**

Disease: gonorrhea

- Male: **urethritis,** proctitis
- Female: **endocervicitis,** PID (contiguous spread), arthritis, proctitis
- Infants: **ophthalmia**(rapidly leads to **blindness if untreated)**
- Disseminated disease: arthritis, skin lesions
- Gonococcal pharyngitis

Key Vignette Clues

Neisseria gonorrhoeae

- Sexually active patient
- Urethral/vaginal discharge (leukorrhea)
- Arthritis possible
- Neonatal ophthalmia
- Gram (–) diplococcus in neutrophils

Diagnosis

- Intracellular **gram-negative diplococci in PMNs** from urethral smear
- Commonly: diagnosis by **genetic probes** with amplification
- Culture (when done) on **Thayer-Martin medium**
  - Oxidase-positive colonies
  - Maltose not fermented
  - No capsule

Treatment: ceftriaxone; test for *C. trachomatis* or treat with macrolide (doxycycline alternative); plasmid-mediated β-**lactamase** produces **high-level penicillin resistance**

Prevention: condoms (adult forms have no vaccine); for neonates, silver nitrate or erythromycin ointment in eyes at birth

Moraxella catarrhalis

Distinguishing Features

- Gram-negative diplococcus
- Close relative of *Neisseria*

Reservoir: normal upper respiratory tract flora

Transmission: respiratory droplets

Pathogenesis: endotoxin may play role in disease

Disease(s): otitis media; sinusitis; bronchitis and bronchopneumonia in elderly patients with COPD

Treatment: amoxicillin and clavulanate, second- or third-generation cephalosporin or TMP-SMX; drug resistance is a problem (most strains produce a β-lactamase)

GRAM-NEGATIVE BACILLI

GENUS: *PSEUDOMONAS*

Genus Features

- **Gram-negative rod**
- **Oxidase-positive**, catalase-positive
- **Aerobic (nonfermenting)**

Species of Medical Importance: *Pseudomonas aeruginosa*

Key Vignette Clues

Pseudomonas

- Gram (–), oxidase (+), aerobic bacillus
- Blue-green pigments, fruity odor
- Burn infections—blue-green pus, fruity odor
- Typical pneumonia—CGD or CF
- UTI—catheterized patients

Note

Pseudomonas **Medical Ecology**

Pseudomonas aeruginosa is a **ubiquitous water** and soil organism that grows to very high numbers overnight in standing water (distilled or tap). Sources for infection include:

- Raw vegetables, respirators, humidifiers, sink drains, faucet aerators, cut and potted flowers, and, if not properly maintained, whirlpools

- Transient colonization of colons in about 10% of people; bacteria get on skin from fecal organisms; requires exquisitely careful housekeeping and restricted diets in burn units

Pseudomonas aeruginosa

Distinguishing Features

- **Oxidase-positive, Gram-negative rods, nonfermenting**
- **Pigments: pyocyanin (blue-green)** and fluorescein
- **Grape-like odor**
- **Slime layer**
- **Non–lactose fermenting** colonies on EMB or MacConkey
- **Biofilm**

Reservoir: ubiquitous in water

Transmission: water aerosols, raw vegetables, flowers

Pathogenesis

- **Endotoxin** causes inflammation in tissues and gram-negative shock in septicemia
- Pseudomonas **exotoxin A ADP ribosylates eEF-2,** inhibiting protein synthesis (like diphtheria toxin)
- **Liver is primary target**
- **Capsule/slime layer** allows formation of pulmonary **microcolonies**; difficult to remove by phagocytosis

Disease(s)

- Healthy people: transient GI tract colonization (loose stool 10% population); hot tub folliculitis; eye ulcer (trauma, coma, prolonged contact wear)
- Burn patients: GI tract colonization → skin → colonization of eschar → **cellulitis (blue-green pus)** → **septicemia**
- Neutropenic patients: **pneumonia** and **septicemia** (often **superinfection,** i.e., infection while on antibiotics)
- Chronic granulomatous disease: pneumonias, septicemias (*Pseudomonas* is catalase-positive); [diabetic] osteomyelitis (diabetic foot)
- Otitis externa: swimmers, diabetics, those with pierced ears
- Septicemias: fever, shock ± skin lesions (black, necrotic center, erythematous margin, **ecthyma gangrenosum)**
- Catheterized patients: urinary tract infection
- Cystic fibrosis: early pulmonary colonization, recurrent pneumonia; **always** high **slime-producing strain**

Diagnosis: Gram stain and culture

Treatment: antipseudomonal penicillin and an aminoglycoside or fluoroquinolone

Prevention: pasteurize or disinfect water-related equipment, hand washing; prompt removal of catheters; avoid flowers and raw vegetables in burn units

Burkholderia cepacia

Distinguishing Features: oxidase-positive, catalase-positive; non-fermenting

Transmission: water aerosols, person-person (respiratory droplets)

Disease(s): cystic fibrosis (recurrent pneumonia); CGD (pneumonia, septicemia)

Treatment: trimethoprim-sulfamethoxazole

Acinetobacter baumannii

Distinguishing Features: oxidase-negative; non-fermenting; biofilm

Transmission: wound infection or nosocomial

Disease(s): wound infection and pneumonia in military personnel; 'Iraqibacter'

Treatment: highly drug-resistant; carbapenem or polymyxin

GENUS: *LEGIONELLA*

Legionella pneumophila

Distinguishing Features

- **Stain poorly** with standard Gram stain; **gram-negative**
- **Fastidious** requiring increased **iron and cysteine** for laboratory culture (BCYE, buffered charcoal, yeast extract)
- **Facultative intracellular**

Reservoir: rivers/streams/amebae; air-conditioning water cooling tanks

Transmission: aerosols from contaminated **air-conditioning; no human-to-human transmission**

Predisposing Factors: smokers age >55 with **high alcohol** intake; **immunosuppressed patients** such as renal transplant patients

Pathogenesis: facultative intracellular pathogen; **endotoxin**

Note

Drug Resistance in
P. aeruginosa

Susceptibilities important and drug resistance very common.

Intrinsic resistance (missing high affinity porin some drugs enter through); plasmid-mediated

β-lactamases and acetylating enzymes.

Key Vignette Clues

Legionella pneumophila

- Elderly smoker, heavy drinker, or Immunosuppressed
- Exposure to aerosols of water
- Atypical pneumonia
- Triad of atypical pneumonia, diarrhea, and hyponatremia

Disease(s)

- Legionnaires disease ("atypical pneumonia"): associated with air-conditioning systems (now routinely decontaminated); pneumonia; hyponatremia; mental confusion; diarrhea (no *Legionella* in GI tract)

- Pontiac fever: pneumonitis; no fatalities

Diagnosis

- **Urinary antigen test (serogroup 1)**
- **DFA** (direct fluorescent antibody) on biopsy, (+) by Dieterle silver stain
- Fourfold increase in antibody

Treatment: fluoroquinolone (levofloxacin) or macrolide (azithromycin) with rifampin (immunocompromised patients); drug must penetrate human cells.

Prevention: routine decontamination of air-conditioner cooling tanks

GENUS: *FRANCISELLA*

Francisella tularensis

Distinguishing Features

- Small gram-negative rod
- **Potential biowarfare agent**
- **Zoonosis**

Reservoir: many species of wild **animals**, especially rabbits, deer, and rodents; endemic in every state of the U.S. but highest in Arkansas and Missouri

Transmission

- **Tick bite** *(Dermacentor)* → **ulceroglandular** disease, characterized by **fever**, ulcer at bite site, and regional lymph node enlargement and necrosis
- **Traumatic implantation** while skinning rabbits → ulceroglandular disease
- Aerosols (skinning rabbits) → pneumonia
- Ingestion (of undercooked, infected meat or contaminated water) produces typhoidal tularemia.

Pathogenesis: facultative intracellular pathogen (localizes in reticuloendothelial cells); granulomatous response

Disease: ulceroglandular tularemia (open wound contact with rabbit blood; tick bite); pneumonic tularemia (bioterrorism; atypical pneumonia)

Diagnosis: serodiagnosis (culture is hazardous); DFA; grows on BCYE

Treatment: streptomycin

Prevention: protection against tick bites; glove use while butchering rabbits; live, attenuated vaccine (for those at high risk)

GENUS: *BORDETELLA*

Genus Features
- **Gram-negative small rods**
- **Strict aerobes**

Species of Medical Importance: *Bordetella pertussis*

Bordetella pertussis

Distinguishing Features: small **gram-negative,** aerobic **rods**; encapsulated organism

Reservoir: **human** (vaccinated)

Transmission: respiratory droplets

Pathogenesis
- ***B. pertussis* is mucosal surface pathogen**
- **Attachment** to nasopharyngeal ciliated epithelial cells is via filamentous hemagglutinin; pertussis toxin (on outer membrane) aids in attachment
- **Toxins** damage respiratory epithelium.
  - **Adenylate cyclase toxin:** impairs leukocyte chemotaxis → inhibits phagocytosis and causes local edema
  - **Tracheal cytotoxin:** interferes with ciliary action; kills ciliated cells
  - Endotoxin
  - **Pertussis toxin** (A and B component, OM protein toxin): **ADP ribosylation of G$_i$** (inhibiting negative regulator of adenylate cyclase) interferes with transfer of signals from cell surface to intracellular mediator system: lymphocytosis; islet-activation leading to hypoglycemia; blockin of immune effector cells (decreased chemotaxis); increased histamine sensitivity

Key Vignette Clues

Bordetella pertussis
- Unvaccinated child (immigrant family or religious objections)
- Cough with inspiratory "whoop"

In a Nutshell

B. pertussis Immunity
- Vaccine immunity lasts 5–10 yrs (and is primarily IgA)
- Babies born with little immunity
- Vaccinated humans >10 yrs serve as reservoir
- 12–20% of afebrile adults with cough >2 wks have pertussis
- Vaccine (DTaP)
- Acellular
- Components: immunogens vary by manufacturer; pertussis toxoid; filamentous hemagglutinin; pertactin (OMP); 1 other

Table II-2-18. Stages of Whooping Cough (Pertussis) vs. Results of Bacterial Culture

	Incubation	Catarrhal	Paroxysmal	Convalescent
Duration	7–10 days	1–2 weeks	2–4 weeks	3–4 weeks (or longer)
Symptoms	None	Rhinorrhea, malaise, sneezing, anorexia	Repetitive cough with whoops, vomiting, leukocytosis	Diminished paroxysmal cough, development of secondary complications (pneumonia, seizures, encephalopathy)
Bacterial Culture				

Diagnosis

- Fastidious/delicate: **Regan-Lowe** or Bordet-Gengou media; either direct cough plates or nasopharyngeal cultures

- Difficult to culture from middle of paroxysmal stage on

- Direct immunofluorescence (**DFA**) on nasopharyngeal smear

- PCR and serologic tests available

Treatment: supportive care, i.e., hospitalization if age <6 months; erythromycin for 14 days including all household contacts

Prevention: vaccine DTaP (acellular pertussis: filamentous hemagglutin plus pertussis toxoid); immunity wanes 5–7 years; babies are born with little or no immunity (IgA) from mother

GENUS: *BRUCELLA*

Brucella Species

Distinguishing Features

- Small **gram-negative** rods, aerobic

- Facultative intracellular

- **Zoonosis**

- Culture is hazardous

- **Potential bioterrorism agent**

Reservoir: domestic livestock

Transmission

- **Unpasteurized dairy products** (California and Texas highest number of cases; most associated with travel to Mexico)
- **Direct contact with the animal,** work in slaughterhouse
  - *Brucella abortus*: cattle
  - *Brucella melitensis*: goats
  - *Brucella suis*: pigs
  - *Brucella canis*: dogs

Pathogenesis

- **Endotoxin**
- **Facultative intracellular parasite** (localizes in cells of reticuloendothelial system) → **septicemia**
- **Granulomatous response** with central necrosis

Disease: brucellosis (undulant fever)

- Acute septicemias
- Fever 100–104°F (often in evening)
- Influenza-like symptoms, including arthralgias, anorexia, myalgia, back pain
- **Profuse sweating**
- Hepatomegaly

Diagnosis: culture is hazardous; serum agglutination test, fourfold increase in titer; antibodies against *Brucella* >1:160 considered positive

Treatment: rifampin and doxycycline minimum 6 weeks (adults); rifampin and cotrimoxazole (children)

Prevention: vaccinate cattle; pasteurize milk (especially goat milk)

GENUS: *HAEMOPHILUS*

Haemophilus influenzae

Distinguishing Features

- Encapsulated, **gram-negative rod; 95%** of invasive disease caused by capsular type b
- **Requires growth factors X (hemin) and V (NAD) for growth** on nutrient or blood agar (BA)
- Grows near *S. aureus* on BA = "satellite" phenomenon
- Chocolate agar provides both X and V factors

Note

Zoonotic Organisms

- *Brucella*
- *Bacillus anthracis*
- *Listeria monocytogenes*
- *Salmonella enteritidis*
- *Campylobacter*
- *Chlamydophila psittaci*
- *Francisella tularensis*
- *Yersinia pestis*

Key Vignette Clues

Haemophilus influenzae

- Unvaccinated child 3 mo–2 y: meningitis, pneumonia, epiglottitis
- Smokers with COPD: bronchitis, pneumonia
- Gram (–) rod, requires factors X and V

Reservoir: human nasopharynx

Transmission: respiratory droplets, shared toys

Pathogenesis

- **Polysaccharide capsule (type b capsule is polyribitol phosphate)** most important virulence factor
- Capsule important in diagnosis; **antigen screen on CSF** (e.g., latex particle agglutination); serotype all isolates by quellung.
- **IgA protease** is a mucosal colonizing factor.

Diseases

- Meningitis

  - **Epidemic in unvaccinated children ages 3 months to 2 years**

  - After maternal antibody has waned and before immune response of child is adequate

  - Up to 1990, *H. influenzae* was most common cause of meningitis age 1–5 (mainly <2); is still a problem if child age <2 and not vaccinated

- Otitis media: usually nontypeable strains
- Bronchitis: exacerbations of acute bronchitis in smokers with COPD
- Pneumonia: 1–24 months; rare in vaccinated children; smokers
- Epiglottitis: rare in vaccinated children; seen in unvaccinated toddlers; *H. influenzae* **was major causal agent**

Diagnosis: blood or CSF culture on chocolate agar; PCR; antigen detection of capsule (latex particle agglutination)

Treatment: cefotaxime or ceftriaxone for empirical therapy of meningitis; check nasal carriage before releasing; use rifampin if still colonized

Prevention

- **Conjugate capsular polysaccharide-protein vaccine**
- **Vaccination effective** to prevent type b disease

  - **Polyribitol capsule conjugated to protein:** (diphtheria toxoid or *N. meningitidis* outer membrane proteins), making it a **T-cell dependent vaccine**

  - Vaccine: 2, 4, 6 months; booster 15 months; 95% effective

- Rifampin reduces oropharynx colonization and prevents meningitis in unvaccinated, close contacts age <2 years

Haemophilus ducreyi

Reservoir: human genitals

Transmission: sexual transmission and direct contact

Diseases

- Chancroid

- Genital ulcers: **soft, painful chancre** ("You do cry with ducreyi.")

- **Slow to heal without treatment**

- **Open lesions increase transmission of HIV.**

Diagnosis: DNA probe, 'school of fish' appearance on Gram stain

Treatment: azithromycin, ceftriaxone, or ciprofloxacin

GENUS: *PASTEURELLA*

Pasteurella multocida

Distinguishing Features: small gram-negative rods; facultative anaerobic rods

Reservoir: mouths of many animals, especially cats and dogs

Transmission: animal bites; **particularly from cat bites**

Pathogenesis: **endotoxin, capsule;** spreads rapidly within skin, no exotoxins known

Disease: cellulitis with lymphadenitis (rapidly spreading wound infections, frequently polymicrobial infections)

Diagnosis: rarely cultured because routine prophylaxis is common

Treatment: amoxicillin/clavulanate for cat bites; resistant to macrolides

Prevention: amoxicillin/clavulanate is standard prophylaxis and treatment for most bites (including human), along with thorough cleaning

Key Vignette Clues

Pasteurella multocida

- Patient with animal (cat) bite

- Cellulitis/lymphadenitis

Table II-2-21. Additional Organisms Associated with Animal/Human Bites

Organism	Characteristics	Reservoir/ Transmission	Disease	Treatment
Eikenella corrodens	Gram-negative rods **"corrodes" agar; bleach-like odor**	Human oro-pharynx **human bites or fist fight injuries**	Cellulitis	Third-generation cephalosporins; fluoroquinolones
Capnocytophaga canimorsus	Gram-negative filamentous rods	Dog oropharynx/**dog bite wounds**	Cellulitis splenectomy → overwhelming sepsis	Third-generation cephalosporins; fluoroquinolones resistant to aminoglycosides
Bartonella henselae	Gram-negative rods	Cats and dogs/ bites, scratches, fleas	Cat scratch fever; **bacillary angio-matosis (AIDS)**	Azithromycin; doxycycline

HACEK Group Infections

- Group of gram-negative fastidious rods
  - *Aggregatibacter aphrophilus* (formerly *Haemophilus aphrophilus*)
  - *Aggregatibacter actinomycetemcomitans*
  - *Cardiobacterium hominis*
  - *Eikenella corrodens*
  - *Kingella kingae*
- HACEK organisms responsible for 5–10% of infective endocarditis cases (usually subacute)
- Most common cause of gram-negative endocarditis in non–IV drug users
- All part of normal oral flora
- Difficult to diagnose, with mean diagnosis time 3 months
- Treat with third-generation cephalosporin or fluoroquinolone

GENUS: *CAMPYLOBACTER*

Campylobacter jejuni

Distinguishing Features: Gram-negative curved rods with polar flagella ("gulls' wings"); oxidase-positive; microaerophilic; **grows at 42°C** on Campy or Skirrow agar

Reservoir: intestinal tracts of humans, cattle, sheep, dogs, cats, **poultry**

Transmission: fecal-oral, Skirrow agarprimarily from **poultry**

Pathogenesis: low infectious dose (as few as 500); invades mucosa of the colon, destroying mucosal surfaces; blood and **pus** in stools (inflammatory diarrhea); rarely penetrates to cause septicemia

Key Vignette Clues

Campylobacter jejuni

- Patient with inflammatory diarrhea
- Gram (–), curved rod, microaerophilic, oxidase (+), grows at 42°C

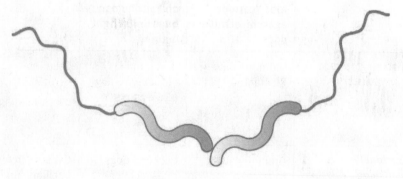

Campylobacter

Disease: gastroenteritis

- Common cause of infectious diarrhea worldwide

- In U.S., *Campylobacter* enteritis > (*Salmonella* plus *Shigella*)

- **≥10 stools/day** (may be **frankly bloody**)

- Abdominal pain, fever, malaise, nausea, and vomiting

- Generally **self-limiting in 3–5 days** but may last longer

- Complications

  ◦ **Guillain-Barré syndrome (GBS)** → 30% of GBS in U.S. Serotype O:19, antigenic cross-reactivity between *Campylobacter* oligosaccharides and glycosphingolipids on neural tissues

  ◦ Reactive arthritis (HLA-B27)

Diagnosis: culture on Campylobacter or Skirrow agar at 42°C; microaerophilic

Treatment: mostly supportive, i.e., fluid and electrolyte replacement; erythromycin, fluoroquinolones; resistant to penicillins

GENUS: *HELICOBACTER*

Helicobacter pylori

Distinguishing Features: Gram-negative spiral gastric bacteria with flagella; oxidase-positive, urease-positive; microaerophilic, grows at 37˚C on Campy or Skirrow agar

Reservoir: humans

Transmission: fecal-oral; oral-oral

Pathogenesis

- **Motile**

- **Urease-positive:** ammonium cloud neutralizes stomach acid, allowing survival in stomach acid during transit to border

- **Mucinase** aids in penetration of mucous layer (rapid shift down to neutral as it penetrates)

- **Invasive** into stomach lining where pH is neutral

- Inflammation is prominent

- Two biotypes (I and II); type I produces vacuolating cytotoxin

Diseases: chronic gastritis and duodenal ulcers

- Associated with several forms of **stomach cancer** (gastric adenocarcinoma, gastric mucosa-associated lymphoid tissue lymphoma [MALToma], B-cell lymphomas)

- Now classed by WHO as **type I carcinogen**

Key Vignette Clues

Helicobacter pylori

- Patient with gastritis, ulcers, stomach cancer

- Gram (–), helical bacilli, oxidase (+), microaerophilic, urease (+)

Diagnosis

- Biopsy with culture; histology with Giemsa or silver stain
- Urea breath test: ^{13}C-urea swallowed; ammonia+^{13}C-CO_2 exhaled
- Serology

Treatment: myriad of regimens

- Omeprazole + amoxicillin + clarithromycin is one example of triple therapy
- Treat for 10–14 days
- Quadruple therapy is used in areas where clarithromycin resistance is ≥15%, e.g., PPI + bismuth + 2 antibiotics (metronidazole + tetracycline)

GENUS: *VIBRIO*

Genus Features

- **Gram-negative curved rod with polar flagella**
- Oxidase positive
- Vibrionaceae
- Growth on **alkaline,** but not acidic, media (**TCBS, t**hiosulfate **c**itrate **b**ile salt **s**ucrose medium)

Species of Medical Importance

- *Vibrio cholerae*
- *Vibrio parahaemolyticus*
- *Vibrio vulnificus*

Vibrio cholerae

Distinguishing Features: rice-water diarrhea; growth on TCBS

Reservoir

- Human colon; **no vertebrate animal carriers** (copepods or shellfish may be contaminated by water contamination)
- Human carriage may persist after untreated infection for months after infection; permanent carrier state is rare.

Key Vignette Clues

Vibrio cholerae

- Patient with noninflammatory diarrhea
- Rice-water stool
- Dehydration from choleraDehydration
- Travel to endemic area
- Gram (–) curved rods, polar flagellae, oxidase (+)
- Alkaline growth

Transmission

- Fecal-oral spread; sensitive to stomach acid
- Requires high dose ($>10^7$ organisms), if stomach acid is normal

Pathogenesis

- Motility, mucinase, and toxin coregulated pili (TCP) aid in attachment to the intestinal mucosa.
- **Cholera enterotoxin (choleragen) similar to *E. coli* LT; ADP ribosylates (G_s alpha) activating adenylate cyclase → increased cAMP → efflux of Cl⁻ and H_2O (persistent activation of adenylate cyclase)**

Disease: cholera

- **Rice water stools**, tremendous fluid loss
- Hypovolemic shock if not treated

Diagnosis: culture stool on TCBS; **oxidase positive**

Treatment: **fluid and electrolyte replacement;** doxycycline or ciprofloxacin to shorten disease and reduce carriage; resistance to tetracycline reported

Prevention: proper sanitation; new vaccine

Other *Vibrio* Species

Table II-2-19. Additional *Vibrio* Species

Species	Reservoir	Transmission	Disease	Symptoms	Treatment
V. parahaemolyticus	Marine life	Consumption of undercooked or raw seafood	Gastroenteritis	Watery diarrhea with cramping and abdominal pain	Self-limiting
V. vulnificus	Brackish water, oysters	Consumption of undercooked or raw seafood	Gastroenteritis	As above	As above
		Swimming in brackish water, shucking oysters	Cellulitis	Rapidly spreading; difficult to treat	Tetracycline; third-generation cephalosporins

FAMILY: ENTEROBACTERIACEAE

Family Features

- **Gram-negative rods**
- **Facultative anaerobes**
- Ferment glucose
- **Cytochrome C oxidase negative**
- **Reduce nitrates to nitrites**
- Catalase positive

Family Pathogenesis

- **Endotoxin**; some also produce **exotoxins**
- **Antigens**

    - O: cell envelope or O antigen
    - H: flagellar (motile cells only) antigen
    - K: capsular polysaccharide antigen
    - Vi (virulence): *Salmonella* capsular antigen

Lab Diagnosis

- Blood agar
- Eosin methylene blue or MacConkey agar (differentiate lactose fermentation)
- **Lactose fermenters** (colored colonies)
- **Non–lactose fermenters** (colorless colonies)

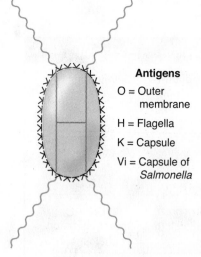

Antigens

O = Outer membrane

H = Flagella

K = Capsule

Vi = Capsule of *Salmonella*

Antigens of Enterobacteriacae

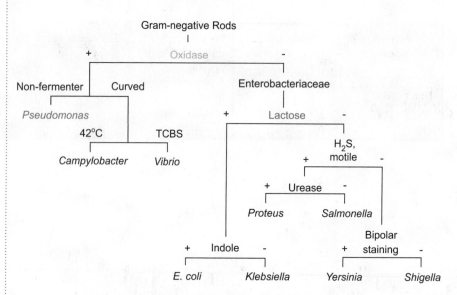

Figure II-2-4. Differentiaion of Gram-Negative Rods

GENUS: *ESCHERICHIA*

Genus Features

- **Gram-negative rods**
- **Enterobacteriaceae**
- **Ferments lactose**

Species of Medical Importance—*Escherichia coli*

Escherichia coli

Distinguishing Features

- **Gram-negative rod**
- **Facultative anaerobic, oxidase negative**
- *E.coli* is a **lactose fermenter:** colonies with iridescent green sheen on EMB

Reservoir: human colon; may colonize vagina or urethra; contaminated crops where human fecal fertilizer is used; **enterohemorrhagic strains: bovine feces**

Transmission

- Endogenous
- Fecal-oral
- Maternal fecal flora
- Enterohemorrhagic strains: bovine fecal contamination (raw or undercooked beef, milk, apple juice from fallen apples)

Pathogenesis: listed under specific diseases

Note

E. coli identification from stool

- **Isolation of *E. coli* from feces is not by itself significant.**
- **Sorbitol MacConkey screen**
- Most *E. coli* ferment sorbitol.
- Most EHEC do not (colorless)

E. coli from normal flora are more commonly:

- **Immunoassay** looking for specific protein antigens (on or excreted by the bacterium)
- **Serotyping** since certain serotypes are more often pathogenic
- **DNA probes** for specific genes in a culture
- **PCR** on clinical specimen

Mnemonic

Toxins ↑cAMP

    c = cholera

    A = anthrax

    Σ = ETEC LT

    P = pertussis

Mnemonic

PITcH

EPEC	P = pediatric
EIEC	I = inflammatory
ETEC	T = traveler
	C = coli
EHEC	H = hamburger

Table II-2-20. Disease Syndromes Caused by *Escherichia coli*

Transmission	Mechanism of Pathogenesis	Clinical Clues	Treatment
UTIUrinary tract infection (most common cause)			
Endogenous fecal flora contaminate and ascend	Motility Adherence to uroepithelium pyelonephritis associated pili, X-adhesins, β hemolytic (many)	Gram (–) bacilli, $\geq 10^5$ CFU/ml	Fluoroquinolone or sulfonamides
Neonatal septicemia/ meningitis (second most common cause)			
Maternal fecal flora contaminate during parturition	Capsule: K1 serotype, endotoxin	Blood, cerebrospinal fluid culture, gram (–) bacilli	Ceftriaxone
Septicemia			
Indwelling IV lines, cytotoxic drugs damage intestinal mucosa, allow escape	Endotoxin	Blood culture, gram (–) bacilli, oxidase (–)	Fluoroquinolones, third-generation cephalosporins
Gastroenteritis			
ETEC (travelers' diarrhea) Fecal/oral	LT: heat-labile toxin stimulates adenylate cyclase by ADP ribosylation of Gs ST: stimulates guanylate cyclase; capsule impedes phagocytosis; colonizing factor adhesins bind to mucosa	Noninflammatory diarrhea, identify enterotoxin by immunoassay, bioassay, DNA probe	Rehydration, TMP/SMX may shorten symptoms
EPEC (second most common infantile diarrhea) Fecal/oral	Adherence to M cells → rearrangement of actin and effacement of brush border microvilli	Noninflammatory diarrhea in babies in developing countries	Beta-lactams
EIEC Fecal/oral	Invades large bowel Inflammatory diarrhea; similar to shigellosis, induces formation of actin jet trails	Inflammatory diarrhea, blood, pus, fever, abdominal pain	
EAEC Fecal/oral	Adherence fimbriae can induce IL-8	Noninflammatory diarrhea in adults and children in United States	Ciprofloxacin if warranted
EHEC (VTEC): O157:H7 most common Bovine feces, petting zoos	Verotoxin: Shigella-like toxins 1 and 2, decreased protein synthesis by interfering with 60S ribosomal subunit	No fever, no PMNs, blood in stool, nonfermenters of sorbitol; may progress to hemorrhagic colitis and HUS; most common in children age <5 years	Antibiotics ↑ risk of hemolytic uremic syndrome

Definition of abbreviations: EIEC, enteroinvasive *E. coli*; EHEC, enterohemorrhagic *E. coli*; EPEC, enteropathogenic *E. coli*, EAEC, enteroaggregative *E. coli*

GENUS: *KLEBSIELLA*

Klebsiella pneumoniae

Distinguishing Features

- **Gram-negative rods** with **large** polysaccharide **capsule**
- **Mucoid, lactose-fermenting** colonies on MacConkey agar
- Oxidase negative

Reservoir: human colon and upper respiratory tract

Transmission: endogenous

Pathogenesis : **capsule** (impedes phagocytosis); **endotoxin** (causes fever, inflammation, and shock [septicemia])

Disease(s)

- Pneumonia

    - Community-acquired, most often older males; most commonly **those with chronic lung disease, alcoholism, or diabetes** (but this is not the most common cause of pneumonia in alcoholics; *S. pneumoniae* is.)

    - Endogenous; assumed to reach lungs by inhalation of respiratory droplets from upper respiratory tract

    - Frequent **abscesses** make it hard to treat; fatality rate high

    - **Sputum is generally thick and bloody (currant jelly)** but not foul-smelling as in anaerobic aspiration pneumonia

- Urinary tract infection: **catheter-related (nosocomial)** from fecal contamination of catheters

- Septicemia: in immunocompromised patients, may originate from bowel defect or invasion of IV line

Diagnosis: culture of sputum or clean catch urine sample; lactose fermenter

Treatment: third-generation cephalosporin with or without an aminoglycoside; carbapenem for ESBL-producing strains; KPC strains becoming more predominant

Prevention: good catheter care, limit use

Klebsiella granulomatis

Distinguishing Features: previously called *Calymmatobacterium granulomatis*; facultative-intracellular

Transmission: sexual contact

Key Vignette Clues

Klebsiella pneumoniae

- Elderly patient with typical pneumonia: currant-jelly sputum

- UTI (catheter associated)

- Septicemia: immunocompromised or nosocomial

- Gram (–) bacilli, oxidase (–), encapsulated, lactose fermenters

In a Nutshell

Comparative Microbiology

Major encapsulated organisms

Some **K**illers **H**ave **P**retty **N**ice **C**apsules:

Strep pneumoniae

Klebsiella pneumoniae

Haemophilus influenzae Type b (a-d)

Pseudomonas aeruginosa

Neisseria meningitidis

Cryptococcus neoformans (the yeast)

(Not a complete list, just the big ones)

Disease(s): granuloma inguinale (Donovanosis): small painless nodules that burst and ulcerate; beefy red painless genital ulcers

Diagnosis: Donovan bodies seen on Wright-Giemsa stain; not seen on Gram stain

Treatment: doxycycline

GENUS: *SHIGELLA*

Species of Medical Importance

- *Shigella sonnei* (**most common in U.S.**)
- *Shigella flexneri*
- *Shigella dysenteriae* (**most severe disease**)
- *Shigella boydii*

Shigella Species

Distinguishing Features

- **Gram-negative rods,** nonmotile, non-lactose fermenters

Reservoir: human colon only (no animal carriers)

Transmission: fecal-oral spread, person to person

Pathogenesis

- **Endotoxin** triggers inflammation
- No H antigens
- Shigellae **invade M cells** (membrane ruffling and macropinocytosis), get into the cytoplasm, replicate, and then **polymerize actin jet trails to go laterally** without going back out into the extracellular milieu. This produces **very shallow ulcers** and rarely causes invasion of blood vessels.
- **Shiga toxin:**
  - Produced by *S. dysenteriae*, type 1
  - Three activities: **neurotoxic, cytotoxic, enterotoxic**
  - **AB component toxin** is internalized in human cells; **inhibits protein synthesis by clipping 60S ribosomal subunit**

Disease(s): enterocolitis/shigellosis (most severe form is dysentery)

- Few organisms required to start infection (1–10) (extremely acid-resistant)
- 1–4 day incubation
- Organisms invade, producing bloody diarrhea

Note

Comparative Microbiology

- Invasive bacteria: PMN in stool: *Shigella, Salmonella, Campylobacter*, EIEC.
- Toxigenic bacteria: ETEC, *V. cholerae, Cl. perfringens*, EHEC.

Key Vignette Clues

Shigella

- Patient with acute bloody diarrhea and fever
- Gram (–) bacilli, which are nonmotile, nonlactose fermenters, do not produce H$_2$S

- Fever (generally >101.0°F); lower abdominal cramps; tenesmus; diarrhea first watery, then bloody; invasive but rarely causes septicemia; shallow ulcers
- Severity depends on age of patient and strain; *S. dysenteriae* type 1 with toxin most severe

Diagnosis: isolation from stool during illness and culture on selective media

Treatment: fluid and electrolyte replacement (mild cases); antibiotics (severe cases); resistance is mediated by plasmid-encoded enzymes; many strains are ampicillin-resistant

Prevention: proper sanitation (sewage, clean drinking water, hand washing)

Aeromonas spp.

Distinguishing Features: oxidase-positive; not Enterobacteriaceae

Transmission: contaminated water or food

Disease(s): inflammatory diarrhea similar to shigellosis (blood and PMNs)

Diagnosis: oxidase-positive, flagellated, glucose-fermenting, gram-negative rods

Treatment: cefixime

GENUS: YERSINIA

Yersinia pestis

Distinguishing Features

- Small **gram-negative** rods with **bipolar staining**
- **Facultative intracellular parasite**
- **Coagulase positive**

Reservoir: zoonosis; U.S. desert southwest: rodents (e.g., prairie dogs, chipmunks, squirrels); potential **biowarfare agent**

Transmission: wild rodents **flea bite** lead to sylvatic plague; human-to-human transmission by **respiratory droplets**

Pathogenesis

- **Coagulase**-contaminated mouth parts of flea
- **Endotoxin** and exotoxin
- **Envelope antigen (F-1) inhibits phagocytosis.**
- Type III secretion system suppresses cytokine production and resists phagocytic killing

Key Vignette Clues

Yersinia pestis

- Patient with high fever, buboes, conjunctivitis, pneumonia
- Exposure to small rodents, desert Southwest
- Bioterrorism

Disease(s)

- Bubonic plague
  - Flea bites infected animal and then later uninfected human
  - Symptoms: **rapidly increasing fever, regional buboes, conjunctivitis**; if untreated, leads to septicemia and death
- Pneumonic plague
  - Arises from septic pulmonary emboli in bubonic plague or **inhalation of organisms from infected individual**
  - **Highly contagious**
  - Bioterrorism
  - Hemoptysis, chest pain, dyspnea

Diagnosis

- Clinical specimens and **cultures** are hazardous
- **Serodiagnosis** or direct **immunofluorescence**
- **"Safety pin" staining** on blood stain (Wright or Wayson)

Treatment: aminoglycosides

Prevention: animal control and avoidance of sick/dead animals; **killed vaccine** (military)

Yersinia enterocolitica

Distinguishing Features: motile at 25.0°C, nonmotile at 37.0°C; cold growth

Reservoir: zoonotic

Transmission: unpasteurized milk, pork; prominent in northern climates (Michigan, Scandinavia)

Pathogenesis

- Enterotoxin, endotoxin
- **Multiplies in the cold**

Disease(s)

- Enterocolitis: presentations may vary with age
  - Very young: febrile diarrhea (blood and pus)
  - Older kids/young adults: **pseudoappendicitis** (also caused by *Yersinia pseudotuberculosis*)
  - Adults: enterocolitis with postinfective sequelae like reactive arthritis
- Blood transfusion–associated infections

Key Vignette Clues

Yersinia enterocolitica

- Patient with inflammatory diarrhea or pseudoappendicitis
- Cold climates
- Unpasteurized milk, pork
- Gram (–) bacilli, non–lactose fermenters, non–H_2S producers

Diagnosis: stool culture, 25°C, cold enrichment

Treatment: supportive care; fluoroquinolone or third-generation cephalosporin for immunocompromised

GENUS: *PROTEUS*

Proteus mirabilis/Proteus vulgaris

Distinguishing Features

- Gram-negative rods, non-lactose fermenting
- **Highly motile;** "swarming" motility on surface of blood agar
- **Urease** produced
- Facultative anaerobe (Enterobacteriaceae), oxidase negative

Reservoir: human colon and environment (water and soil)

Transmission: endogenous

Pathogenesis

- **Urease raises urine pH to cause kidney stones** (staghorn renal calculi)
- **Motility** may aid entry into bladder
- Endotoxin causes fever and shock when septicemia occurs

Disease(s): urinary tract infection; septicemia

Diagnosis: culture of blood or urine for lactose-negative organisms with swarming motility

Treatment: fluoroquinolone, TMP-SMX, or third-generation cephalosporin for uncomplicated UTI; remove stones if present

Prevention: promptly remove urinary tract catheter

GENUS: *SALMONELLA*

Species of Medical Importance

There are >2,400 serotypes of salmonellae.

- *S. typhi*
- *S. enteritidis*
- *S. typhimurium*
- *S. choleraesuis*
- *S. paratyphi*
- *S. dublin*

Key Vignette Clues

Proteus mirabilis/Proteus vulgaris

- Patient with UTI or septicemia
- Swarming motility
- Staghorn renal calculi (struvite stones)
- Gram (–), non–lactose fermenting, urease (+)

Note

Weil-Felix test: antigens of OX strains of *Proteus vulgaris* cross-react with rickettsial organisms.

Key Vignette Clues

Salmonella typhi

- Patient with fever, abdominal pain

- Travel to endemic area

- Gram (–), encapsulated, nonlactose fermenter, produces H$_2$S gas

- Widal test

Salmonella enterica typhi

Distinguishing Features

- **Gram-negative rods,** highly motile with the **Vi capsule**

- Facultative anaerobe, **non–lactose fermenting**

- **Produces H$_2$S**

- Species identification with biochemical reactions

- **Sensitive to acid**

Reservoir: humans only; no animal reservoirs

Transmission: fecal-oral route from **human carriers (gall bladder); decreased stomach acid or** impairment of mononuclear cells as in **sickle cell disease predisposes** to *Salmonella* infection

Pathogenesis and Disease: typhoid fever (enteric fever), *S. typhi* (milder form: paratyphoid fever; *S. paratyphi*)

- **Infection begins in ileocecal region; constipation** common

- Host cell membranes "ruffle" from *Salmonella* contact.

- *Salmonella* reach basolateral side of M cells, then **mesenteric lymph nodes and blood** (transient 19 septicemia)

- At 1 week: patients have 80% **positive blood cultures**; 25% have **rose spots** (trunk/abdomen), signs of **septicemia** (mainly fever)

- *S. typhi* survives intracellularly and replicates in macrophages; **resistant to macrophage killing** because of **decreased fusion of lysosomes with phagosomes** and **defensins** (proteins) allow it to withstand oxygen-dependent and oxygen-independent killing

- **By week 3: 85% of stool cultures** are positive

- Symptoms: **fever,** headache, abdominal pain, constipation more common than diarrhea

- Complications if untreated: **necrosis of Peyer patches** with perforation (local endotoxin triggered damage), thrombophlebitis, cholecystitis, pneumonia, abscess formation, etc.

Diagnosis: organisms can be isolated from blood, bone marrow, urine, and tissue biopsy from the rose spots if present; antibodies to O, Vi, and H antigens in patient's serum can be detected by agglutination (**Widal test**)

Treatment: fluoroquinolones or third-generation cephalosporins

Prevention: sanitation; 3 vaccines (attenuated oral vaccine of *S. typhi* strain 21 (Ty21a), parenteral heat-killed *S. typhi* (no longer used in U.S.), and parenteral ViCPS polysaccharide capsular vaccine)

Salmonella Subspecies other than *typhi* (*S. enteritidis, S. typhimurium*)

Distinguishing Features

- Facultative gram-negative rods, non–lactose-fermenting on EMB, MacConkey medium
- Produces H_2S, **motile** (unlike *Shigella*)
- Speciated with biochemical reactions and serotyped with O, H, and Vi antigens

Reservoir: enteric tracts of humans and domestic animals, e.g., **chickens** and turtles

Transmission: raw chicken and eggs in kitchen; food-borne outbreaks (peanut butter, produce, eggs); reptile pets (snakes, turtles)

Pathogenesis

- Sensitive to stomach acid (infectious dose 10^5 organisms)
- Lowered stomach acidity (antacids or gastrectomy) increases risk
- Endotoxin in cell wall; no exotoxin
- **Invades** mucosa in ileocecal region, invasive to lamina propria $\rightarrow$ **inflammation** $\rightarrow$ **increased PG** $\rightarrow$ **increased cAMP** $\rightarrow$ loose diarrhea; shallow ulceration
- Spread to septicemia not common with *S. enterica* subsp. *enteritidis* (the most common) but may occur with others

Disease(s)

- Enterocolitis/gastroenteritis (second most common bacterial cause after *Campylobacter*): **6–48 hour incubation; nausea; vomiting; only occasionally bloody, loose stools; fever; abdominal pain; myalgia; headache**
- Septicemia (*S. enterica* subsp. *choleraesuis*, *S. enterica* subsp. *paratyphi*, and *S. enterica* subsp. *dublin*): usually in very young or elderly when it occurs; endocarditis or arthritis complicates 10% of cases
- Osteomyelitis: sickle cell disease predisposes to osteomyelitis; salmonella is **most common causal agent of osteomyelitis in sickle cell disease** (not trait) **patients** (>80%)

Diagnosis: culture on Hektoen agar, H_2S production

Treatment: antibiotics are contraindicated for self-limiting gastroenteritis; ampicillin, third-generation cephalosporin, fluoroquinolone, or TMP-SMX for invasive disease

Prevention: properly cook foods and wash hands, particularly food handlers

Key Vignette Clues

Salmonella enterica Subspecies Other Than *typhi*

- Enterocolitis—inflammatory, follows ingestion of poultry products or handling pet reptiles
- Septicemia—very young or elderly
- Osteomyelitis—sickle cell disease
- Gram (–) bacillus, motile, non–lactose fermenter, produces H_2S

GENUS: *GARDNERELLA*

Gardnerella vaginalis

Distinguishing Features

- Gram-variable rod; has Gram-positive cell envelope
- Facultative anaerobe
- Catalase-negative and oxidase-negative

Reservoir: human vagina

Transmission: endogenous (normal flora gets disturbed, increased pH)

Pathogenesis

- Polymicrobial infections
- Works synergistically with other normal flora organisms including *Lactobacillus, Mobiluncus, Bacteroides, Peptostreptococcus*
- Thought to flourish when the vaginal pH increases, reduction of vaginal *Lactobacillus*
- Follows menses or antibiotic therapy

Disease: bacterial vaginosis (**vaginal odor, increased discharge** (thin, gray, adherent fluid)

Diagnosis: pH >4.5, **clue cells** (epithelial cells covered with bacteria) on vaginal saline smear; for Whiff test, add KOH to sample and assess for "fishy" amine odor

Treatment: metronidazole or clindamycin

GENUS: *BACTEROIDES*

Bacteroides fragilis

Distinguishing Features: anaerobic gram-negative rods; modified LPS with reduced activity

Reservoir: human **colon**; the genus *Bacteroides* is predominant anaerobe

Transmission: **endogenous** from bowel defects (e.g., cytotoxic drug use, cancer), surgery, or trauma

Pathogenesis: modified LPS (missing heptose and 2-keto-3 deoxyoctonate) has reduced endotoxin activity; capsule is antiphagocytic

Diseases: **septicemia, peritonitis (often mixed infections), and abdominal abscess**

Diagnosis: anaerobes are identified by biochemical tests and gas chromatography

Treatment

- Metronidazole, clindamycin, or cefoxitin; **abscesses should be surgically drained**
- **Antibiotic resistance** common (penicillin G, some cephalosporins, and aminoglycosides); 7–10% of all strains now clindamycin-resistant

Prevention: prophylactic antibiotics for GI or biliary tract surgery

Porphyromonas, Prevotella, Fusobacterium spp.

Distinguishing Features: Gram-negative rods, anaerobic, normal oral flora

Transmission: endogenous

Pathogenesis: *Porphyromonas* has gingipains: act as proteases, adhesins, degrades IgG antibodies and inflammatory cytokines

Disease: periodontal disease

Diagnosis: anaerobic, gram-negative rods isolated from abscess

Treatment: metronidazole

SPIROCHETES

GENUS: *TREPONEMA*

Treponema pallidum

Distinguishing Features

- **Thin spirochete,** not reliably seen on Gram stain (basically a gram-negative cell envelope)
- Outer membrane has endotoxin-like lipids
- Axial filaments = endoflagella = periplasmic flagella
- Cannot culture in clinical lab; serodiagnosis
- Is an **obligate pathogen (but not intracellular)**

Reservoir: human genital tract

Transmission: transmitted **sexually** or **across the placenta**

Pathogenesis: disease characterized by **endarteritis resulting in lesions**; strong tendency to chronicity

Key Vignette Clues

Treponema pallidum

- Sexually active patient or neonate of IV drug-using female
- **Primary**: nontender, indurated genital chancre
- **Secondary**: maculopapular, copper-colored rash, condylomata lata
- **Tertiary**: gummas in CNS and cardiovascular system
- Spirillar, gram (–) bacteria visualized by dark-field or fluorescent antibody
- Specific and nonspecific serologic tests

Table II-2-22. Stages of Syphilis

Stage	Clinical	Diagnosis
Primary (10 d to 3 mo post-exposure)	Nontender chancre; clean, indurated edge; contagious; heals spontaneously 3–6 weeks	**Fluorescent microscopy of lesion** 50% of patients will be negative by nonspecific serology
Secondary (1 to 3 mo later)	Maculopapular (copper-colored) rash, diffuse, includes palms and soles, patchy alopecia Condylomata lata: flat, wartlike perianal and mucous membrane lesions; highly infectious	**Serology nonspecific and specific;** both positive
Latent	None	Positive serology
Tertiary (30% of untreated, years later)	Gummas (syphilitic granulomas), aortitis, CNS inflammation (tabes dorsalis)	**Serology: specific tests** Nonspecific may be negative
Congenital (babies of IV drug–using)	Stillbirth, keratitis, 8th nerve damage, notched teeth; most born asymptomatic or with rhinitis → widespread desquamating maculopapular rash	Serology: should revert to negative within 3 mo of birth if uninfected

Diagnosis

- **Visualize organisms by immunofluorescence or microscopy** (dark field microscopy was standard but no longer used)

- **Serology** important: 2 types of antibody:

  1. **Nontreponemal antibody (= reagin) screening tests**

     - **Ab binds to cardiolipin**: antigen found in mammalian mitochondrial membranes and treponemes; cheap source of antigen is cow heart, used in screening tests (VDRL, RPR, ART); very sensitive in primary (except early) and secondary syphilis; titer may decline in tertiary and with treatment; not specific so confirm with FTA-ABS

     - **Examples:** venereal disease research lab (VDRL), rapid plasma reagin (RPR), automated reagin test (ART), recombinant antigen test (ICE)

  2. **Specific tests for treponemal antibody (more expensive)**

     - **Earliest** antibodies; **bind to spirochetes**: these tests are more specific and positive earlier; usually remain positive for life, but positive in those with other treponemal diseases (bejel) and may be positive in Lyme disease; fluorescent treponemal antibody-absorption (**FTA-ABS; most widely used test**); *Treponema pallidum* microhemagglutination (MHA-TP)

Treatment

- **Benzathine penicillin** (long-acting form) for primary and secondary syphilis (no resistance to penicillin); penicillin G for congenital and late syphilis

- Jarisch-Herxheimer reaction: starts during first 24 hours of antibiotic treatment; increased temperature and decreased BP; rigors, leukopenia; may occur during treatment of **any spirochete disease**

Prevention: benzathine penicillin given to contacts; no vaccine available

GENUS: *BORRELIA*

Genus Features

- **Larger spirochetes**
- **Gram negative**
- **Microaerophilic**
- **Difficult to culture**

Borrelia burgdorferi

Reservoir: white-footed mice (nymphs) and **white-tailed deer (adult ticks)**

Transmission: *Ixodes* (deer) ticks and nymphs; worldwide but in 3 main areas of U.S.:

- ***Ixodes scapularis (I. dammini)*** in Northeast (e.g., Connecticut), Midwest (e.g., Wisconsin, Minnesota)
- ***Ixodes pacificus*** on West Coast (e.g., California)
- Late spring/early summer incidence

Pathogenesis: *B. burgdorferi* **invades skin and spreads via bloodstream** to involve primarily the heart, joints, and CNS; arthritis is caused by immune complexes

Disease: Lyme disease (#1 vector-borne disease in U.S.)

Key Vignette Clues

Borrelia burgdorferi

- Patient with influenza-like symptoms and erythema migrans
- Spring/summer seasons
- Northeast, Midwest, West Coast
- Later: neurologic, cardiac, arthritis/arthralgias

Stage 1: early localized (3 days to 1 month)	Target rash
	Flu-like symptoms
Stage 2: early disseminated (days to weeks) **(organism spreads hematogenously)**	Swollen lymph nodes
	Secondary annular skin lesions
	Bell palsy, headache, meningitis, extreme fatigue, conjunctivitis
	Palpitations, arrhythmias, myocarditis, pericarditis
Stage 3: late persistent (months to years)	Arthritis (mostly knees), immune complex-mediated

Diagnosis: **serodiagnosis** by ELISA (negative early); Western blot for confirmation

Treatment: doxycycline, amoxicillin, or azithromycin/clarithromycin for primary; ceftriaxone for secondary; doxycycline or ceftriaxone for arthritis

Prevention: DEET; avoid tick bites; vaccine (OspA flagellar antigen) not used in U.S.

Borrelia recurrentis and B. hermsi

Distinguishing Features: spirochetes, cause relapsing fever

Transmission: human body louse for *B. recurrentis*; soft ticks from mice for *B. hermsi* (and 13 other species of Borrelia)

Pathogenesis: antigenic variation leads to return of fever/chills

Disease(s): relapsing fever (tick-borne relapsing fever in U.S. is caused mainly by *B. hermsi*); associated with camping in rural areas of Colorado

Diagnosis: spirochetes seen on dark-field microscopy of blood smear when patient is febrile

Treatment: doxycycline; Jarisch-Herxheimer reaction possible

GENUS: *LEPTOSPIRA*

Leptospira interrogans

Distinguishing Features: **spirochetes with tight terminal hooks or coils** (seen on **dark-field microscopy** but not light; can be cultured in vitro; aerobic); generally diagnosed by serology

Reservoir: wild and domestic animals (zoonosis)

Transmission

- **Contact with animal urine in water; organism penetrates mucous membranes or enters small breaks in epidermis**
- In U.S., **viadog, livestock,** and **rat urine** through contaminated **recreational waters (jet skiers) or occupational exposure (sewer workers)**
- **Hawaii highest incidence state**

Pathogenesis: no toxins or virulence factors known

Disease: leptospirosis (swineherd's disease, swamp or mud fever); **influenza-like disease ± GI tract symptoms (Weil disease)**; if not treated, can progress to hepatitis and renal failure

Diagnosis: serodiagnosis (agglutination test); culture (blood, CSF, urine) available in few labs; dark-field microscopy insensitive

Treatment: penicillin G or doxycycline

Prevention: doxycycline for short-term exposure; vaccination of domestic livestock and pets; rat control

---

Key Vignette Clues

Leptospira interrogans

- Patients with influenza-like symptoms ± GI symptoms
- Occupational or recreational exposure to water aerosols
- Hawaii
- Spirochetes with terminal hook

UNUSUAL BACTERIA

Table II-2-23. Comparison of *Chlamydiaceae*, *Rickettsiaceae*, and *Mycoplasmataceae* with Typical Bacteria

	Typical Bacteria (*S. aureus*)	Chlamydiaceae	Rickettsiaceae	Mycoplasmataceae
Obligate intracellular parasite?	Mostly no	Yes	Yes	No
Make ATP?	Normal ATP	No ATP	Limited ATP	Normal ATP
Peptidoglycan layer in cell envelope?	Normal peptidoglycan	Modified* peptidoglycan	Normal peptidoglycan	No peptidoglycan

*Chlamydial peptidoglycan lacks muramic acid and is considered by some as modified, by others as absent.

FAMILY: CHLAMYDIACEAE

Family Features

- Obligate intracellular bacteria
- Elementary body/reticulate body
- Not seen on Gram stain
- Cannot make ATP
- Cell wall lacks muramic acid

Genera of Medical Importance

- *Chlamydia trachomatis*
- *Chlamydophila pneumoniae*
- *Chlamydophila psittaci*

Chlamydia trachomatis

Distinguishing Features

- Obligate intracellular bacterium; cannot make ATP
- Found **in cells as metabolically active, replicating reticulate bodies**
- **Infective form:** inactive, extracellular **elementary body**
- Not seen on Gram stain; peptidoglycan layer lacks muramic acid

Key Vignette Clues

Chlamydia trachomatis

- Sexually active patient or neonate
- **Adult:** urethritis, cervicitis, PID, inclusion
- conjunctivitis
- **Neonate:** inclusion conjunctivitis/pneumonia
- Immigrant from Africa/Asia, genital lymphadenopathy
- Cytoplasmic inclusion bodies in scrapings

Reservoir: human genital tract and eyes

Transmission: sexual contact and **at birth;** trachoma is transmitted by **hand-to-eye contact** andflies.

Pathogenesis: infection of nonciliated columnar or cuboidal epithelial cells of mucosal surfaces leads to **granulomatous response and damage**

Diseases

- STDs in U.S.

    - **Serotypes D-K** (most common **bacterial** STD in U.S., though overall herpes and HPV are more common in prevalence)

    - **Nongonococcal urethritis, cervicitis, PID,** and major portion of infertility (no resistance to reinfection)

    - **Inclusion conjunctivitis** in adults (with NGU and reactive arthritis)

    - **Inclusion conjunctivitis** and/or **pneumonia in neonates/infants (staccato cough)** with eosinophilic infiltrate

- Lymphogranuloma venereum

    - **Serotypes L1, 2, 3** (prevalent in Africa, Asia, South America); painless ulcer at site of contact; swollen lymph nodes (buboes) around inguinal ligament (groove sign); tertiary includes ulcers, fistulas, genital elephantiasis

- Trachoma

    - Leading cause of preventable infectious blindness: **serotypes A, B, Ba, and C**

    - **Follicular conjunctivitis** leading to **conjunctival scarring,** and **inturned eyelashes** leading to **corneal scarring** and **blindness**

Diagnosis

- NAAT; DNA probes in U.S. (rRNA) and PCR

- **Cytoplasmic inclusions seen on Giemsa-, iodine-, or fluorescent-antibody-stained smear or scrapings**

- **Cannot be cultured on inert media**

- Is cultured in **tissue cultures or embryonated eggs**

- Serodiagnosis: DFA, ELISA

Treatment: azithromycin or doxycycline

Prevention: erythromycin for infected mothers to prevent neonatal disease; systemic erythromycin for neonatal conjunctivitis to prevent pneumonia

GENUS: *CHLAMYDOPHILA*

Table II-2-24. Diseases Caused by *Chlamydophila* Species

Organism	C. pneumoniae	C. psittaci
Distinguishing characteristics	Potential association with atherosclerosis	No glycogen in inclusion bodies
Reservoir	Human respiratory tract	Birds, **parrots,** turkeys (major U.S. reservoir)
Transmission	Respiratory droplets	Dust of dried bird secretions and feces
Pathogenesis	Intracellular growth; infects smooth muscle, endothelial cells, or coronary artery and macrophages	Intracellular growth
Disease	Atypical "walking" pneumonia; single lobe; bronchitis; scant sputum, prominent dry cough and hoarseness; sinusitis	Psittacosis (ornithosis); atypical pneumonia with hepatitis, possible CNS and GI symptoms
Diagnosis	Serology (complement fixation or microimmunofluorescence) Cold-agluttinin negative	Serology, complement fixation Cold-agluttinin negative
Treatment	Macrolides and tetracycline	Doxycycline
Prevention	None	Avoid birds

Key Vignette Clues

Chlamydophila

- *C. pneumoniae:* atypical pneumonia: sputum with intracytoplasmic inclusions

- *C. psittaci:* atypical pneumonia: exposure to parrots

GENUS: *RICKETTSIA*

Table II-2-25. Infections Caused by Rickettsiae and Close Relatives

Group Disease	Bacterium	Arthropod Vector	Reservoir Host
Rocky Mountain Spotted Fever	*R. rickettsii*	Ticks	Ticks, dogs, rodents
Epidemic Typhus	*R. prowazekii*	Human louse	Humans
Endemic Typhus	*R. typhi*	Fleas	Rodents
Scrub Typhus	*Orientia tsutsugamushi*	Mites	Rodents
Ehrlichiosis	*E. chafeensis* *A. phagocytophilum*	Tick	Small mammals

Genus Features

- Aerobic, gram-negative bacilli (too small to stain well with Gram stain)
- Obligate intracellular bacteria (do not make sufficient ATP for independent life)

Species of Medical Importance

- *Rickettsia rickettsii*
- *Rickettsia prowazekii*
- *Rickettsia typhi*
- *Orientia tsutsugamushi* (formerly *R. tsutsugamushi*)
- *Ehrlichia spp.*
- *Coxiella burnetii*

Rickettsia rickettsii

Reservoir: small wild rodents and larger wild and domestic animals (dogs)

Transmission: hard ticks: *Dermacentor* **(also reservoir hosts** because of trans-ovarian transmission)

Pathogenesis: invade endothelial cells lining capillaries, causing vasculitis in many organs including brain, liver, skin, lungs, kidney, and GI tract

Disease: Rocky Mountain spotted fever (RMSF)

- Prevalent on **East Coast (OK, TN, NC, SC)**; 2–12 day incubation
- **Headache, fever (102°F)**, malaise, myalgias, toxicity, vomiting, and confusion
- **Rash** (maculopapular → **petechial) starts** (by day 6 of illness) **on ankles and wrists** and then spreads to the trunk, **palms, soles, and face (centripetal rash)**
- **Ankle and wrist swelling** also occur
- Diagnosis may be confused by GI symptoms, periorbital swelling, stiff neck, conjunctivitis, and arthralgias

Diagnosis

- Clinical symptoms (above) and tick bite
- **Start treatment** without laboratory confirmation
- **Serological IFA test most widely used; fourfold increase in titer is diagnostic**
- Weil-Felix test (cross-reaction of *Rickettsia* antigens with OX strains of *Proteus vulgaris*) is no longer used (but may still be asked!)

Treatment: doxycycline, even in children age <8 years

Prevention: tick protection and prompt removal; doxycycline for exposed persons

GENUS: *EHRLICHIA*

Genus Features

- Gram-negative bacilli
- Obligate intracellular bacteria of mononuclear or granulocytic phagocytes

Species of Medical Importance

- *Ehrlichia chaffeensis*
- *Anaplasma phagocytophilum*

Ehrlichia chaffeensis/Anaplasma phagocytophilum

Table II-2-26. Diseases Caused by *Ehrlichia* Species

Organism	Reservoir	Transmission	Pathogenesis	Disease	Diagnosis	Treatment
E. chaffeensis	Ticks and deer	Lone star tick (*Amblyomma*)	Infects monocytes and macrophages	Ehrlichiosis (monocytic) similar to RMSF without rash; leukopenia, low platelets, morulae	IFA PCR Blood film **Morulae**	Doxycycline
A. phagocytophilum	Ticks, deer, mice	*Ixodes* ticks Coinfection with *Borrelia*	Infects neutrophils	Ehrlichiosis (granulocytic) similar to RMSF without rash; leukopenia, low platelets, morulae	IFA PCR Blood film **Morulae**	Doxycycline

Disease

- Similar to Rocky Mountain spotted fever but generally without rash
- Leukopenia
- Thrombocytopenia
- Morulae: mulberry-like structures inside infected cells

Diagnosis: Giemsa-stained blood film (**morulae**); serology; DNA probe

Treatment: doxycycline (begin before lab confirmation)

Prevention: no vaccine, avoid ticks

Key Vignette Clues

Ehrlichia chaffeensis/Anaplasma phagocytophila

- Patient with influenza-like symptoms, no rash, leukopenia, thrombocytopenia
- Same geographic range as Lyme disease
- Spring/summer seasons
- Exposure to outdoors
- Morulae inside monocytes or granulocytes

Coxiella burnetii

Distinguishing Features: obligate intracellular, spore-like characteristics

Transmission: inhalation from dried placental material; zoonosis (sheep and goats); possible bioterrorism agent

Pathogenesis: obligate intracellular, live inside phagolysosomes

Disease(s): Q fever: atypical pneumonia, hepatitis, or endocarditis

Diagnosis: serologic detection of Phase II LPS antigen (for acute disease) and Phase I and Phase II LPS antigens (for chronic disease)

Treatment: doxycycline

FAMILY: MYCOPLASMATACEAE

Family Features

- **Smallest free-living (extracellular) bacteria**
- **Missing peptidoglycan (no cell wall)**
- **Sterols in membrane**
- **Require cholesterol for in vitro culture**
- **"Fried-egg" colonies on *Mycoplasma* or Eaton's media**

Genera of Medical Importance

- *Mycoplasma pneumoniae*
- *Ureaplasma urealyticum*

Mycoplasma pneumoniae

Distinguishing Features

- Extracellular, tiny, flexible
- No cell wall; not seen on Gram-stained smear
- Membrane with cholesterol but **does not synthesize cholesterol**
- Requires cholesterol for in vitroculture

Reservoir: human respiratory tract

Transmission: respiratory droplets; close contact: families, military recruits, medical school classes, college dorms

Key Vignette Clues

Mycoplasma pneumoniae

- Young adult with atypical pneumonia
- Mulberry-shaped colonies on media containing sterols
- Positive cold agglutinin test

Pathogenesis

- Surface parasite: not invasive
- **Attaches to respiratory epithelium via P1 protein**
- **Inhibits ciliary action**
- **Produces hydrogen peroxide, superoxide radicals, and cytolytic enzymes,** which damage the respiratory epithelium, leading to necrosis and a bad, hacking cough (walking pneumonia)
- *M. pneumoniae* functions as superantigen, elicits production of IL-1, IL-6, and TNF-α

Disease: walking pneumonia

- **Pharyngitis**
- May develop into atypical pneumonia with persistent hack (**little sputum produced**)
- **Most common atypical pneumonia (along with viruses) in young adults**

Diagnosis

- Primarily clinical diagnosis; PCR/nucleic acid probes
- **ELISA and immunofluorescence sensitive and specific**
- **Fried-egg-shaped colonies on sterol-containing media, 10 days**
- **Positive cold agglutinins** (autoantibody to RBCs) test is nonspecific and is positive in only 65% of cases

Treatment: erythromycin, azithromycin, clarithromycin; **no cephalosporin or penicillin**

Prevention: none

Ureaplasma urealyticum

Distinguishing Features: member of family Mycoplasmataceae

Pathogenesis: urease positive

Diseases: urethritis, prostatitis, renal calculi

Diagnosis: non-Gram-staining, urease(+)

Treatment: erythromycin or tetracycline

Key Vignette Clues

Ureaplasma urealyticum

- Adult patient with urethritis, prostatitis, renal calculi
- Alkaline urine
- Non–Gram-staining, urease (+)

Microbial Genetics/Drug Resistance

Learning Objectives

❏ Explain information related to rearrangement of DNA within a bacterium

❏ Answer questions about bacterial gene transfer

❏ Solve problems concerning mechanisms of bacterial DNA exchange and conjugal crosses

❏ Demonstrate understanding of drug resistance

❏ Explain information related to antibiotic susceptibility testing

THE BACTERIAL GENETIC MATERIAL

Three different types of DNA may be found in a bacterial cell: bacterial chromosomal DNA, plasmid DNA, or bacteriophage DNA.

Bacterial Chromosome (Genome)

- Most bacteria have only **one chromosome but often multiple copies** of it in the cell.

- Most bacterial chromosomes are a **large, covalently closed, circular DNA molecule** (about 1,000 times the diameter of the cell).

- The chromosome is **organized into loops** around a proteinaceous center. A single-stranded topoisomerase (1 nick) will relax only the nicked loop, allowing DNA synthesis or transcription.

- Most have **around 2,000 genes**. (*E. coli* has about 4,500 kbases.)

- All **essential genes** are on the bacterial chromosome.

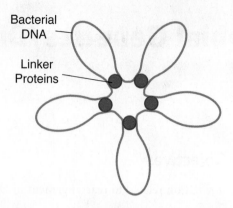

Figure II-3-1. The Bacterial Chromosome

Plasmids

- Are **extrachromosomal genetic elements** found in bacteria (and eukaryotes)

- Are generally covalently closed, **circular DNA**

- Are **small** (1.5–400 kB)

- Can **replicate autonomously** in bacterial cells

- One subclass of plasmids, called **episomes**, may be integrated into the bacterial DNA. Episomes have insertion sequences matching those on the bacterial chromosome.

- Plasmids carry the genetic material for a variety of genes, e.g., the **fertility genes** directing conjugation (*tra* operon), many of the genes for **antibiotic resistance**, and most **bacterial exotoxins**.

- They contain genes that are **nonessential** for bacterial life.

Bacteriophage (= Phage = Bacterial Virus) Genome

- **Stable pieces of bacteriophage DNA** may be present in the bacterial cell.

- These are **generally repressed temperate phage (called prophage)** inserted into the bacterial chromosome.

- Besides the repressor protein, prophage DNA may also direct synthesis of other proteins. Most notable are gene products that make bacteria more pathogenic. This enhanced virulence is called **lysogenic conversion.**

REARRANGEMENT OF DNA WITHIN A BACTERIUM

Homologous Recombination

- Homologous recombination is a gene exchange process that may **stabilize genes** introduced into a cell by transformation, conjugation, or transduction.

- Imported bacterial DNA (transferred into a cell by transformation, conjugation, or transduction) is on short linear pieces of DNA called **exogenotes**. Most linear DNA is not stable in cells because it is broken down by exonucleases.

- Homologous recombination produces an **"exchange"** of DNA between the linear exogenote of DNA and a homologous region on the stable (circular) bacterial chromosome.

- Homologous recombination requires:

  - Several genes worth of homology or near homology between the DNA strands.

  - A series of recombination enzymes/factors coded for by the recombination genes recA, recB, recC, and recD (with recA generally an absolute requirement).

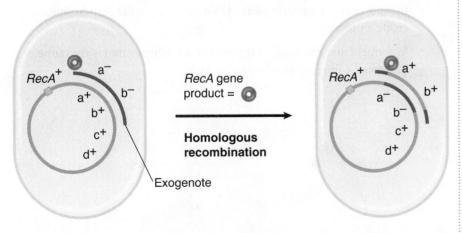

Genes ending up on the linear piece of DNA are lost. Those on the circular molecule become part of the cell's permanent genetic make up.

Figure II-3-2. Homologous Recombination

Site-Specific Recombination

Site-specific recombination is the integration of one DNA molecule into another DNA molecule with which it has **no homology** except for a small site on each DNA (called an **attachment, integration, or insertion site**).

- Requires **restriction endonucleases** and restriction endonuclease sites on each DNA

- Because this process **integrates** rather than exchanges pieces of DNA, the end result is a molecule the **sum of the two original molecules**.

In a Nutshell

Site-Specific Recombination

- Is the mechanism used to combine **circular pieces** of DNA:
    - Plasmids
    - Temperate phage
    - Transposons

- It requires **no homology**.

- **No DNA is lost**.

- It **requires restriction endonucleases**.

■ = Integration sites

Figure II-3-3. Site-Specific Recombination

Three major roles of site-specific integration

- Integration of a **fertility factor** to make an Hfr cell

- Integration of **temperate phage** DNA into a bacterial chromosome to create a prophage

- Movement and insertion of **transposons** (transposition is the name of site-specific integration of transposons)

GENE TRANSFER

Overview

Bacterial reproduction is asexual, so progeny are identical to parent cell with only rare mutations.

How do you get new genetic combinations in bacteria?

Answer: Gene transfer followed by stabilization of genes (recombination)

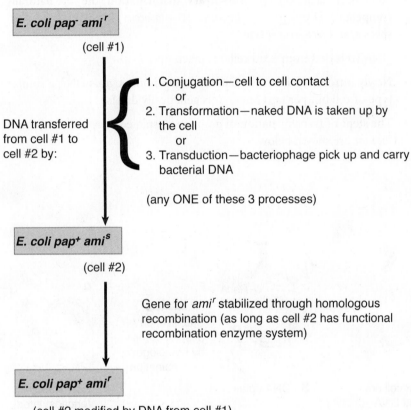

· Now *pap*⁺ (initially linked to *ami*ˢ) is linked to *ami*ʳ instead, producing a new combination of genes and more significantly, a cell that can cause pyelonephritis and is amikacin resistant.
· (Could also have yielded *E. coli* that was *pap*⁻ *ami*ˢ or *pap*⁻ *ami*ʳ or the cell could have stayed *pap*⁺ *ami*ˢ.)

Figure II-3-4. The Classic Experiment Demonstrating That Bacteria Are Capable of Genetic Exchange

Any DNA that is transferred between bacterial cells must be stabilized by recombination or it will be lost.

MECHANISMS OF DNA EXCHANGE

Transformation

Transformation is the uptake of naked DNA from the environment by competent cells.

- Cells become **competent (able to bind short pieces of DNA to the envelope and import them into the cell)** under certain environmental conditions (which you do not need to know).

- Some bacteria are capable of **natural transformation** (they are naturally competent): *Haemophilus influenzae*, *Streptococcus pneumoniae*, *Bacillus* species, and *Neisseria* species.

- DNA (released from dead cells) is taken up.

- Newly introduced DNA is generally linear, homologous DNA a similar type of cell but perhaps one that is genetically diverse.

- The steps of transformation of a nonencapsulated *Streptococcus pneumoniae* are shown below.

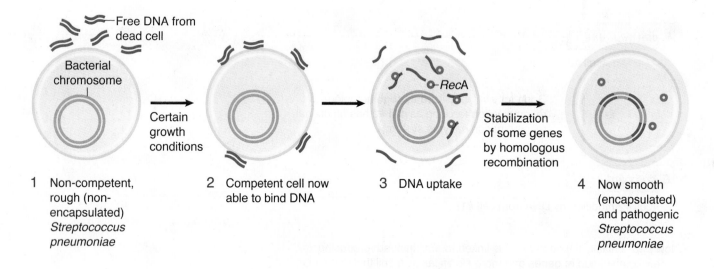

Figure II-3-5. Transformation

Conjugation

Conjugation is gene transfer from one bacterial cell to another involving direct cell-to-cell contact.

- **Fertility factors control** conjugation.
- **Sex pili** (genes on F factor) play a role in establishing cell-to-cell contact.
- A **single strand** (or a portion thereof) of the double helix of DNA is transferred from the donor (or male) cell to the recipient or female cell.
- Chromosomal genes transferred in by conjugation have to be stabilized by **homologous recombination** (in an Hfr × F^- cross). Plasmid genes transferred by conjugation circularize and are stable without recombination (in an F^+ × F^- cross).
- Conjugation with recombination may produce new genetic combinations.

Donor (male) cells

- All have fertility plasmids known as **F factors.** F factors have a series of important plasmid "fertility" genes called the transfer or ***tra* region,** which code for:
  - Sex pili
  - Genes whose products stabilize mating pairs
  - Genes that direct conjugal DNA transfer, and other genes.
- Have a region called ***oriT* (origin of transfer)** where a single strand break in the DNA will be made and then *oriT* begins the transfer of one strand of the double helix.
- Many have **insertion sequences** where the plasmid can be inserted into the bacterial chromosome combining to make one larger molecule of DNA.
- A genetic map of an F factor is shown below.

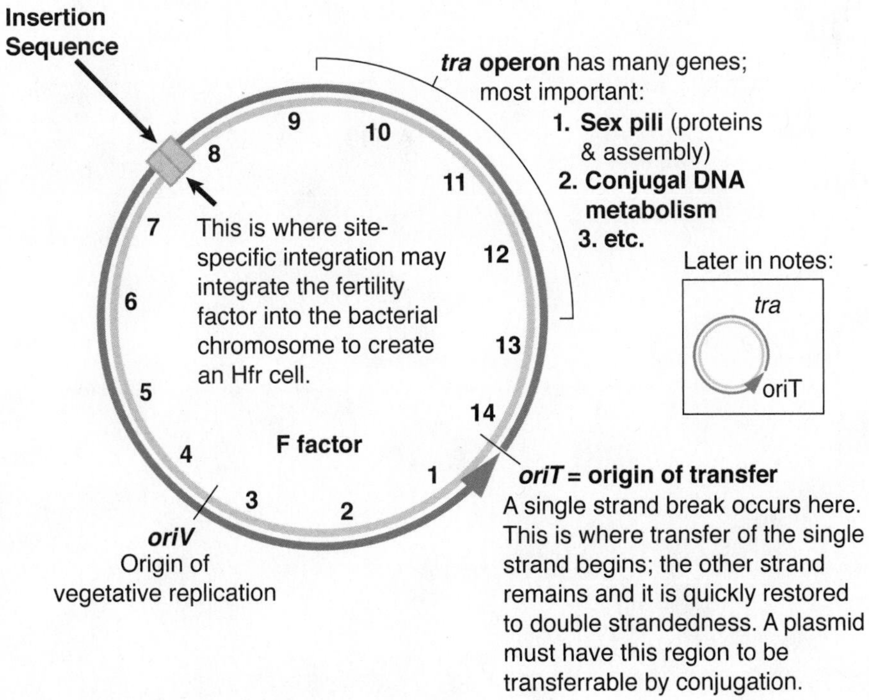

Figure II-3-6. Fertility Factor

In a Nutshell

- **Conjugation:** gene transfer from donor (F^+ or Hfr cell) to recipient (F^- cell) during cell-to-cell contact
- **Fertility factors** (in plasmid or episome form) **control conjugation.**
- A single strand of DNA is transferred to recipient from donor.

- Donor cells in which the **fertility plasmid** is in its **free state** are called **F⁺ cells**.

- Donor cells in which the **fertility factor has inserted** itself into the bacterial chromosome are called **Hfr cells**. An integrated plasmid is called an episome.

Recipient (female) cells: F– cells

- Recipient cells **lack fertility factors**.

- In every cross, one cell must be an F⁻ cell.

Mating types of bacterial cells

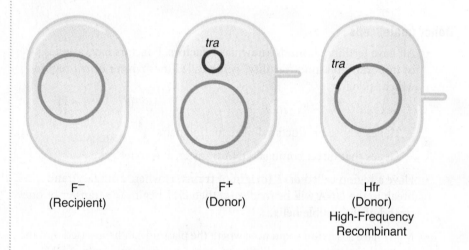

Figure II-3-7. Mating Types of Bacteria

CONJUGAL CROSSES

There are two major types of crosses:

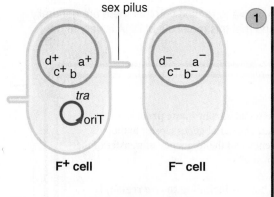

① Important points: In the male or F$^+$ parent, the fertility factor is present but free from the bacterial chromosome. Transfer is uni-directional from male to female. *OriT*, as in every cross, will be transferred first and then the rest of the plasmid genes.

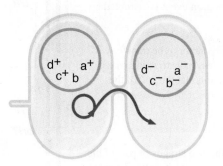

② Only a single strand of the plasmid DNA duplex is transferred. The area that is lost is reduplicated so that the donor always stays the same genotype. The last genes to be transferred are the *tra* region.

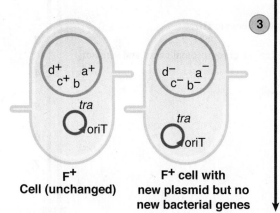

③ The transfer of the plasmid is fairly quick so assume it is transferred in its entirety 100% of the time unless otherwise told. Note that the F$^-$ cell undergoes a sex change, becoming F$^+$ (male). These two F$^+$ cells can no longer mate, but no BACTERIAL genes are transferred.

Figure II-3-8. The F$^+$ by F$^-$ Conjugal Cross

In a Nutshell

In the F$^+$ × F$^-$ cross:

- One strand of the entire plasmid is transferred

- Recipient becomes F$^+$

Integrated Fertility Factor

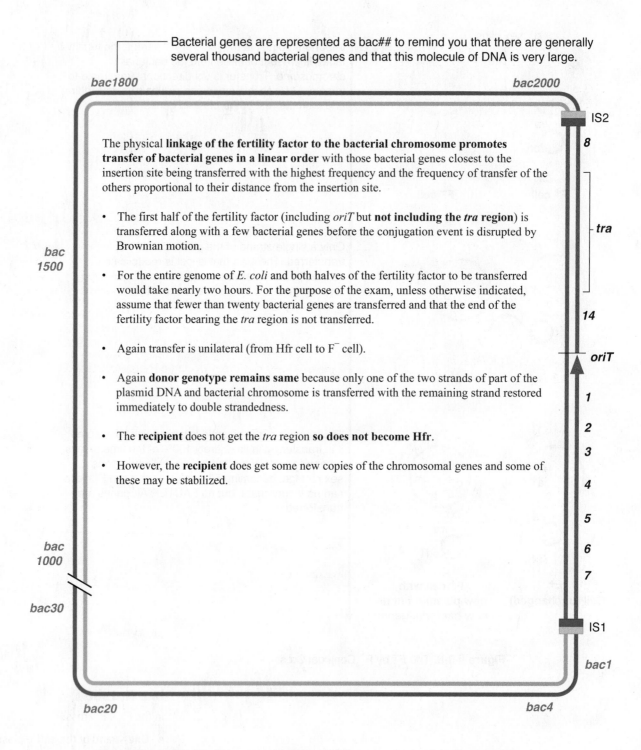

Bacterial genes are represented as bac## to remind you that there are generally several thousand bacterial genes and that this molecule of DNA is very large.

The physical **linkage of the fertility factor to the bacterial chromosome promotes transfer of bacterial genes in a linear order** with those bacterial genes closest to the insertion site being transferred with the highest frequency and the frequency of transfer of the others proportional to their distance from the insertion site.

- The first half of the fertility factor (including *oriT* but **not including the *tra* region**) is transferred along with a few bacterial genes before the conjugation event is disrupted by Brownian motion.

- For the entire genome of *E. coli* and both halves of the fertility factor to be transferred would take nearly two hours. For the purpose of the exam, unless otherwise indicated, assume that fewer than twenty bacterial genes are transferred and that the end of the fertility factor bearing the *tra* region is not transferred.

- Again transfer is unilateral (from Hfr cell to F⁻ cell).

- Again **donor genotype remains same** because only one of the two strands of part of the plasmid DNA and bacterial chromosome is transferred with the remaining strand restored immediately to double strandedness.

- The **recipient** does not get the *tra* region **so does not become Hfr**.

- However, the **recipient** does get some new copies of the chromosomal genes and some of these may be stabilized.

Figure II-3-9. The Hfr Chromosome (Bacterial Chromosome with Integrated F Factor)

Conjugation: 2nd type of cross Hfr × F⁻

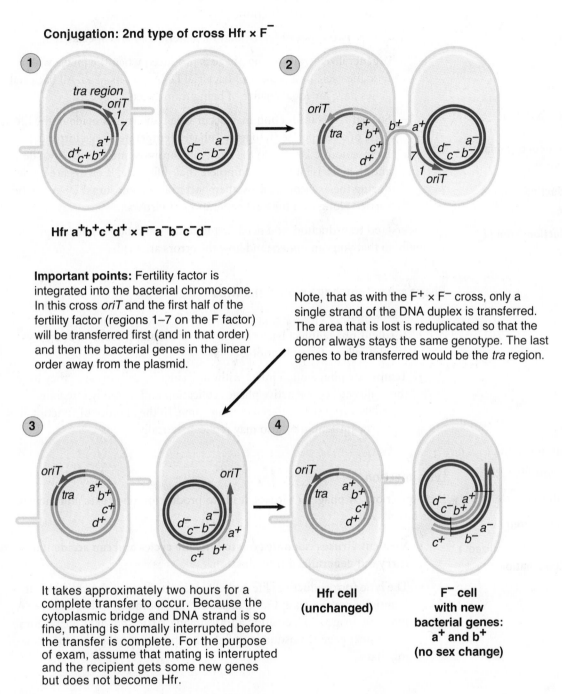

Hfr a⁺b⁺c⁺d⁺ × F⁻a⁻b⁻c⁻d⁻

Important points: Fertility factor is integrated into the bacterial chromosome. In this cross *oriT* and the first half of the fertility factor (regions 1–7 on the F factor) will be transferred first (and in that order) and then the bacterial genes in the linear order away from the plasmid.

Note, that as with the F⁺ × F⁻ cross, only a single strand of the DNA duplex is transferred. The area that is lost is reduplicated so that the donor always stays the same genotype. The last genes to be transferred would be the *tra* region.

It takes approximately two hours for a complete transfer to occur. Because the cytoplasmic bridge and DNA strand is so fine, mating is normally interrupted before the transfer is complete. For the purpose of exam, assume that mating is interrupted and the recipient gets some new genes but does not become Hfr.

Hfr cell (unchanged)

F⁻ cell with new bacterial genes: a⁺ and b⁺ (no sex change)

Figure II-3-10. The Hfr by F⁻ Conjugal Cross

In a Nutshell

In the **Hfr × F⁻ cross:**

- Chromosomal genes **closest to oriT** are transferred.

- Transferred genes must be stabilized by **homologous recombination.**

- The bridge does not remain long enough to transfer the *tra* operon; recipient remains F⁻.

Transduction

- **Transduction** is the transfer of bacterial DNA by a phage vector.

- During transduction, the phage picks up the bacterial DNA through an error in phage production.

- There are **two types of transduction: generalized and specialized**.

  - A generalized transducing phage is produced when the phage with a lytic life cycle puts a piece of bacterial DNA into its head. All bacterial genes have an equal chance of being transduced.

  - Specialized transduction may occur when an error is made in the life cycle of a temperate (lysogenic) phage. Temperate phage introduce their genomic DNA into the bacterial chromosome at a specific site and then excise it later to complete their life cycle. If errors are made during the excision process, then bacterial chromosomal DNA can be carried along into the next generation of viruses.

To understand transduction, you need first to understand how a phage replicates normally so that you can understand how the errors are made.

Phage = bacteriophage = bacterial virus

Come in two major types:

- **Virulent phage** infect bacterial cells, always making more virus and lysing the cells (lytic replication).

- **Temperate phage** often infect without lysing the cells because they have the ability to repress active phage replication and to stably integrate their DNA into the bacterial chromosome. In the absence of functional repressor protein, they also may replicate lytically.

Lytic infection

Lytic infection, by phage or viruses, leads to production of viruses and their release by cell lysis.

- **Virulent viruses can only go into lytic life cycles and can accidentally carry out generalized transduction.**

- The lytic (or productive) life cycle of virulent phage is shown below. It is entirely normal except for a mistaken incorporation of bacterial DNA into one phage head, creating a transducing virus, shown at the bottom of the next page. Transduction of another bacterial cell is shown following that.

In a Nutshell

- **Transduction:** transfer of bacterial DNA via phage vector

- **Generalized transduction:** error of **lytic virus** life cycle

- **Specialized transduction:** error of **temperate virus** life cycle

In a Nutshell

Generalized transduction

- Requires virus with **lytic life cycle**

- It is an **accident** of the life cycle

- **Any** genes can be transferred

- Transferred genes must be stabilized by **homologous recombination**

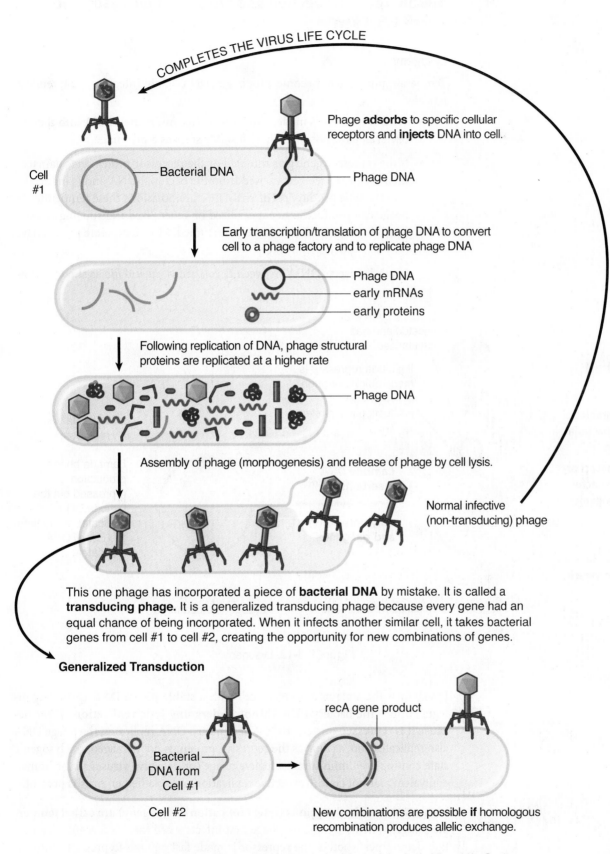

COMPLETES THE VIRUS LIFE CYCLE

Phage **adsorbs** to specific cellular receptors and **injects** DNA into cell.

Cell #1

Bacterial DNA

Phage DNA

Early transcription/translation of phage DNA to convert cell to a phage factory and to replicate phage DNA

Phage DNA
early mRNAs
early proteins

Following replication of DNA, phage structural proteins are replicated at a higher rate

Phage DNA

Assembly of phage (morphogenesis) and release of phage by cell lysis.

Normal infective (non-transducing) phage

This one phage has incorporated a piece of **bacterial DNA** by mistake. It is called a **transducing phage.** It is a generalized transducing phage because every gene had an equal chance of being incorporated. When it infects another similar cell, it takes bacterial genes from cell #1 to cell #2, creating the opportunity for new combinations of genes.

Generalized Transduction

recA gene product

Bacterial DNA from Cell #1

Cell #2

New combinations are possible **if** homologous recombination produces allelic exchange.

Figure II-3-11. Generalized Transduction as an Accident of the Lytic Virus Life Cycle

Specialized Transduction as a Sequela to the Lysogenic Phage Life Cycle

Lysogeny

Temperate phage may become prophage (DNA stably integrated) or replicate lytically.

- When repressor is made, temperate phage insert their DNA into the bacterial chromosome where it stably stays as a **prophage**.

- If the repressor gene gets mutated or the repressor protein gets damaged then the prophage gets excised from the bacterial DNA and is induced into the lytic production of virus. On rare occasions these temperate phage can produce either specialized or generalized transducing viruses. Lambda phage of *E. coli* is the best studied. Most temperate phages have only a single insertion site.

- **Lambda inserts ONLY between *E. coli* genes *gal* and *bio* as shown below.**

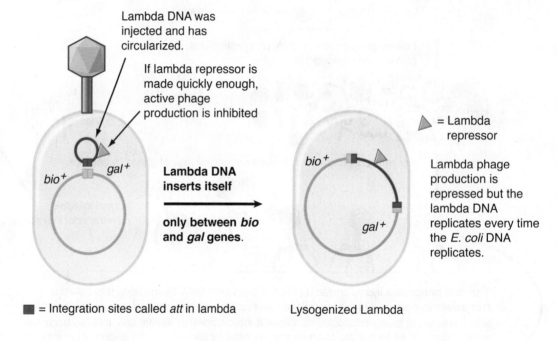

Figure II-3-12. Lysogeny

Lysogeny is the state of a bacterial cell with a **stable phage DNA** (generally integrated into the bacterial DNA), **not undergoing lytic replication either because it is repressed or defective**. When the cell DNA replicates, the phage DNA also replicates and, as long as the repressor protein is not damaged, the lysogenic state continues ad infinitum. Defective phage (or defective viruses in the human equivalent) cannot go into an active replication unless a helper virus is present.

Phage that have both options (lytic replication or lysogeny) are called temperate phage. When a temperate phage first infects a cell there is a regulatory race that determines whether the repressor is made fast enough to prevent synthesis of phage components.

The lysogenized cell will replicate to produce two identical cells each with a prophage as long as the repressor gene product is present.

Lysogeny can confer new properties on a genus such as toxin production or antigens (**lysogenic conversion**):

> C: Cholera toxin
>
> O: Presence of specific prophage in *Salmonella* can affect <u>O</u> antigens.
>
> B: Phage CE β or DE β cause *Clostridium botulinum* to produce <u>B</u>otulinum toxin.
>
> E: <u>E</u>xotoxins A–C (erythrogenic or pyogenic) of *Streptococcus pyogenes*
>
> D: Prophage beta causes *Corynebacterium diphtheriae* to make <u>D</u>iphtheria toxin.
>
> S: <u>S</u>higa toxin

- (Mnemonic for phage-mediated pathogenic factors = COBEDS)
- Model for retrovirus provirus
- Allows specialized transduction

Induction

If the repressor is damaged (by UV, cold, or alkylating agents), then the prophage is excised and the cell goes into lytic replication phase. This process is called **induction**.

Most of the time this process is carried out **perfectly**, recreating the figure 8 of DNA that was the product of viral site-specific recombination, and normal (**nontransducing**) **phage** are produced.

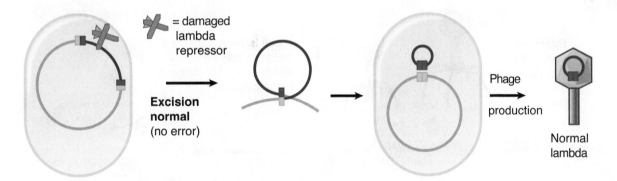

Figure II-3-13. Normal Excision of a Lysogenic Phage

Rarely, in the excision process, an **excisional error** is made and **one of the bacterial genes next to the insertion site is removed attached to the lambda DNA, and a little bit of lambda DNA is left behind**. Only genes on one side *or* the other side of the virus insertion site can be incorporated by excisional error.

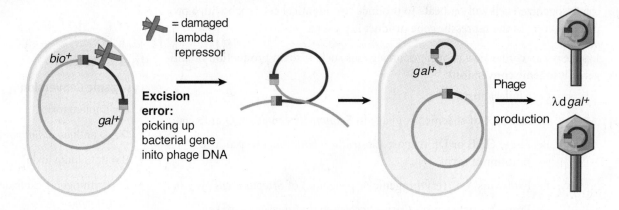

Figure II-3-14. Excision Error of a Lysogenic Phage

In a Nutshell

Specialized Transduction

- Requires a **temperate phage and lysogeny**

- Requires an **error in excision**

- Only genes **near the virus insertion site** can be transferred.

- Any transferred genes must be stabilized by **homologous recombination.**

Because lambda has only one insertion site (between *gal* or *bio*), only *gal* <u>or</u> *bio* can be incorporated by excisional error.

Because all of the phage genes are still in the cell, phage are still made with the circular defective phage genome copied and put in each phage head. These are **specialized transducing phage** (only able to transduce *bio* or *gal*).

Specialized Transduction

Bacterial genes picked up by error in the excision process are transferred to another closely related but often genetically distinct cell. If any genes on the exogenote are stabilized by recombinational exchange, then new genetic combinations occur.

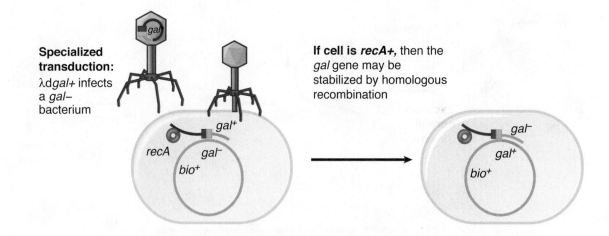

Figure II-3-15. Specialized Transduction

Only those genes next to the phage insertion site can be transduced by specialized transduction.

Table II-3-1. Comparison of Transformation, Conjugation, and Transduction

Requirement	Transformation	Conjugation	Transduction
Is cell-to-cell contact required?	No	Yes	No
Does it require an antecedent phage infection?	No	No	Yes
Is competency required?	Yes	No	No
Is naked (free) DNA involved?	Yes	No	No
Is recombination required to stabilize new genes?	Yes	No for F⁺ × F⁻ Yes for Hfr × F⁻	Yes

Table II-3-2. Comparison of Generalized and Specialized Transduction

	Generalized	Specialized
Mechanism	**Error in assembly**	**Error of excision** Requires stable insertion of prophage DNA (lysogeny)
What genes may be transferred?	**Any**	Only **genes next to the insertion site**

DRUG RESISTANCE

Drug resistance is becoming such a significant problem that there are bacteria for which most antibiotics no longer work. We are entering a "post-antibiotic era."

- Drug resistance can be transferred from one genus of bacteria to another, e.g., from normal flora to a pathogen.

- Three general types of antibiotic resistance exist: intrinsic, chromosome-mediated, and plasmid-mediated.

Intrinsic Drug Resistance

Bacteria are intrinsically resistant to an antibiotic if they lack the target molecule for the drug or if their normal anatomy and physiology makes them refractory to the drug's action.

- Bacteria that lack mycolic acids are intrinsically resistant to isoniazid.

- Bacteria such as *Mycoplasma* that lack peptidoglycan are intrinsically resistant to penicillin.

In a Nutshell

Drug resistance may be:

- **Intrinsic**
- **Chromosomal**
- **Plasmid mediated**

Intrinsic mechanisms:

innate to organism

Chromosome-Mediated Antibiotic Resistance

The genes that determine this resistance are located on the bacterial chromosome.

- Most commonly these genes modify the **receptor for a drug** so that the drug can no longer bind (e.g., a mutation in a gene for a penicillin binding protein).

- In general, causes **low-level drug resistance** rather than high

- In methicillin-resistant *Staphylococcus aureus* a major penicillin-binding protein was mutated.

- Even low-level resistance may be clinically significant, e.g., in *Streptococcus pneumoniae* meningitis.

Plasmid-Mediated Drug Resistance

The genes that determine this resistance are located on plasmids.

- Plasmid-mediated resistance is created by a variety of mechanisms but often genes code for **enzymes that modify the drug**.

- R factors are conjugative plasmids carrying genes for drug resistance.

    - One section of the DNA (containing oriT and the tra gene region) mediates conjugation.

    - The other section (R determinant) carries genes for drug resistance. Multiple genes seem to have been inserted through transpositional insertion into a "hot spot."

How Do Multiple Drug-Resistance Plasmids Arise?

Gene cassettes/integrons/transposons:

- Are mobile genetic elements (DNA) that can move themselves or a copy from one molecule of DNA to another ("jumping genes")

- Are found in eukaryotic and bacterial cells and viruses

- Have at least one gene for a **transposase** (enzyme involved in the movement)

- Create additional **mutations** with their insertion into another totally unrelated gene

A typical genetic map of an R factor (a conjugative drug-resistant plasmid) is shown:

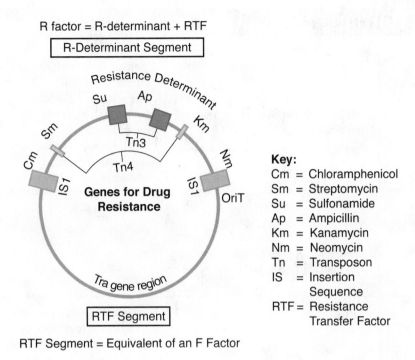

R factor = R-determinant + RTF

R-Determinant Segment

Genes for Drug Resistance

Key:
Cm = Chloramphenicol
Sm = Streptomycin
Su = Sulfonamide
Ap = Ampicillin
Km = Kanamycin
Nm = Neomycin
Tn = Transposon
IS = Insertion Sequence
RTF = Resistance Transfer Factor

RTF Segment

RTF Segment = Equivalent of an F Factor

Figure II-3-16. A Resistance Transfer Factor

Table II-3-3. Plasmid-Mediated Mechanisms of Bacterial Drug Resistance

Antimicrobial Agent	Mechanism
Penicillins and cephalosporins	Production of β-**lactamase**; cleavage of β-lactam rings
Aminoglycosides	Production of acetyltransferase, adenosyltransferase, or phosphotransferase; **inactivation of drug by acetylation**, adenosylation, or phosphorylation
Chloramphenicol	Production of acetyltransferase; **inactivation of drug by acetylation**
Tetracyclines	Increased **efflux** out of cell
Sulfonamides	Active **export** out of cell and lowered affinity of enzyme
Vancomycin	Ligase produces cell wall pentapeptides that terminate in D-alanine-D-lactate, which will not bind to drug

Table II-3-4. Summary of Emerging Bacterial Resistances to Antimicrobial Agents

Antimicrobic	Mechanism		
Inhibitors of Cell Wall Synthesis			
	Altered Accumulation	**Altered Target**	**Enzymatic Inactivation**
β-lactams	Variable outer membranes (chromosome mediated): gram (–), e.g., *Pseudomonas aeruginosa* (ceftazidime)	Mutant and new PBPs (chromosome mediated): *Streptococcus pneumoniae* (penicillin); *Haemophilus influenzae* (ampicillin); *Staphylococcus aureus* (methicillin); *Neisseria gonorrhoeae* (penicillin)	β-lactamases* (plasmid mediated), *Staphylococcus aureus* (penicillin); *Haemophilus influenzae* (ampicillin); *Neisseria gonorrhoeae* (penicillin); *Klebsiella* and *Enterobacter* spp. (third-generation cephalosporins)
Glycopeptides	↑ cell-wall thickness (chromosome mediated), vancomycin intermediate *Staphylococcus aureus* (VISA)	Amino acid substitution (chromosome- or plasmid-mediated transposon), *Enterococcus faecalis* and *E. faecium* (vancomycin); *Staphylococcus aureus* (plasmid mediated), vancomycin, VRSA[†]	—
Isoniazid	—	—	Mutation of catalase-peroxidase gene needed to activate the drug (chromosome mediated), *Mycobacterium tuberculosis*
Ethambutol	—	Mutation of arabinosyl transferase gene (chromosome mediated), *Mycobacterium tuberculosis*	—
Inhibitors of Protein Synthesis			
Aminoglycosides	Oxidative transport required (plasmid mediated), *Pseudomonas aeruginosa*, gentamicin	Ribosomal binding site mutations (chromosome mediated), *Enterococcus*, gentamicin	Adenylases, acetylases, phosphorylases (plasmid mediated), *Klebsiella* and *Enterobacter* spp., gentamicin
Macrolides, lincosamides	Minimal outer membrane penetration (chromosome mediated), gram (–); efflux pump (plasmid mediated), gram (+) cocci; erythromycin	Methylation of 23S rRNA (plasmid mediated), *Bacteroides fragilis*, *Staphylococcus aureus*, MLS resistance[‡]	Phosphotransferase, esterase (plasmid mediated), gram (+) cocci
Chloramphenicol	—	—	Acetyltransferase (plasmid mediated), *Salmonella*, chloramphenicol
Tetracycline	Efflux pump (transposon in plasmid), widespread due to use in animal feed	New protein protects ribosome site (transposon in chromosome or plasmid), *Staphylococcus aureus*	—

(Continued)

Table II-3-4. Summary of Emerging Bacterial Resistances to Antimicrobial Agents (*Cont'd*)

Antimicrobic	Mechanism		
Inhibitors of Nucleic Acid Synthesis			
	Altered Accumulation	**Altered Target**	**Enzymatic Inactivation**
Fluoroquinolones	Efflux pump (plasmid mediated), *Enterococcus*; permeability mutation (chromosomal), *Pseudomonas*	Mutant topoisomerase (chromosome mediated), *Escherichia coli* and *Pseudomonas aeruginosa*, ciprofloxacin	—
Rifamycins	—	Mutant RNA polymerase (chromosome mediated), *Mycobacterium tuberculosis*, *Staphylococcus* spp., and *Neisseria meningitidis*, rifampin	—
Folate inhibitors	—	New dihydropteroate synthetase, altered dihydrofolate reductase (chromosome mediated), Enterobacteriaceae sulfonamides	—

* Gram (+) β-lactamases are exoenzymes with little activity against cephalosporins, methicillin, or oxacillin. Gram (−) β-lactamases act in the periplasmic space and may have both penicillinase and cephalosporinase activity. Extended spectrum β-lactamases (ESBLs) are inducible and may not be detected by susceptibility testing. The range of ESBLs includes multiple cephalosporins. *TEM-1* is the most common of the plasmid β-lactamase genes.

† The most common vancomycin resistance genes, *vanA* and *vanB*, are found in a transposon. These have been transferred from *Enterococcus* to a multidrug resistance plasmid in *Staphylococcus aureus*. The super multidrug resistance plasmid now contains resistance genes against β-lactams, vancomycin, aminoglycosides, trimethoprim, and some disinfectants.

‡ MLS, macrolide-lincosamine-streptogramin resistance. Methylation of the 23S rRNA will impart resistance to erythromycin, lincomycin, and clindamycin.

Transfer of Drug Resistance

Conjugation

Gram-negative bacilli

Plasmid mediated, transferred by conjugation.

Staphylococcus aureus (Methicillin Resistant = MRSA)

Resistance to methicillin is chromosomal, transferred by transduction. Most of the other antibiotic resistance is transferred by plasmids.

S. aureus recently acquired the genes for vancomycin resistance (van A and van B) from *Enterococcus faecalis* via a transposon on a multi-drug resistant conjugative plasmid. In *S. aureus*, the transposon moved from the *E. faecalis* plasmid to a multi-drug resistant plasmid in *S. aureus*. The new *S. aureus* super multi-drug resistant plasmid now contains resistance genes against β-lactams, vancomycin, aminoglycosides, trimethoprim, and some disinfectants and can be transferred to other strains via conjugation.

Enterococcus faecalis and *faecium*

Resistance to vancomycin is carried on a multi-drug–resistant conjugative plasmid.

Note

- **Conjugation is the most common means of exchange of drug resistance genes (DRGs), which are encoded in plasmids.**

- Accumulation of DRGs into multiple drug resistance plasmids can be detected by the identification of characteristic flanking sequences (direct and indirect repeats).

- Plasmids can be easily exchanged between members of the same or different species, or even different genera (between normal flora in the intestine).

- Although it is the most rapid and efficient means of transfer in any bacteria, it is most common in gram (–) bacilli.

Neisseria gonorrhoeae

In *Neisseria gonorrhoeae*, two plasmids are required to transfer drug resistances. In this bacterial species, drug resistance genes are located on **nonconjugative plasmids**. These are plasmids that have lost their *tra* operon but retained *oriT*. Nonconjugative plasmids may be transferred by conjugation as long as there is another fertility factor in the same cell with a functional *tra* operon. The process is referred to as **mobilization**.

Transformation

It is difficult to mark the movement of drug resistance genes through the process of transformation, but epidemiologic studies suggest that the spread of **penicillin-binding protein mutations of *Streptococcus pneumoniae* occurs via transformation.**

Transduction

The high host cell specificity of bacteriophage limits transduction to a transfer mechanism between members of the same bacterial species. Nevertheless, in *Staphylococcus aureus* **resistance to methicillin is chromosome mediated and transferred by transduction**. In *Pseudomonas aeruginosa*, imipenem resistance is transferred from one member of the species to another during transduction by wild-type bacteriophage.

ANTIBIOTIC SUSCEPTIBILITY TESTING

Kirby-Bauer Agar Disk Diffusion Test

- Solid medium with patient's isolate swabbed on the entire plate surface.

- Multiple paper disks, each with a single dried drug placed on plate.

- Hydration and diffusion of drug sets up a concentration gradient during incubation and growth of the bacteria.

- The diameter of the zones of inhibition must be measured to determine significance.

- Advantages: relatively cheap, easy, can test numerous antibiotics on one plate, wealth of information based on clinical correlation.

- Disadvantage: qualitative. Bacterial isolate is classified as resistant, intermediate, or susceptible to each drug.

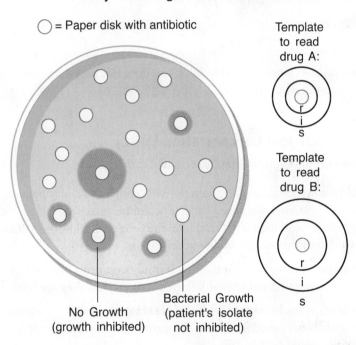

**Antibiotic Susceptibility Testing
Kirby Bauer Agar Diffusion Plate**

Figure II-3-17. The Kirby-Bauer Agar Disk Diffusion Technique

E-Test (Agar Diffusion)

E-test uses a strip of plastic marked with a gradient unique to each antibiotic that has dried antibiotic on the underside. This is placed on an agar plate already swabbed with the patient's isolate and read after incubation. It produces a µg/ml value that is much more quantitative than the results of the Kirby-Bauer.

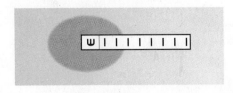

Figure II-3-18. The E Test

"Rapid" Methods

Testing for specific enzymes and a very few probes for genes determining drug resistance are currently available but still require a culture of the patient's pathogen. One current example is β-lactamase testing, shown below.

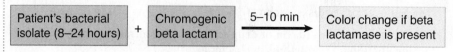

Minimal Inhibitory Concentration (MIC)

MIC measures antibiotic inhibition of bacterial multiplication.

- This is a dilution technique where **each container** (well of microtiter plate, test tube, or automated system bottle) **has one concentration of an antibiotic** with the patient's isolate. Always one control container has just the patient's isolate and growth medium with no antibiotic to make sure the inoculum is viable.

- **Lowest concentration showing no visible growth is the MIC.**

- In the example, MIC = 2 μg/ml.

- This indicates levels needed to inhibit; it does not necessarily indicate killing levels, which is done with the MBC.

Minimal Bactericidal Concentration (MBC)

This measures the antibiotic killing (bactericidal activity).

- A dilution technique starting with the MIC containers and subplating onto solid medium. Because a small inoculum is used on the plate with a large volume of medium, this dilutes the drug way below the MIC and allows determination of viability of cells.

- Important to determine for treating immunocompromised patients whose immune system cannot kill the bacteria while they are inhibited.

- **The MBC is the lowest antibiotic concentration showing no growth on subculture to media without the antibiotic.** In the example below, the MBC would be 4 μg/ml.

Minimal Inhibitory Concentration = MIC
1. Each container has one concentration of a drug.
2. Each container has identical inoculum of the patient's bacterial isolate
3. Must run a no drug control.
4. Lowest concentration showing no visible growth = MIC
   (in example, MIC = 2 µg/ml)

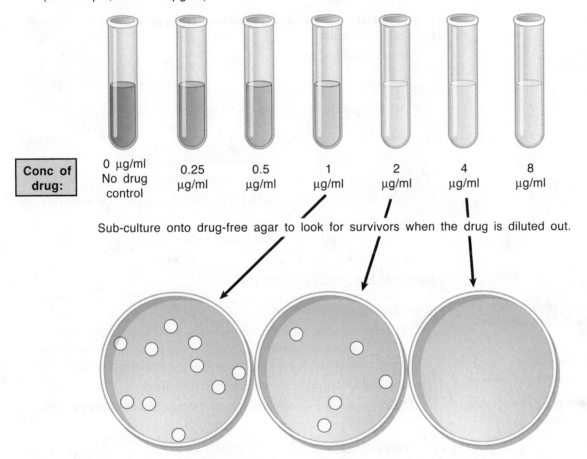

Sub-culture onto drug-free agar to look for survivors when the drug is diluted out.

Minimal Bactericidal Concentration (MBC)
(Not routinely done in many hospitals but ordered when necessary)

The lowest drug concentration showing no growth on sub-culture to media without drugs = MBC
MBC in example would be 4 µg/ml.

Figure II-3-19. The Minimal Inhibitory Concentration (MIC) and
the Minimal Bactericidal Concentration (MBC) for a Drug

Sterilization, Disinfection, Pasteurization

Sterilization: complete removal or killing of all viable organisms.

Disinfection: the removal or killing of disease-causing organisms. Compounds for use on skin: antiseptics.

Pasteurization: the rapid heating and cooling of milk designed to kill milk-borne pathogens such as *Mycobacterium bovis*, *Brucella*, and *Listeria*.

Physical Methods of Control

Heat = saturated steam

- **Autoclaving (steam under pressure): 15 lbs pressure → 121°C 15–20 min** (sterilizing)
- Dry heat—2 hr 180°C

Radiation

- UV: formation of thymine–thymine pairs on adjacent DNA bases

Filtration

- HEPA (High Efficiency Particulate Air) filters for air
- Nitrocellulose or other known pore-size filters
  - 0.45 μm filters out most bacteria except mycoplasmas and other cell-wall–less forms.
  - 0.22 μm will filter out all bacteria and spores.

Chemical Methods of Control

Agents damaging membranes

- **Detergents:** surface active compounds—most notable the quaternary ammonium compounds like benzalkonium chloride—interact with membrane through hydrophobic end disrupting membrane.
- **Alcohols:** disrupt membrane and denature proteins.
- **Phenols** and derivatives: damage membrane and denature proteins.

Agents modifying proteins

- **Chlorine:** oxidizing agent inactivating sulfhydryl-containing enzymes
- **Iodine and iodophors** (that have reduced toxicity): also oxidation of sulfhydryl-containing enzymes
- **Hydrogen peroxide:** oxidizing agent (sulfhydryl groups); catalase inactivates
- **Heavy metals:** (silver and mercury)—bind to sulfhydryl groups inhibiting enzyme activity
- **Ethylene oxide:** alkylating agent (sterilizing agent)
- **Formaldehyde** and glutaraldehyde: denatures protein and nucleic acids and alkylates amino and hydroxyl groups on both

Modification of nucleic acids

- **Dyes:** like crystal violet and malachite green whose positively charged molecule binds to the negatively charged phosphate groups on the nucleic acids

In a Nutshell

The choice of disinfectant depends on the **outer surface** of the infectious agent.

- Use **membrane-denaturing** compounds on **enveloped** viruses
- Use **protein-denaturing** compounds on **naked capsid** viruses

Medically Important Viruses 4

Learning Objectives

- ❑ Demonstrate understanding of structure, morphology, and replication of medically important viruses
- ❑ Answer questions related to patterns of infection, resistance, and treatment of DNA viruses, positive-stranded RNA viruses, negative-stranded RNA viruses, double-stranded RNA viruses, onco-viruses, and prions
- ❑ Explain information related to viral hepatitis

STRUCTURE AND MORPHOLOGY

DNA or RNA*	+	Structural proteins (capsomers, etc.)	=	Nucleocapsid	=	Naked capsid virus
Enzymes e.g., polymerase						

Nucleocapsid	+	Host membrane with viral-specified glycoproteins (critical for infectiousness of viral progeny)	=	Enveloped virus

Figure II-4-1. Basic Virion

Bridge to Biochemistry

Positive-sense = coding strand
Negative-sense = template strand

*Positive-sense RNA = (+)RNA (can be used itself as mRNA)

*Negative-sense RNA = (–)RNA

- Complementary to mRNA
- Cannot be used as mRNA
- Requires virion-associated, RNA-dependent RNA polymerase (as part of the mature virus)

VIRAL STRUCTURE

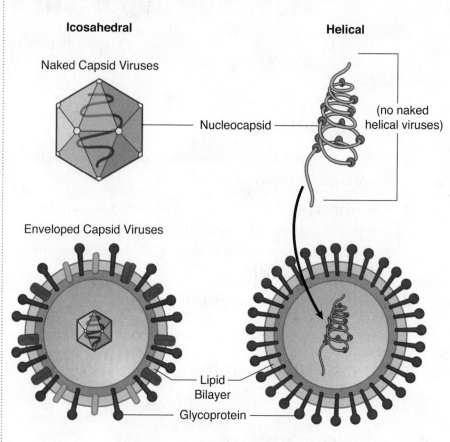

Figure II-4-2. Morphology of Viruses

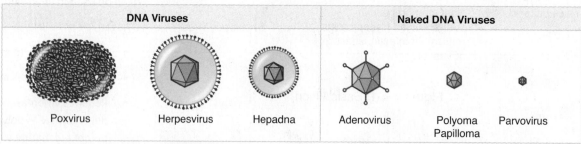

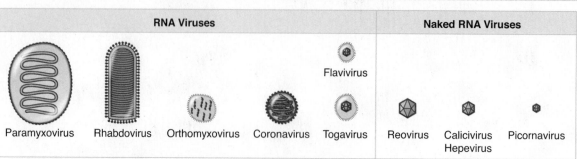

Figure II-4-3. Relative Sizes and Shapes of Different Viruses

VIRAL REPLICATION

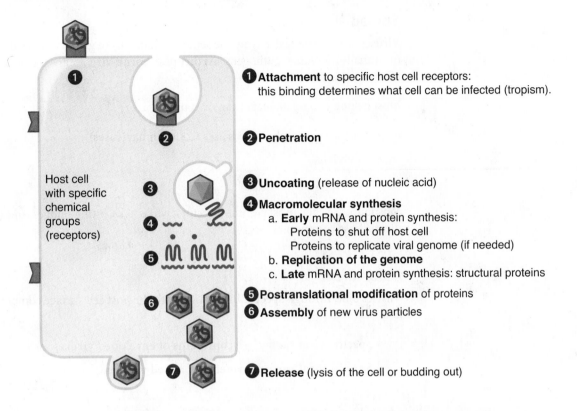

Figure II-4-4. Generalized Viral Replication Scheme

The following are drugs that target viral replication:

Number from Figure Above	Stages of Viral Replication	Examples of Drugs that Target	Mechanism of Action	Use to Treat
1	Attachment	Maraviroc	CCR5 antagonist	HIV
2	Penetration	Enfuviritide	Fusion inhibitor	HIV
3	Uncoating (no longer used; only had activity against influenza A)	Amantadine/ rimantadine	Blocks uncoating via M2 protein	Influenza
4	Macromolecular synthesis (just examples; largest list of antivirals)	Acyclovir. zidovudine, etc.	Nucleic acid synthesis	Many
5	Post-translational modification of proteins	Ritonavir	Protease inhibitor	HIV
6	Assembly	N/A	N/A	N/A
7	Release	Oseltamavir	Neuraminidase inhibitor	Influenza
Retrovirus specific	Integration	Raltegravir	Integrase inhibitor	HIV

IMPORTANT STEPS IN VIRAL REPLICATION

Spread

Viruses are spread basically by the same mechanisms (e.g., respiratory droplets or sexually) as other pathogens. **Arthropod-borne** viruses are referred to as **arboviruses**.

Most belong to 3 formal taxonomic groups:

- Togavirus encephalitis viruses (a.k.a. alphaviruses)
- Flavivirus
- Bunyavirus

Mosquitoes are the most common vectors, while ticks, biting midges, and sand-flies are less common.

Attachment

Viruses bind through specific interaction with the host cell surface components **and**

- Specific **viral surface glycoproteins** of **enveloped viruses**, or
- Specific **viral surface proteins** of **naked viruses**.

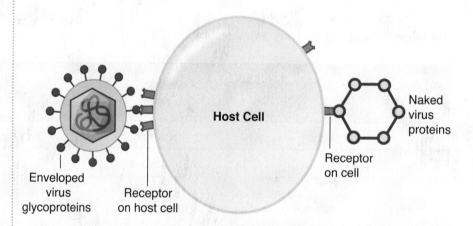

Figure II-4-5. Attachment

These **interactions** (and the distribution of the receptors) **determine viral host range** (e.g., horses or humans) and **tissue specificity** (e.g., liver versus heart; **tropism**).

Table II-4-1. Specific Viral Receptors to Know

Virus	Target Cell	Receptor on Host Cell
HIV	Th cells, macrophages, microglia	CD4 plus CCR5 or CXCR4
EBV	B lymphocytes	CD21 = CR2
Rabies	Neurons	Acetylcholine receptor
Rhinovirus	Respiratory epithelial cells	ICAM-1

Table II-4-2. Difference Between Naked and Enveloped Viruses

	Naked	Enveloped
Inactivated by heat, detergents, acid and organic solvents like ether and alcohols?	No	Yes, since the lipid envelope holds the glycoproteins essential for attachment. Dissolving the envelope inhibits attachment and therefore uptake.

Viral Entry Into Host Cell

Viral entry takes place by receptor-mediated endocytosis, uptake via coated pits, or for those enveloped viruses with fusion proteins via fusion of the cell membrane with the viral envelope.

Replication of the Genomic Nucleic Acid (NA)

Progeny viruses have a nucleic acid sequence **identical to the parent virus.** All single-stranded **RNA viruses replicate through a replicative intermediate.**

Table II-4-3.   Strategy for Viral Genome Replication

Virus Type	Parental Genome	Intermediate Replicative Form	Progeny Genome
Most dsDNA viruses	dsDNA		dsDNA
Hepatitis B	dsDNA	ssRNA →	dsDNA
Most +ssRNA viruses	+ssRNA	−ssRNA	+ssRNA
Retroviruses	+ssRNA →	dsDNA	+ssRNA
−ssRNA viruses	−ssRNA	+ssRNA	−ssRNA

+ means an RNA which can serve as mRNA (or for the retroviruses has the same sequence.)
→ = RNA-dependent DNA polymerase
- Called reverse transcriptase for the retroviruses.
- Called the DNA polymerase for hepatitis B.
- Both actually make the first strand of the DNA using the RNA original and then break down the RNA and use the single strand of DNA as template to make the second strand.

Release of Viruses

Naked viruses lyse the host cells. Thus, there are **no persistent productive infections** with naked viruses (only cytolytic productive or latent infections).

Release of enveloped viruses: Budding leads to cell senescence (aging), but cells may produce a low level of virus for years as occurs in chronic hepatitis B.

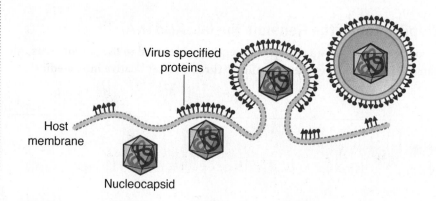

Figure II-4-7. Release of Enveloped Virus

The glycoproteins on the enveloped viral surface are essential for viral infectivity.

PATTERNS OF VIRAL INFECTION

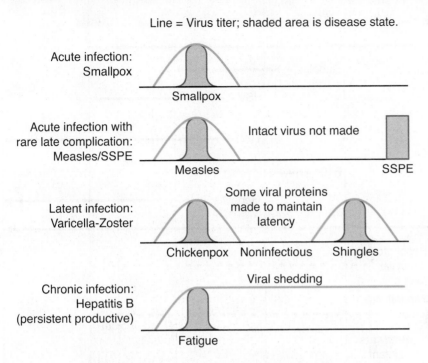

Figure II-4-8. Time Courses of Viral Infections

Table II-4-4. Cellular Effects

Infection Type	Virus Production	Fate of Cell
Abortive	−	No effect: No virus is made nor is latency established; Virus is terminated
Cytolytic Naked viruses lyse host cells. Some enveloped viruses also are cytolytic, killing the cell in the process of replication.	+	Lysis of the host cell (death)
Persistent Productive (enveloped viruses) Latent Transforming	+ − ±	Senescence (premature aging) No overt damage to host; no production of virus, but viral production may be turned on later. Immortalization

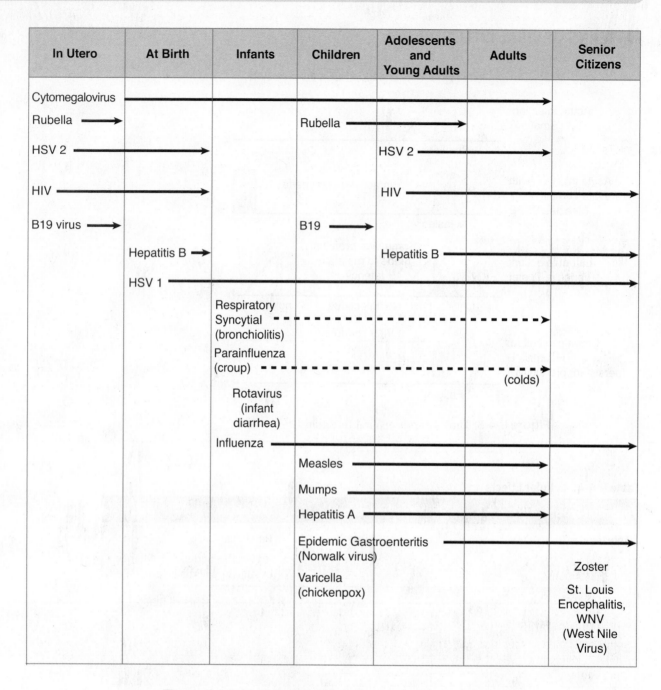

Figure II-4-9. Most Common Age Groups for Viral Infection

VIRAL HEPATITIS

Symptoms of Hepatitis

Fever, malaise, headache, anorexia, vomiting, dark urine, jaundice.

Table II-4-5. Hepatitis Viruses (Hepatotropic)

	Hepatitis A	Hepatitis B	Hepatitis C	Hepatitis D	Hepatitis E
	"Infectious" (HAV)	"Serum" (HBV)	"Post-transfusion Non A, Non B" (HCV)	"Delta" (HDV)	"Enteric" (HEV)
Family	Picornavirus	Hepadnavirus	Flavivirus	N/A	Hepevirus
Features	RNA Naked Capsid	DNA Enveloped	RNA Enveloped	Viroid Circular RNA Enveloped	RNA Naked capsid
Transmission	Fecal-oral	Parenteral, sexual	Parenteral, sexual	Parenteral, sexual	Fecal-oral
Disease presentation	Mild acute No chronic No sequellae	Acute; occasionally severe Chronic: 5–10% adults 90% infants Primary hepatocellular carcinoma, cirrhosis	Acute is usually subclinical 80% become chronic Primary hepatocellular carcinoma, cirrhosis	Co-infection with HBV: occasionally severe Superinfection with HBV: often severe Cirrhosis, fulminant hepatitis	Normal patients mild Pregnant patients severe Chronic in IC patients
Mortality	<0.5%	1–2%	0.5–1%	High to very high	Normal patients 1–2% Third-trimester pregnant patients 25%
Diagnosis	IgM to HAV	HBsAg, IgM to HBcAg	Antibody to HCV, ELISA	Hepatitis D Ab, HBsAg	Antibody to HEV, ELISA
Treatment	Symptomatic	IFN-α+RTI (NT analogs)	Elbasavir/ grazoprevir* Ledipasvir/ sofosbuvir	N/A	Mostly symptomatic**

*ribavirin, $\pm$pegylated IFN-α for patients with cirrhosis

**ribavirin and pegylated IFN-α can be used for chronic

Note: Hepatitis also may occur in other viral diseases (e.g., CMV and EBV infections, congenital rubella, yellow fever).

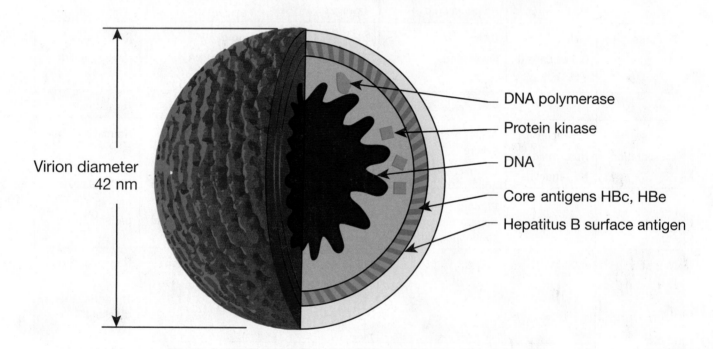

Virion diameter
42 nm

DNA polymerase

Protein kinase

DNA

Core antigens HBc, HBe

Hepatitus B surface antigen

Figure II-4-10 Dane Particle

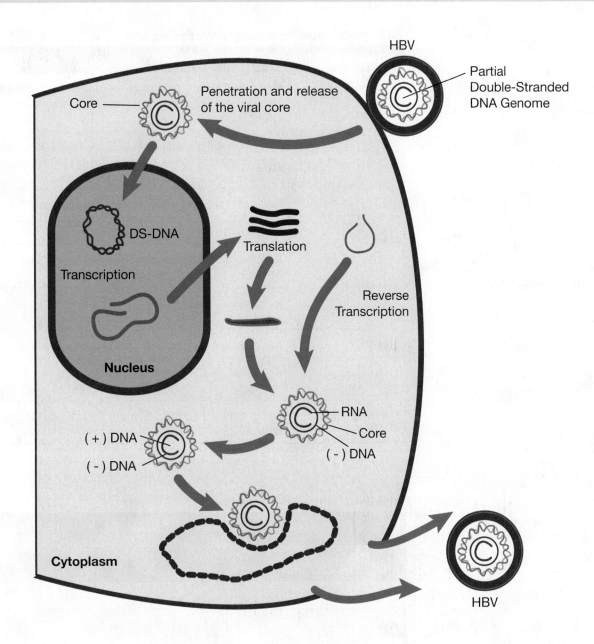

Figure II-4-11 Hepatitis B Virus Replication

Table II-4-6. Hepatitis B Terminology and Markers

Abbreviation	Name and Description
HBV	Hepatitis B virus, a hepadnavirus (enveloped, partially double-stranded DNA virus); Dane particle = infectious HBV
HBsAg	Antigen found on surface of HBV; also found on spheres and filaments in patient's blood: positive during acute disease; continued presence indicates carrier state
HBsAb	Antibody to HBsAg; provides immunity to hepatitis B
HBcAg	Antigen associated with core of HBV
HBcAb	Antibody to HBcAg; positive during window phase; IgM HBcAb is an indicator of recent disease
HBeAg	A second, different antigenic determinant on the HBV core; important indicator of transmissibility
HBeAb	Antibody to e antigen; indicates low transmissibility
Delta agent	Small RNA virus with HBsAg envelope; defective virus that replicates only in HBV-infected cells
Window period	Period between end of detection of HBsAg and beginning of detection HBsAb

Table II-4-7. Hepatitis B Serology

	HBsAg HBeAg* HBV-DNA	HBcAb IgM	HBcAb IgG	HBeAb	HBsAb
Acute infection	+	+	−	−	−
Window period	−	+/−	+	+	−
Prior infection	−	−	+	+	+
Immunization	−	−	−	−	+
Chronic infection	+	−	+	+/−	−

*HBeAg: correlates with viral proliferation and infectivity

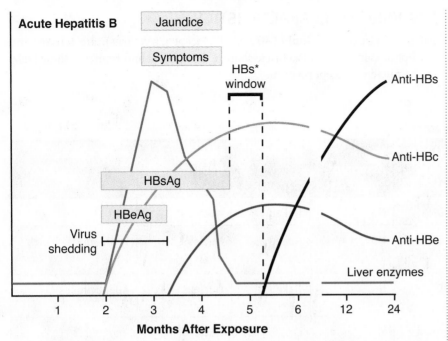

Acute Hepatitis B

*The window is the time between the disappearance of the HBsAg and before HBsAb is detected.

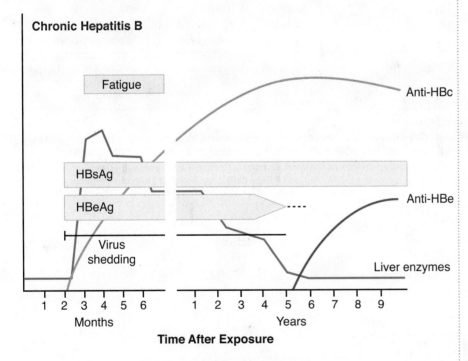

Chronic Hepatitis B

Figure II-4-11. Hepatitis B

DNA VIRUSES: CHARACTERISTICS

All DNA viruses are **double-stranded** (except parvovirus); are **icosahedral** (except poxvirus which is a brick-shaped "complex"); and **replicate their DNA in the nucleus** (except poxvirus).

Table II-4-8. DNA Viruses*

Virus Family	DNA type	Virion-Associated Polymerase	Envelope	DNA Replicates in:	Major Viruses
Parvovirus	ssDNA	No	Naked	Nucleus	B19
Papillomavirus Polyomavirus	dsDNA, circular	No	Naked	Nucleus	Papilloma, Polyoma
Adenovirus	dsDNA, linear	No	Naked	Nucleus	Adenoviruses
Hepadnavirus	Partially dsDNA, circular	Yes***	Enveloped	Nucleus, RNA intermediate	Hepatitis B
Herpes virus	dsDNA, linear	No	Enveloped (nuclear)	Nucleus; virus assembled in nucleus	HSV, Varicella-zoster, Epstein-Barr, Cytomegalovirus
Poxvirus	dsDNA, linear	Yes**	Enveloped	Cytoplasm	Variola, Vaccinia, Molluscum contagiosum

* Mnemonic: Pardon Papa As He Has Pox

** **Poxviruses** have a **virion-associated transcriptase** (DNA dependent RNA polymerase), so it can transcribe its own DNA in the cytoplasm and make all of the enzymes and factors necessary for replication of the poxvirus DNA in the cytoplasm.

*** Hepadnaviruses: DNA viruses that carry a DNA polymerase with reverse transcriptase activity to synthesize an RNA intermediate that is then used to make the genomic DNA. Hepatitis B is partially double-stranded with one complete strand.

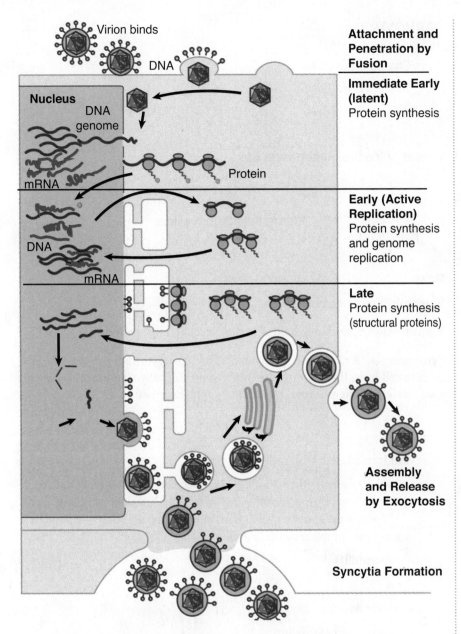

Figure II-4-12. DNA Virus: Life Cycle of Herpes

PARVOVIRIDAE

Virus Characteristics

- ssDNA virus, linear
- Naked, icosahedral

Viruses of Medical Importance: B19

Figure II-4-13. Parvovirus

B19

Reservoir: human respiratory tract

Transmission: respiratory route, fomites, vertical transmission

Pathogenesis: B19 infects immature (cycling) erythroid progenitor cells, causing cell lysis; the resulting **anemia** is only clinically significant in patients with **sickle-cell anemia**, and may result in **aplastic crisis**

Diseases

- Children/adults:
  - Fifth disease, erythema infectiosum, slapped cheek fever: 7–10 day incubation; nonspecific "flu-like" symptoms followed by raised, indurated facial rash; rash and arthralgias (mostly adults) are due to immune complexes in skin and joints
  - Myocarditis
- Fetus
  - Severe anemia
  - Congestive heart failure
  - Hydrops fetalis
  - Spontaneous abortion

Diagnosis: serology and molecular analysis

Treatment: supportive care

Key Vignette Clues

B19

- School-aged child with fever and indurated facial rash
- Pregnant woman with flu-like symptoms → hydrops fetalis or spontaneous abortion

PAPILLOMAVIRIDAE

Virus Characteristics

- dsDNA virus, circular
- Naked, icosahedral

Viruses of Medical Importance

- Human papilloma virus (HPV)

Figure II-4-14. Papillomavirus

Human Papilloma Virus (HPV)

Distinguishing Characteristics

- Over 100 serotypes
- Different serotypes are associated with different clinical presentations

Reservoir: human skin and genitals

Transmission: direct contact, fomites

Pathogenesis

- Virus infects basal layer of the skin and mucous membranes
- Hyperkeratosis leads to the formation of the "wart"
- Malignancy may result: **E6 and E7 inhibit tumor-suppressor genes p53 and Rb, respectively.**

Diseases

- Cutaneous warts
  - **Common warts** (serotypes 2 and 4) are predominantly found on hands and fingers
  - **Plantar warts** (serotype 1) are predominantly found on soles of feet; tend to be deeper and more painful
- Anogenital warts (Condylomata acuminata)
  - **Over 90% are serotypes 6 and 11 (benign)**
  - Also cause laryngeal papillomas in infants and sexually active adults
  - **Serotypes 16 and 18** are preneoplastic (cervical intraepithelial neoplasia or CIN), **31, 33, 35, 45, 52, 58** (16 and 18 >70% of cases)

Key Vignette Clues

HPV

- Warts
- Cervical intraepithelial neoplasia
- Biopsy or Pap smear—koilocytic cells

- Malignancy
  - Viral genes E6 and E7 inactivate tumor-suppresor genes
  - 95% of CIN cases contain HPV DNA
  - Also cause anal, vaginal, vulvar, penile, and laryngeal cancer

Diagnosis

- Cutaneous: clinical grounds
- Genital: finding of koilocytic cells (cells with perinuclear cytoplasmic vacuolization and nuclear enlargement) in Pap smear
- In situ DNA probes and PCR can be used to confirm any diagnosis and type the HPV strain involved

Treatment

- Antiviral: cidofovir
- Surgical: cryotherapy, laser therapy, excisional
- Chemical: podophyllin, trichloroacetic acid, 5-fluorouracil
- Immune-mediated: imiquimod, interferon-alpha
- Recurrence rates 30–70% within 6 months

Prevention: safe sex; vaccines composed of HPV capsid proteins produced by recombinant DNA technology: Gardasil™ quadrivalent (6, 11, 16, 18), Gardasil™ 9 (6, 11, 16, 18, 31, 33, 45, 52, 58), Cervarix™ (16, 18)

POLYOMAVIRIDAE

Table II-4-9. Summary of Polyomaviridae

Virus	Reservoir/ Transmission	Pathogenesis	Disease	Diagnosis	Treatment
BK	Respiratory	Latent infection in kidney	Renal disease in AIDS patients	ELISA, PCR	Supportive
JC	Respiratory	Infection in oligodendrocytes = demyelination	Progressive multifocal leukoencephalopathy (PML) in AIDS and transplant patients	ELISA, PCR	Supportive

ADENOVIRIDAE

Virus Characteristics

- dsDNA, nonenveloped
- Hexons, pentons, and fibers

Viruses of Medical Importance

- Adenovirus
- Over 50 serotypes
- Subgroups A–F

Adenovirus

Reservoir: ubiquitous in humans and animals

Transmission: respiratory, fecal-oral, direct contact

Pathogenesis

- Penton fibers act as hemagglutinin
- Purified penton fibers are toxic to cells
- **Lytic, latent**, or **transforming**: virus is lytic in permissive cells and can be chronic or oncogenic in nonpermissive hosts; the adenoviruses are standard example of permissive host (where virus is produced) and nonpermissive host (where virus is not produced but transformed)

Disease

- Acute respiratory disease (ARD) and pneumonia: spring and winter peak incidence; children, young military recruits, college students serotypes 4 and 7; cough, conjunctivitis, fever, pharyngitis, hoarseness
- Pharyngoconjunctivitis: swimming pool conjunctivitis, pink eye; fever, sore throat, coryza, red eyes; nonpurulent
- Acute hemorrhagic cystitis: mostly boys age 5–15; dysuria, hematuria
- Gastroenteritis: daycare (not as common as rotavirus); serotypes 40 and 41
- Myocarditis
- Transplant patients

Diagnosis: serology; ELISA

Treatment: supportive care for otherwise healthy patients; cidofovir and alpha globulins for immunocompromised or severely diseased

Prevention: live, nonattenuated vaccine

Key Vignette Clues

Adenovirus

- Young adults: ARD
- Swimmers and shipyard workers: nonpurulent conjunctivitis
- Daycare: viral gastroenteritis

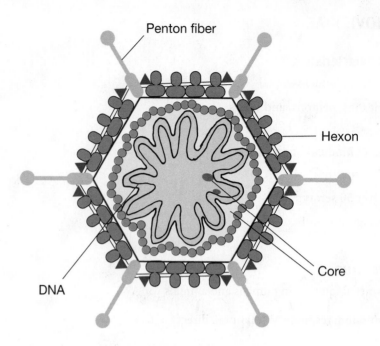

Figure II-4-15. Adenovirus

HEPADNAVIRIDAE (see previous discussion)

HERPESVIRIDAE

Virus Characteristics

- Large dsDNA
- Enveloped, icosahedral
- Derives envelope from nuclear membrane
- **Intranuclear inclusion bodies**
- **Establishes latency**

Viruses of Medical Importance

- Herpes simplex virus 1 and 2 (HSV)
- Varicella-zoster virus (VZV)
- Epstein-Barr virus (EBV)
- Cytomegalovirus (CMV)
- Human herpesvirus 6 (HHV-6)
- Human herpesvirus 8 (HHV-8)

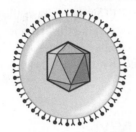

Figure II-4-16. Herpesvirus

HSV-1 and HSV-2

Reservoir: human mucosa and ganglia

Transmission: close personal contact (i.e., kissing, sexual contact)

Pathogenesis: HSV establishes infection in the mucosal epithelial cells and leads to formation of vesicles; virus travels up the ganglion to establish lifelong latent infection; stress triggers reactivation of virus in nerve and recurrence of vesicles

Diseases: Rule of thumb is that **HSV-1** infections generally **occur above the waist** and **HSV-2** infections generally **occur below the waist.**

HSV-1

- Gingivostomatitis and cold sores: blister-like lesions on oral mucosa; **latent in trigeminal ganglion**

- Keratoconjunctivitis: generally with lid swelling and vesicles; possible dendritic ulcers; if untreated and repeat attacks, possible blindness

- Encephalitis: fever, headache, confusion; **focal temporal lesions** and perivascular cuffing; if untreated, 70% mortality rate; **most common cause of viral encephalitis in U.S.**

HSV-2

- Genital infections: painful genital vesicles; systemic effects include fever, malaise, myalgia; **latency in sacral nerve ganglia**

- Neonatal herpes: infection occurs during passage through infected birth canal; usually **severe**, i.e., disseminated with liver involvement and high mortality; encephalitis, high mortality; skin, eyes, mouth)

Diagnosis

- Oral lesions: clinical

- Encephalitis: PCR on CSF; large numbers of RBCs in CSF

- Genital infections: Tzank smear to show formation of multinucleated giant cells and Cowdry type A intranuclear inclusions has been largely replaced by immunofluorescent staining, which can distinguish HSV-1 from HSV-2

Key Vignette Clues

HSV-1 and HSV-2

- Cold sores/genital vesicles

- Keratoconjunctivitis

- Meningoencephalitis/ encephalitis

- Neonatal disseminated/encephalitis

- Tzanck smear, Cowdry type A inclusion bodies

Treatment: Acyclovir, a nucleoside analog that is only activated in cells infected with HSV-1, HSV-2 or VZV. (This is because the virus thymidine kinase is required to activate the drug by placing the first phosphate on the drug, followed by the phosphorylation via cellular enzymes.) In cases of acyclovir resistance (caused by a mutation in the thymidine kinase), use famciclovir, valacyclovir, or penciclovir.

Varicella Zoster Virus (VZV)

Reservoir: human mucosa and nerves

Transmission: respiratory droplets

Pathogenesis: VZV enters the respiratory tract → replicates in local lymph nodes → primary viremia → spleen and liver → secondary viremia → skin (rash) → **latent in the dorsal root ganglia.** Reactivation of virus due to stress or immunocompromise causes vesicular lesions and severe nerve pain.

Diseases

- Chickenpox
  - Fever, pharyngitis, malaise, rhinitis
  - **Asynchronous rash**
  - One of 5 "classic" childhood exanthems; less common due to vaccination
- Shingles
  - Zoster
  - Pain and vesicles restricted to one dermatome
  - Fifth or sixth decade of life
  - **Reactivation of latent infection**

Diagnosis

- Tzanck smear—Cowdry type A, intranuclear inclusions
- Antigen detection by PCR

Treatment

- Healthy adults with shingles—oral acyclovir
- Immunocompromised—IV acyclovir
- Aspirin contraindicated due to association with Reye syndrome

Prevention

- Live, attenuated vaccine, booster for 60-year-old to prevent shingles
- VZIG (varicella-zoster immunoglobulin) for postexposure prophylaxis of the immunocompromised

Key Vignette Clues

VZV

- Chickenpox: unvaccinated child with asynchronous rash
- Shingles: elderly with unilateral vesicular rash that follows dermatome
- Tzank smear with Cowdry type A intranuclear inclusions and syncytia

Epstein-Barr Virus (EBV)

Reservoir: humans

Transmission: saliva, 90% of adult population is seropositive

Pathogenesis

- Virus infects nasopharyngeal epithelial cells, salivary and lymphoid tissues → latent infection of B cells (EBV binds to CD21 and acts as a B-cell mitogen) → results in production of atypical reactive T cells (Downey cells), which may constitute up to 70% of WBC count

- Heterophile antibodies are produced (due to B cell mitogenesis)

Diseases

- Heterophile-positive mononucleosis, "kissing disease": fatigue, fever, sore throat, lymphadenopathy, splenomegaly; **latency in B cells**

- Lymphoproliferative disease: occurs in immunocompromised patients; T cells can't control B-cell growth

- Hairy oral leukoplakia: hyperproliferation of lingual epithelial cells; occurs in AIDS patients

Malignancies

- Burkitt lymphoma: cancer of the maxilla, mandible, abdomen; Africa; malaria cofactor; AIDS patients; translocation juxtaposes c-myc onco-gene to a very active promoter such as mmunoglobulin gene promoter

- Nasopharyngeal carcinoma: Asia (most common cancer in southern China); tumor cells of epithelial origin

- Hodgkin and non-Hodgkin lymphoma

Diagnosis: heterophile-antibody positive (IgM antibodies that recognize Paul-Bunnell antigen on sheep and bovine RBCs)

Treatment: symptomatic, for uncomplicated mononucleosis

Cytomegalovirus (CMV)

Cytomegalovirus **Reservoir:** humans

Transmission: saliva, sexual, parenteral, in utero

Pathogenesis: CMV infects salivary gland epithelial cells and establishes a persistent infection in fibroblasts, epithelial cells, and macrophages; **latency in mononuclear cells**

Disease

- Cytomegalic inclusion disease: **most common in utero infection in U.S.**; ranges from infected with no obvious defects to severe disease characterized by jaundice, hepatosplenomegaly, thrombocytic purpura ("blueberry muffin baby"), pneumonitis, and CNS damage to death

Key Vignette Clues

EBV

- Young adult with fever, lymphadenopathy, splenomegaly

- Downey type II atypical T lymphocytes reach 70% in blood

- Heterophile (monospot) positive

Key Vignette Clues

CMV

- Heterophile-negative mononucleosis in children and adults

- Neonate with jaundice, hepatosplenomegaly, thrombocytic purpura

- Owl-eye intranuclear inclusion bodiesOwl-eye intranuclear inclusion bodies in biopsy

- Mononucleosis (children and adults): heterophile-negative mononucleosis
- Immunocompromised patients
  - Interstitial pneumonitis to severe systemic infection (due to reactivation in transplanted organ or AIDS patient)
  - CMV retinitis common in AIDS patients
  - GI disease common in AIDS patients

Diagnosis

- Owl-eye inclusion ("sight-o-megalo-virus") in biopsy material and urine
- Basophilic intranuclear inclusions
- Serology, DNA detection, virus culture

Treatment: supportive for healthy patients; ganciclovir/foscarnet ± human immunoglobulin for immunocompromised (AIDS and transplant patients) (resistance to ganciclovir through hL97 gene)

Prevention: safe sex; screening of blood and organ donors

Key Vignette Clues

HHV-6

Infant with fever → lacy body rash

HHV-6/7

Reservoir: humans

Transmission: respiratory droplets

Pathogenesis: replicates in peripheral blood mononuclear cells

Disease: roseola (exanthem subitum); fever for 3–5 days followed by lacy body rash

Diagnosis: clinical

Treatment: symptomatic

Key Vignette Clues

HHV-8

AIDS patient with sarcoma

HHV-8 (Kaposi sarcoma-associated herpesvirus KSHV)

Reservoir: humans

Transmission: sexual contact, saliva, vertical, transplantation

Pathogenesis: gene turns on vascular endothelial growth factor (VEGF); plays direct role in development of Kaposi sarcoma; latent in B cells and glandular epithelial cells

Disease: Kaposi sarcoma

Diagnosis: clinical; serology, PCR

Treatment: none

Table II-4-10. Herpesvirus Infections

Virus	Site of Primary Infection	Clinical Presentation of Primary Infection	Site of Latency	Clinical Presentation of Recurrent Infection
HSV-1	Mucosa	Gingivostomatitis, keratoconjunctivitis, pharyngitis	Trigeminal ganglia	Cold sores
HSV-2	Mucosa	Genital herpes, neonatal herpes	Sacral ganglia	Genital herpes
VZV	Mucosa	Chickenpox	Dorsal root ganglia	Shingles (zoster)
EBV	Mucosal epithelial cells, B cells	Mononucleosis (heterophile ⊕)	B cells	Asymptomatic shedding of virus
CMV	Mononuclear cells, epithelial cells	Mononucleosis (heterophile −), cytomegalic inclusion disease	Mononuclear cells	Asymptomatic shedding of virus
HHV-6	Mononuclear cells	Roseola infantum	Mononuclear cells	Asymptomatic shedding of virus
HHV-8	Dermis	Fever, rash	B cells, glandular epithelial cells	Kaposi sarcoma

POXVIRIDAE

Virus Characteristics

- Large dsDNA, enveloped
- Complex morphology
- Replicates in the cytoplasm
- Potential biowarfare agent

Viruses of Medical Importance

- Variola
- Vaccinia (vaccine strain)
- Molluscum contagiosum
- Orf
- Monkeypox

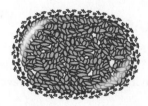

Figure II-4-17. Poxvirus

Variola/Smallpox

- Virus extinct
- Synchronous rash begins in mouth → face and body
- Guarnieri bodies (intracytoplasmic inclusions)

Variola/Smallpox

Reservoir: humans; Variola has 1 serotype making eradication (1979) possible

Transmission: respiratory route

Pathogenesis

- Via inhalation, the virus enters the upper respiratory tract and disseminates via lymphatics → viremia
- After a secondary viremia, the virus infects all dermal tissues and internal organs
- Classic "pocks"

Disease

- 5–17 day incubation
- Prodrome of flu-like illness for 2–4 days
- Prodrome followed by rash, which begins in mouth and spreads to the face, arms and legs, hands, and feet and can cover entire body within 24 hours
- All vesicles are in same stage of development (synchronous rash)

Diagnosis: clinical; Guarnieri bodies found in infected cells (intracytoplasmic)

Treatment: supportive care

Prevention: live, attenuated vaccine

Key Vignette Clues

Molluscum Contagiosum

- Young adult (wrestling, swim team)
- Umbilicated warts
- Eosinophilic cytoplasmic inclusion bodies

Molluscum contagiosum

Reservoir: humans

Transmission: direct contact (sexual) and fomites

Pathogenesis: replication in dermis

Disease: single or multiple (<20) benign, wart-like tumors; molluscum bodies in central caseous material (eosinophilic cytoplasmic inclusion bodies)

Diagnosis: clinical (warts are umbilicated); eosinophilic cytoplasmic inclusion bodies

Treatment: self-limiting in healthy persons; ritonavir, cidofovir for immunocompromised

RNA VIRUSES: CHARACTERISTICS

All RNA viruses are single-stranded (ss) except Reovirus. ss(−)RNA viruses carry RNA-dependent RNA polymerase. A virion-associated polymerase is also carried by Reovirus, Arenavirus, and Retrovirus (reverse transcriptase).

Most RNA are enveloped; the **only naked ones** are Picornavirus, Calicivirus and Hepevirus, and Reovirus.

Some RNA viruses are segmented, i.e., there are different genes on different pieces of RNA:

- **R**eovirus
- **O**rthomyxovirus
- **B**unyavirus
- **A**renavirus

POSITIVE-STRANDED RNA VIRUSES

Table II-4-11. Positive-Stranded RNA Viruses*

Virus Family	RNA Structure	Virion-Associated Polymerase	Envelope	Shape	Multiplies in	Major Viruses
Calicivirus	ss(+)RNA Linear	No polymerase	Naked	Icosahedral	Cytoplasm	Norwalk agent Noro-like virus
Hepevirus	ss(+)RNA Linear	No polymerase	Naked	Icosahedral	Cytoplasm	Hepatitis E
Picornavirus	ss(+)RNA Linear	No polymerase	Naked	Icosahedral	Cytoplasm	Polio** ECHO Enteroviruses Rhino Coxsackie Hepatitis A
Flavivirus	ss(+)RNA Linear	No polymerase	Enveloped	Icosahedral	Cytoplasm	Yellow fever Dengue St. Louis encephalitis Hepatitis C West Nile virus
Togavirus	ss(+)RNA Linear	No polymerase	Enveloped	Icosahedral	Cytoplasm	Rubella WEE, EEE Venezuelan encephalitis
Coronavirus	ss(+)RNA Linear	No polymerase	Enveloped	Helical	Cytoplasm	Coronaviruses SARS-CoV
Retrovirus	Diploid ss (+) RNA Linear	RNA dep. DNA polymerase	Enveloped	Icosahedral or truncated conical	Nucleus	HIV HTLV Sarcoma

*Mnemonic: (+)RNA Viruses: <u>C</u>all <u>H</u>enry <u>P</u>ico and <u>F</u>lo <u>T</u>o <u>C</u>ome <u>R</u>ightaway
**Mnemonic: Picornaviruses: <u>PEE</u> <u>Co</u> <u>Rn</u> <u>A</u> Viruses
Polio, <u>E</u>ntero, <u>E</u>cho, <u>C</u>oxsackie, <u>R</u>hino, Hep <u>A</u>

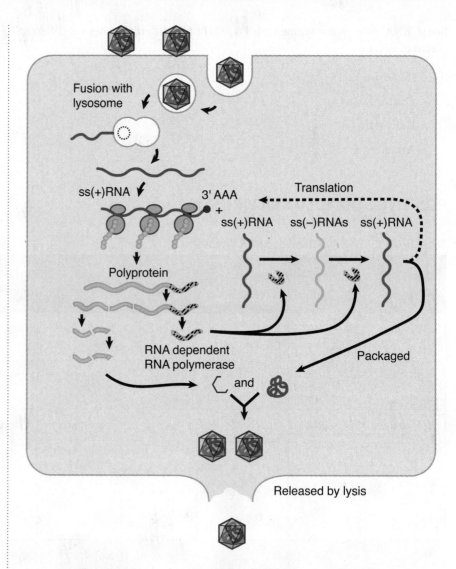

Figure II-4-18. Positive-Sense RNA Virus Life Cycle

CALICIVIRIDAE

Family Characteristics

- Naked, icosahedral
- Positive-sense ssRNA

Viruses of Medical Importance

- Norwalk virus (Norovirus)
- Noro-like virus

Norwalk Virus

Reservoir: human GI tract

Transmission: fecal-oral route, contaminated food and water

Disease: acute gastroenteritis

- Watery; no blood or pus in stools
- Nausea, vomiting, diarrhea
- 60% of all nonbacterial gastroenteritis in U.S.
- Outbreak of viral gastroenteritis in cruise ships attributed to Norovirus

Diagnosis: RIA, ELISA

Treatment: self-limiting; no specific antiviral treatment

Prevention: handwashing

HEPEVIRIDAE

- Naked, icosahedral
- Positive-sense ssRNA

Hepatitis E Virus (previously discussed)

PICORNAVIRIDAE

Family Characteristics

- Small, naked, icosahedral
- Positive-sense ssRNA
- Summer/fall peak incidence
- Resistant to alcohol, detergents (naked capsid)
- Divided into genera:
  - **Enteroviruses**: fecal-oral transmission, do **not** cause diarrhea, peak age <9 years, stable at pH 3
  - **Rhinoviruses**: not stable under acidic conditions, growth at 33°C
  - **Heparnavirus**

Figure II-4-19. Picornavirus

Viruses of Medical Importance

- Enteroviruses (acid-stable): polio virus; coxsackie virus A; coxsackie virus B; D68; echoviruses
- Rhinoviruses (acid labile)
- Heparnaviruses: HAV

Table II-4-12. Summary of Picornaviridae

Virus	Transmission	Pathogenesis	Diseases	Diagnosis	Treatment/Prevention
Enteroviruses					
Polio	Fecal-oral	Virus targets anterior horn motor neurons	Asymptomatic to fever of unknown origin; aseptic meningitis; paralytic polio (flaccid asymmetric paralysis, no sensory loss)	Serology (virus absent from CSF)	No specific antiviral/live vaccine (Sabin); killed vaccine (Salk)
		Neural fatigue	Post-Polio Syndrome	Patient with polio decades earlier, progressive muscle atrophy	
Coxsackie A	Fecal-oral	Fecal-oral spread with potential for dissemination to other organs; often asymptomatic with viral shedding	Hand, foot, and mouth (A16); herpangina; aseptic meningitis; acute lymphoglandular pharyngitis; common cold	Virus isolation from throat, stool, or CSF	No specific treatment/handwashing
Coxsackie B	Fecal-oral	As above	Bornholm disease (devil's grip); aseptic meningitis; severe systemic disease of newborns; **myocarditis**	As above	No specific/handwashing
D68	Fecal-oral, respiratory	Invade mucosa, lymphatics; potential spread to CNS	Motor-neuron disease; respiratory diseases	Serology/RT-PCR	No specific/IVIG/handwashing
Echoviruses	Fecal-oral	As above	Fever and rash of unknown origin; aseptic meningitis	As above	No specific/handwashing
Rhinovirus					
Rhinovirus	Respiratory	Acid labile; grows at 33°C; over 100 serotypes	Common cold; #1 cause, peak summer/fall	Clinical	No specific/handwashing
Heparnavirus					
HAV	Fecal-oral	Virus targets hepatocytes; liver function is impaired	Infectious hepatitis	IgM to HAV serology	No specific/killed vaccine and hyperimmune serum

FLAVIVIRIDAE

Family Characteristics

- Enveloped, icosahedral
- Positive-sense ssRNA
- Arthropod-borne (arboviruses)

Viruses of Medical Importance

- St. Louis encephalitis virus (SLE)
- West Nile encephalitis virus (WNV)
- Dengue virus
- Yellow fever virus (YFV)
- Zika
- Hepatitis C virus (HCV; discussed with the hepatitis viruses)

Table II-4-13. Summary of Flaviviridae

Virus	Transmission	Host(s)	Disease	Diagnosis	Treatment/ Prevention
St. Louis encephalitis virus	Mosquito (*Culex*)	Birds	Encephalitis	Serology, hemagglutination inhibition, ELISA, latex particle agglutination	Symptomatic/ vector control
West Nile encephalitis virus	Mosquito (*Culex*)	Birds (killed by virus)	Encephalitis	As above	Symptomatic/ vector control
Dengue	Mosquito (*Aedes*)	Humans (monkeys)	Break bone fever (rash, muscle and joint pain), reinfection, can result in dengue hemorrhagic shock	As above	Symptomatic/ vector control
Yellow Fever virus	Mosquito (*Aedes*)	Humans (monkeys)	Yellow fever: liver, kidney, heart, and GI (black vomit) damage	As above	Symptomatic/ vector control/ live, attenuated vaccine
Zika	Mosquito (*Aedes*), vertical, sexual	Vertebrates	Mild → febrile illness of rash and arthralgia Congenital: microcephaly and fetal demise	RT-PCR serology	Symptomatic/ vector control

TOGAVIRIDAE

Family Characteristics

- Enveloped, icosahedral
- Positive-sense ssRNA

Viruses of Medical Importance

- **Alphaviruses (arboviruses)**
  - Eastern equine encephalitis virus (EEE)
  - Western equine encephalitis virus (WEE)
  - Venezuelan equine encephalitis virus (VEE)
  - Chikungunya
- **Rubivirus**
  - Rubella

Figure II-4-20. Togavirus

Table II-4-14. Summary of Togaviridae

Virus	Transmission	Host	Disease(s)	Diagnosis	Prevention
Eastern equine encephalitis virus (EEE), Venezuelan equine encephalitis virus (VEE), Western equine encephalitis virus (WEE)	Mosquito	Birds, horses	Encephalitis	Cytopathology, immunofluorescence, RT-PCR, serology	Killed vaccines for EEE and WEE
Chikungunya	Mosquito (*Aedes*)	Primates, rodents, birds	Febrile polyarthralgia, arthritis		
Rubella	Respiratory	humans	German measles (erythematous rash begins on face, progresses to torso)	Serology	Live, attenuated vaccine
	Vertical	humans	Congenital rubella syndrome*		

*Congenital rubella syndrome: patent ductus arteriosis, pulmonary stenosis, cataracts, microcephaly, deafness (effects are more serious if maternal infection is acquired during first 16 weeks' gestation)

CORONAVIRIDAE

Family Characteristics

- Enveloped, helical
- Positive-sense ssRNA
- Hemagglutinin molecules make up peplomers on virus surface, which give shape like sun with corona

Viruses of Medical Importance

- **Coronavirus**
- **Severe acute respiratory syndrome coronavirus (SARS-CoV)**

Coronavirus

- Second most common cause of the common cold
- Winter/spring peak incidence

SARS-CoV

Reservoir: birds and small mammals (civet cats)

Transmission: respiratory droplets; virus also found in urine, sweat, and feces; original case is thought to have jumped from animal to human

Disease: severe acute respiratory syndrome (SARS)

- Atypical pneumonia
- Clinical case definition includes fever of >100.4°F, flu-like illness, dry cough, dyspnea, and progressive hypoxia
- Chest x-ray may show patchy distribution of focal interstitial infiltrates

Diagnosis

- Includes clinical presentation and prior history of travel to endemic area or an association with someone who recently traveled to endemic area
- Lab tests: detection of antibodies to SARS-CoV, RT-PCR, and isolation of the virus in culture

Treatment: supportive; ribavirin and interferon are promising

MERS-CoV (Middle Eastern Respiratory Syndrome)

Reservoir: bats and camels

Disease and transmission: similar to SARS

Key Vignette Clues

SARS-CoV

- Patient with acute respiratory distress
- Travel to Far East or Toronto
- Winter/spring peak incidence

RETROVIRIDAE

Family Characteristics

- Positive-sense ssRNA
- Virion-associated reverse transcriptase
- Enveloped

Viruses of Medical Importance

- **Oncovirus group**
  - **Human T-cell leukemia/lymphotropic (HTLV)**
    - Adult T-cell leukemia, HTLV-1 associated myelopathy (HAM)
    - Causes proliferation of T cells and transformation
    - Tax gene required for transformation
    - Clover leaf nucleus
    - C-type particle (most oncoviruses, centrally located electron-dense nucleocapsid)
    - Japan, Caribbean, South America
- **Lentivirus group: human immunodeficiency virus (HIV);** acquired immunodeficiency syndrome

Figure II-4-21. Retrovirus

Human Immunodeficiency Virus (HIV)

Distinguishing Characteristics

- HIV virion contains:
  - Enveloped, truncated, conical capsid (type D retrovirus)
  - Two copies of ss(+)RNA
  - RNA-dependent DNA polymerase (reverse transcriptase)
  - Integrase
  - Protease

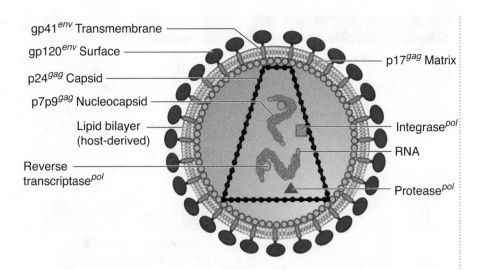

gp41^{env} Transmembrane
gp120^{env} Surface
p24^{gag} Capsid
p7p9^{gag} Nucleocapsid
Lipid bilayer (host-derived)
Reverse transcriptase^{pol}

p17^{gag} Matrix
Integrase^{pol}
RNA
Protease^{pol}

Figure II-4-22. Structure and Genes of HIV

Table II-4-15. Important HIV Genes and Their Functions

Gene	Product(s)	Function
Structural Genes		
Gag	Group-specific antigens	Structural proteins
	p24	Capsid protein
	p7p9	Core nucleocapsid proteins
	p17	Matrix protein
Pol	Reverse transcriptase	Produces dsDNA provirus (extremely error-prone, causes genetic drift of envelope glycoprotein)
	Integrase	Viral DNA integration into host cell DNA
	Protease	Cleaves viral polyprotein
Env	gp120	Surface protein that binds to CD4 and coreceptors CCR5 (macrophages) and CXCR4 (T cells); tropism; genetic drift
	gp41	Transmembrane protein for viral fusion to host cell

Gene	Product(s)	Function
Regulatory Genes		
LTR (U3, U5)	DNA, long terminal repeats	Integration and viral gene expression
Tat	Transactivator	Transactivator of transcription (upregulation); spliced gene
Rev	Regulatory protein	Upregulates transport of unspliced and spliced transcripts to the cell cytoplasm; a spliced gene
Nef	**Regulatory protein**	**Decreases CD4 and MHC I expression on host cells; manipulates T-cell activation pathways; required for progression to AIDS**

The clinical manifestations of mutations of regulatory genes are as follows:

Gene	From	Mutation	Outcome
Nef	HIV	Loss of function	Slow rate of progression to AIDS or no progression to AIDS (non-progressor)
Tat/rev	HIV	Loss of function	Virus unable to replicate
Vif	HIV	Loss of function	Slow rate of progression (non-progressor)
CCR5	HIV	Host cell macrophages/DCs	Homozygous: patient immune to HIV

Heterozygous: slow progression to AIDS |

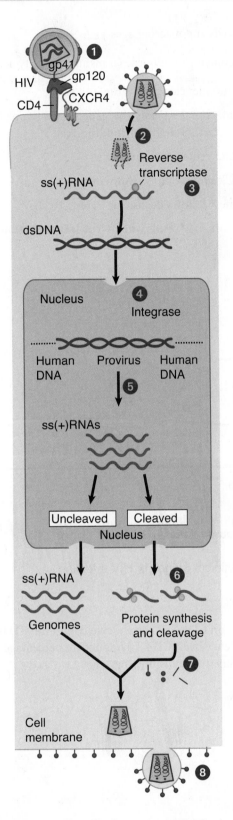

1 Surface gp120 of HIV binds to CD4 of T-helper cells, macrophages, microglia, and coreceptors (*CCR5* and *CXCR4*) found on macrophages and Th cells, respectively.

2 HIV is taken into the cell, losing the envelope; the RNA is uncoated.

3 The RNA is copied using the virion-associated reverse transcriptase; ultimately dsDNA with long terminal repeats is made.

4 The DNA and integrase migrate to nucleus, and the DNA is integrated into host DNA forming the **provirus**. The provirus remains in the host DNA.

The rate of viral replication is regulated by the activity of the regulatory proteins (*tat/rev, nef,* etc). **Tat** upregulates transcription. **Rev** regulates transport of RNA to cytoplasm.

Co-infections (e.g., mycobacterial) stimulate the HIV-infected cells to produce more virus.

5 Transcription produces ss(+)RNA, some cleaved and some remain intact.

- Cleaved RNA will be used as mRNA.
- Uncleaved RNA is used as genomic RNA.

6 Translation produces the proteins, some of which are polyproteins that are cleaved by the HIV protease.

7 Assembly

8 Maturation/release of virus

Figure II-4-23. Retrovirus Life Cycle: HIV

Reservoir: human Th cells and macrophages

Transmission: sexual contact, bloodborne (transfusions, dirty needles), vertical

Disease: acquired immunodeficiency syndrome (AIDS)

- Asymptomatic infection → persistent, generalized lymphadenopathy → symptomatic → AIDS-defining conditions
- Homozygous *CCR5* mutation → immune
- Heterozygous *CCR5* mutation → slow course
- Course of the illness follows decline in CD4+ T cells
- Long-term survivors may result when virus lacks functional *nef* protein

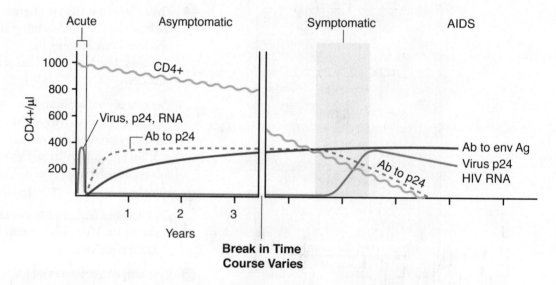

Figure II-4-24. Clinical Stages of HIV Infection

Stage is based primarily on CD4+ T-lymphocyte count; the CD4+ T-lymphocyte count takes precedence over CD4 T-lymphocyte percentage, and the percentage is considered only if count is missing.

Table II-4-16. HIV Infection Stage* based on age-specific CD4+ T-Lymphocyte Count or CD4+ T-Lymphocyte Percentage of Total Lymphocytes

Stage	Age on date of CD4+ T-lymphocyte test		
	Age <1 yr	Age 1–5 yrs	Age ≥6 yrs
1	≥1,500 cells/μL, ≥34%	≥1,000 cells/μL, ≥30%	≥500 cells/μL, ≥26%
2	750–1,499 cells//μL, 26–33%	500–999 cells/μL, 22–29%	200–499 cells/μL, 14-25%
3	<750 cells//μL, <26%	<500 cells/μL, <22%	<200 cells/μL, <14%

There are 3 situations in which stage is not based on table above: 1) if criteria for stage 0 are met, the stage is 0 regardless of criteria for other stages (CD4 T-lymphocyte test results and opportunistic illness diagnoses); 2) if criteria for stage 0 are not met and a stage-3-defining opportunistic illness has been diagnosed, then stage is 3 regardless of CD4 T-lymphocyte test results; or 3) if criteria for stage 0 are not met and information on the above criteria for other stages is missing, then stage is unknown.

Conditions of Early Symptomatic Period

- Bacillary angiomatosis (disseminated bartonellosis)
- Candidiasis (oral or persistent vulvovaginal)
- Cervical dysplasia or carcinoma in situ
- Constitutional symptoms (fever 38.5°C or diarrhea lasting >1 month)
- Hairy leukoplakia
- Idiopathic thrombocytopenic purpura
- Listeriosis
- Pelvic inflammatory disease (especially with abscess)
- Peripheral neuropathy

Conditions Associated with AIDS

- Encephalopathy, HIV-related
- Pneumonia, recurrent (leading cause of death)
- Fungal infections
- Candidiasis of esophagus, bronchi, trachea, or lungs
- Coccidioidomycosis, disseminated or extrapulmonary
- Cryptococcosis, extrapulmonary
- Histoplasmosis, disseminated or extrapulmonary
- *Pneumocystis jirovecii* pneumonia

- Malignancies: invasive cervical carcinoma; Kaposi sarcoma; Burkitt, immunoblastic, or primary CNS lymphoma

- Viral infections: cytomegalovirus retinitis (with loss of vision) or disease (other than liver, spleen, or nodes); herpes simplex: chronic ulcer(s) (>1 month) or bronchitis, pneumonitis, or esophagitis; progressive multifocal leukoencephalopathy; wasting syndrome due to HIV (TNF-α)

- Parasitic infections: cryptosporidiosis, chronic intestinal (>1 month); isosporiasis, chronic intestinal (>1 month); toxoplasmosis of brain

- Bacterial infections

  - *Mycobacterium tuberculosis,* any site (pulmonary or extrapulmonary)

  - *Mycobacterium avium* complex or *M. kansasii* or other species or unidentified species, disseminated or extrapulmonary

  - *Salmonella* septicemia, recurrent

Table II-4-17. Recommended Prophylactic Regimens during HIV Infection

Disease Agent	Begin Prophylaxis
Pneumocystis jirovecii	<200 CD4
Toxoplasma gondii	<100 CD4
Histoplasma capsulatum	<100 CD4 (in endemic area)
Mycobacterium avium intracellulare	<50 CD4
Cytomegalovirus	<50 CD4
Cryptococcus neoformans	<50 CD4

Table II-4-18. Laboratory Analysis for HIV

Purpose	Test
Initial screening	Serologic: ELISA (HIV1 and HIV2 antibodies, p24 antigen)
Confirmation	Nucleic acid test (NAT)
Detection of virus in blood (evaluate **viral load**)	RT-PCR*
Detect HIV infection in newborns of HIV+ mother **(provirus)**	PCR*
Early marker of infection	p24 antigen
Evaluate progression of disease	CD4:CD8 T-cell ratio

*RT-PCR tests for circulating viral RNA and is used to monitor the efficacy of treatment. PCR detects integrated virus (provirus). Viral load has been demonstrated to be the best prognostic indicator during infection.

Table II-4-19. Treatment

Mechanism	Name	Resistance
RT inhibitors Nucleoside or non-nucleoside analogs	End in "ine"	Common, leads to cross-resistance
Protease inhibitors	End in "inavir"	Common via protease mutations, leads to cross-resistance
HAART (highly active anti-retroviral therapy)	2 nucleoside analogs and 1 protease inhibitor	Increasing
Fusion inhibitors	Fuzeon, enfuvirtide	Not yet
CCR5 co-receptor antagonist	Maraviroc	Not yet
Integrase inhibitor	Raltegravir	Not yet

Prevention: safe sex/education; blood/organ screening; infection control; vaccine development (currently none available)

NEGATIVE-STRANDED RNA VIRUSES

Table II-4-20. Negative-Stranded RNA Viruses

Virus	RNA Structure	Virion-Associated Polymerase	Envelope	Shape	Multiplies in	Major Viruses
Paramyxovirus	ss(−)RNA Linear Non-segmented	Yes	Yes	Helical	Cytoplasm	Mumps Measles Respiratory syncytial Parainfluenza
Rhabdovirus	ss(−)RNA Linear Non-segmented	Yes	Yes	Helical, bullet-shaped	Cytoplasm	Rabies Vesicular stomatitis
Filovirus	ss(−)RNA Linear Non-segmented	Yes	Yes	Helical	Cytoplasm	Marburg Ebola
Orthomyxovirus	ss(−)RNA Linear 8 segmented	Yes	Yes	Helical	Cytoplasm & nucleus	Influenza
Bunyavirus	ss(−)RNA Pseudocircular, 3 segments, 1 is ambisense	Yes	Yes	Helical	Cytoplasm	California encephalitis La Crosse encephalitis Hantavirus
Arenavirus	ss(−)RNA Circular 2 segments 1 (−)sense 1 ambisense	Yes	Yes	Helical	Cytoplasm	Lymphocytic choriomeningitis Lassa fever

Mnemonic for ss(−)RNA viruses: Pain Results From Our Bunions Always. Gives them in order of size. Remember that these are the negative ones because pain is a negative thing. Another one: Bring a polymerase or fail replication.

Note that all are enveloped, all have virion-associated polymerase, and all have helical nucleocapsids. The oddballs are the last three:

- The orthomyxoviruses are linear (ortho) but with 8 (ortho/octo) segments, which is one of the reasons they can genetically "mix" it up. The orthomyxoviruses are also odd in that they replicate in both the nucleus and cytoplasm.
- The bunyaviruses are somewhat contortionists (circular): California playboy bunnies in a ménage à trois?
- The arenaviruses have one negative sense and one ambisense strand of RNA.

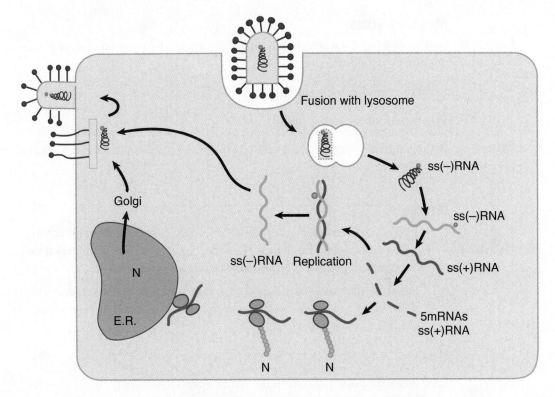

Figure II-4-25. Negative-Sense RNA Virus Life Cycle

PARAMYXOVIRIDAE

Family Characteristics

- Enveloped, helical nucleocapsid
- Negative-sense ssRNA

Viruses of Medical Importance

- Measles
- Mumps
- Parainfluenza
- Respiratory syncytial virus (RSV)
- Human metapneumovirus (human MNV)

Figure II-4-26. Paramyxovirus

Measles Virus

Distinguishing Characteristics: single serotype; H-glycoprotein and fusion protein; no neuraminidase

Reservoir: human respiratory tract

Transmission: respiratory route

Pathogenesis: ability to cause cell: cell fusion → giant cells; virus can escape immune detection

Disease

- Measles: presentation generally 3 Cs (cough, coryza, and conjunctivitis) with photophobia; Koplik spots → maculopapular rash from ears down → giant cell pneumonia (Warthin-Finkeldey cells)
- Subacute sclerosing panencephalitis: rare late complication (mean time 7–10 years); mutant measles virus persists in brain, acts as slow virus; chronic CNS degeneration

Diagnosis: serology

Treatment: supportive, ribavirin (experimental)

Prevention: live, attenuated vaccine, M<u>M</u>R

Mumps Virus

Distinguishing Characteristics: negative-sense ssRNA; helical; enveloped; single HN glycoprotein, also F protein; single serotype

Reservoir: human respiratory tract

Transmission: person to person via respiratory droplets

Pathogenesis: lytic infection of epithelial cells of upper respiratory tract and parotid glands → spread throughout body

Disease: mumps

- Asymptomatic to bilateral parotitis with fever, headache, and malaise
- Complications include pancreatitis, orchitis (leads to sterility in males), and meningoencephalitis

Diagnosis: clinical; serology; ELISA, IFA, hemagglutination inhibition

Treatment: supportive

Prevention: live, attenuated vaccine, M<u>M</u>R

Table II-4-21. Additional Paramyxoviruses

Virus	Transmission	Disease(s)	Diagnosis	Treatment/Prevention
Parainfluenza	Respiratory	Older children and adults: subglottal swelling; hoarse, barking cough Infants: colds, bronchiolitis, pneumonia, **croup**	RT-PCR	Supportive/none
RSV	Respiratory	Adults: colds; infants/**preemies**: bronchiolitis and necrosis of bronchioles, atypical pneumonia (low fever, tachypnea, tachycardia, expiratory wheeze)	Indirect fluorescent antibody, enzyme-linked immunosorbent assay, RT-PCR	Ribavirin and anti-RSV Abs/none Palivizumab blocks fusion protein
Human Metapneumovirus	Respiratory	Common cold (15% in kids), bronchiolitis, pneumonia	RT-PCR	Supportive/none

Definition of abbreviations: RT-PCR, reverse transcriptase-polymerase chain reaction

RHABDOVIRIDAE

Family Characteristics

- Negative-sense ssRNA
- Bullet shaped
- Enveloped, helical

Viruses of Medical Importance

- Rabies

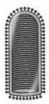

Figure II-4-27. Rhabdovirus

Key Vignette Clues

Rabies

- Patient bitten by bat or dog

- Influenza-like prodrome: hydrophobia, hallucination, coma, death

Rabies Virus

Reservoir: In U.S., most cases are sylvatic (bats, raccoons, foxes, skunks); worldwide, mostly dogs

Transmission: bite or contact with rabid animal

Pathogenesis: After contact, virus binds to peripheral nerves by binding to nicotinic acetylcholine receptor **or** indirectly into the muscle at site of inoculation; virus travels by **retrograde axoplasmic** transport to dorsal root ganglia and spinal cord; once virus gains access to spinal cord, brain becomes rapidly infected

Disease: rabies

- Nonspecific flu-like illness followed by neurologic symptoms of **hydrophobia**, seizures, disorientation, **hallucination**, coma, and death

- With rare exception, rabies fatal unless treated by immunoprophylaxis

Diagnosis: clinical; Negri bodies, intracytoplasmic inclusion bodies (brain biopsy); DFA (impression smears of corneal epithelial cells), PCR (usually too late)

Treatment: none if symptoms are evident; if suspect: postexposure prophylaxis 1 dose of human rabies immunoglobulin (hRIG); 4 doses of rabies vaccine (day of, 3, 7, 14); killed virus vaccine

Prevention: vaccine for high-risk individuals; vaccination program for domestic animals (U.S.)

FILOVIRIDAE

Family Characteristics

- Negative-sense ssRNA

- Enveloped, helical

- Filamentous

Viruses of Medical Importance

- Ebola virus : Zaire species most virulent (2014–2015 outbreak in West Africa), 70% mortality

- Marburg virus

Reservoir

- Ebola: bats suspected

- Marburg: bats confirmed

Transmission (Ebola)

- Contact with body fluids, meat of infected animals
- Direct contact with infected patients, body fluids, blood, skin

Pathogenesis (Ebola)

- Virus infects many cell types (endothelial, epithelial, fibroblasts, etc); macrophages, and dendrite cells first cells likely to be infected
- Virus delivered to regional lymph nodes, then to blood stream
- Systemic inflammatory response induces cytokine storm, which results in tissue damage including vascular leak, SI dysfunction, and eventual multi-organ failure

Ebola

Disease

- Incubation period ~6–12 days
- Non-specific flu-like illness (fever, chills, general malaise)
- Fatigue, headaches, vomiting and diarrhea
- Massive hemorrhage not common, although bleeding via bloody stool, petechiae, or mucosal bleeding can be
- GI manifestations important in severe illness, with vomiting and diarrhea leading to fluid loss
- Rash and meningoencephalitis may occur

Diagnosis

- Determine likelihood of exposure
- RT-PCR (confirmatory); rapid antigen test (screen) must also be confirmed with RT-PCR

Treatment

- Symptomatic
- Non-approved anti-virals (clinical trials): favipiravir, brincidofovir
- Ebola-specific treatments in development include monoclonal antibodies targeting surface GP B and anti-RNA

Prevention

- Infection control precautions: quarantine, travel restrictions
- Vaccines in development

ORTHOMYXOVIRIDAE

Family Characteristics

- Negative-sense ssRNA
- Enveloped
- Segmented (8 segments)
- Helical

Figure II-4-28. Orthomyxovirus

Viruses of Medical Importance

- Influenza A
- Influenza B

Influenza Virus

Key Vignette Clues

Influenza

Patient with headache, malaise, fever, myalgia, cough

Distinguishing Features

- Envelope contains two glycoproteins, H and N
- Used to serotype virus

Reservoir

- Influenza A (birds, pigs, humans)
- Influenza B (humans only)

Transmission

- Direct contact
- Respiratory
- 1997 H5N1 strain jumped directly from birds to humans
- 2009 H1N1 strain—quadruple reassortment virus (North American swine, avian, human; Asian and European swine)

Pathogenesis

- Antigenic drift
  - Influenza A and B
  - Slight changes in antigenicity due to mutations in H and/or N
  - Causes epidemics

- Antigenic shift
  - *Influenza A only*
  - Rare genetic reassortment
  - Coinfection of cells with two different strains of influenza A (H5N1 and H3N2); reassortment of segments of genome
  - Production of a new agent to which population has no immunity
  - Responsible for pandemics

Disease: influenza

- Headache and malaise
- Fever, chills, myalgias, anorexia
- Bronchiolitis, croup, otitis media, vomiting (younger children)
- Pneumonia/secondary bacterial infections
- Can lead to Reye syndrome or Guillain-Barré syndrome

Diagnosis

- Rapid tests (serology)
- Clinical symptoms plus season

Treatment

- Amantadine/rimantadine (current isolates are commonly resistant)
  - Inhibit viral uncoating
  - Administer orally
- Zanamivir/oseltamivir
  - Neuraminidase inhibitors
  - Zanamivir is inhaled
  - Oseltamivir is given orally

Prevention

- Killed vaccine
  - Two strains of influenza A (H3N2, H1N1, for example) and one strain of influenza B are incorporated into the vaccine
- Live, attenuated vaccine
  - Intranasal administration
  - Similar composition
  - No longer recommended

Key Vignette Clues

Hantavirus

- Patient with acute respiratory distress
- Four-corners region
- Exposure to rodent excrement
- Spring/early sumer incidence

BUNYAVIRIDAE

Family Characteristics

- Negative-sense ssRNA
- Enveloped viruses
- Three segments, one ambisense
- Mostly arboviruses, except Hantavirus

Viruses of Medical Importance

- California encephalitis
- LaCrosse encephalitis
- Hantavirus (sin nombre)

Table II-4-22. Bunyaviridae

Virus	Transmission	Disease	Diagnosis
California and LaCrosse encephalitis	Mosquito	Viral encephalitis	Serology
Hantavirus (sin nombre)	Rodent excrement, four-corners region, rainy season	Hantavirus pulmonary syndrome (cough, myalgia, dyspnea, tachycardia, pulmonary edema and effusion, and hypotension [mortality 50%])	RT-PCR

ARENAVIRIDAE

Family Characteristics

- Negative-sense ssRNA
- Pleomorphic, enveloped
- Virions have a sandy appearance (ribosomes in virion)
- Two segments, one ambisense

Viruses of Medical Importance

- Lymphocytic choriomeningitis virus (LCMV)
- Lassa fever virus

Table II-4-23. Arenaviridae

Virus	Transmission	Disease	Diagnosis	Treatment
Lymphocytic choriomen-ingitis virus	Mice and pet hamsters (U.S.)	Influenza-like with meningeal signs	Serology, level 3 isolation	Supportive, ribavirin
Lassa fever	Rodents, human-to-human (West Africa)	Hemorrhagic fever with 50% fatality rate	Serology, level 4 isolation	Supportive, ribavirin

DOUBLE-STRANDED RNA VIRUSES

REOVIRIDAE

Table II-4-24. Double-Stranded RNA Viruses

	RNA Structure	Polymerase	Envelope	Shape	Major Viruses
Reovirus	Linear dsRNA 10-11 segments	Yes	Naked	Icosa-hedral Double shelled	Reovirus Rotavirus Colorado Tick Fever Virus

Figure II-4-29. Reovirus

Table II-4-25. Reoviridae

Virus	Transmission	Disease	Diagnosis	Treatment/Prevention
Reovirus	Fecal-oral, respiratory	Common cold, gastroenteritis	Serology	Self-limiting/none
Rotavirus	Fecal-oral	Gastroenteritis, no blood or pus	Enzyme-linked immunosorbent assay (stool)	Live, attenuated vaccine, oral

PRION DISEASES

Table II-4-26. Prion Diseases

Disease	Infectious agent	Host	Comments
Kuru	Prion	Human	Subacute spongiform encephalopathy (SSE); Fore Tribe, New Guinea; cannibalism
Creutzfeldt-Jakob disease (and variant)	Prion	Human	SSE PrPSc: humalog of normal protein PrPC found in normal brain and tissue Genetic predisposition; ingestion of infected cow brains
Gerstmann-Sträussler-Scheinker	Prion	Human	SSE
Fatal familial insomnia	Prion	Human	SSE
Scrapie	Prion	Sheep	SSE: scraping their wool off on fences

Table II-4-27. Slow Conventional Viruses (Viruses)

Disease	Infectious agent	Host	Comments
Measles SSPE	Virus	Human having had measles	Subacute sclerosing panencephalitis
AIDS dementia	HIV	Human	Dementia
PML	JC virus	Human	Progressive multifocal leukoencephalopathy

Medically Important Fungi 5

Learning Objectives

❏ Demonstrate understanding of mycology and fungal morphology

❏ Differentiate between non-systemic fungal infections and deep fungal infections

MYCOLOGY

Mycology is the **study of fungi (molds, yeasts, and mushrooms).**

All fungi are

- **Eukaryotic** (e.g., true nucleus, 80S ribosomes, mitochondria, as are humans).

- **Complex carbohydrate cell walls: chitin, glucan, and mannan.**

- **Ergosterol = Major membrane sterol**
  Imidazole antifungals inhibit synthesis of ergosterol.
  Polyene antifungals bind more tightly to **ergosterol** than cholesterol.

FUNGAL MORPHOLOGY

Hyphae = filamentous cellular units of molds and mushrooms

Nonseptate Hyphae

- No cross walls
- Broad hyphae with **irregular width**
- **Broad angle of branching**

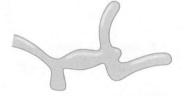

Figure II-5-1. Nonseptate Hyphae

Septate Hyphae

- With **cross walls**
- Width is fairly regular (tube-like).

Hyphal Coloration

- **Dematiaceous: dark colored** (gray, olive)
- **Hyaline: clear**

Mat of hyphae = mycelium

Yeasts = single celled (round to oval) fungi

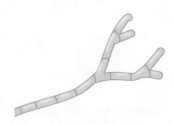

Figure II-5-2. Septate Hyphae

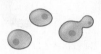

Figure II-5-3. Yeasts

Dimorphic Fungi

- Fungi able to convert from hyphal to yeast or yeast-like forms.
- Thermally dimorphic: in the "cold" are the mold form.

Key Dimorphic Fungi

- *Histoplasma*
- *Blastomyces*
- *Coccidioides*
- *Sporothrix*

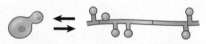

Figure II-5-4. Dimorphic Fungi

Pseudohyphae (Candida albicans)

Hyphae with constrictions at each septum

Spore types

Conidia

- **Asexual spores**
- Formed off of hyphae
- Common
- Airborne

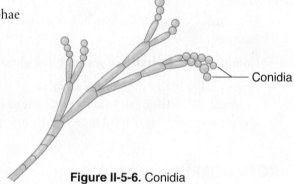

Figure II-5-5.
Candida Pseudohyphae

Note

Mnemonic

Body **H**eat **C**hanges **S**hape
for the dimorphic fungi.

Blastomyces

Histoplasma

Coccidioides

Sporothrix

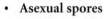

Conidia

Figure II-5-6. Conidia

Blastoconidia: "Buds" on yeasts (asexual budding daughter yeast cells)

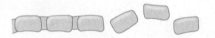

Figure II-5-7. Blastoconidia

Arthroconidia: Asexual spores formed by a **"joint"**

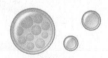

Figure II-5-8. Arthroconidia

Spherules and Endospores (*Coccidioides*): Spores inside the spherules in tissues

Figure II-5-9. Endospores
and Spherules

Diagnosis

Table II-5-1. Microscopic Methods/Special Fungal Stains

Preparation	Fungal Color	Notes
KOH wet mount (KOH degrades human tissues leaving hyphae and yeasts visible)	Colorless (hyaline) refractive green or light olive to brown (dematiaceous) fungal elements	Heat gently; let sit 10 minutes; dissolves human cells
PAS	Hot pink	
Silver stain	Gray to black	*Pneumocystis*
Calcofluor white (can be done on wet mounts)	Bright blue-white on black	Scrapings or sections; fluorescent microscope needed
India ink wet mount of CSF sediment	Colorless cells with halos (capsule) on a black particulate background (*Cryptococcus neoformans*)	Only "rules in"; insensitive; misses 50% **Figure II-5-10.** *Cryptococcus neoformans*

Culture

(May take several weeks.) Special fungal media: inhibitory mold agar is modification of Sabouraud with antibiotics.

- **Sabouraud agar**
- Blood agar
- Both of the above with antibiotics

Identification from cultures

- Fungal **morphology**
- PCR with nucleic acid probes

Serology

(E.g., antibody screen, complement fixation, etc.) Looking for patient antibody.

Fungal antigen detection: (CSF, serum)

Cryptococcal capsular polysaccharide detection by latex particle agglutination (LPA) or counter immunoelectrophoresis.

Key Vignette Clues

Malassezia furfur

- Patient with blotchy hypopigmentation of skin

- KOH scraping shows "spaghetti and meatballs"

Skin tests

- Most useful for **epidemiology** or **demonstration of anergy** to an agent you know patient is infected with (grave prognosis)

- Otherwise, like tuberculosis, a skin test **only indicates exposure** to the agent.

NONSYSTEMIC FUNGAL INFECTIONS

Superficial Infections (Keratinized Tissues)

Malassezia furfur

Normal skin flora (lipophilic yeast)

Diseases

- **Pityriasis or tinea versicolor**

  - Superficial infection of keratinized cells

  - Moist, warm climates predispose

  - Hypopigmented spots on the chest/back (blotchy suntan)

  - KOH mount of skin scales: spaghetti and meatballs (bacon and eggs) Yeast clusters & short curved septate hyphae

  - Coppery-orange fluoresence under Wood lamp (UV)

  - Treatment is topical selenium sulfide; recurs.

- **Fungemia in premature infants** on intravenous lipid supplements

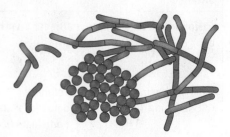

Figure II-5-11. *Malassezia furfur*

Cutaneous Fungal Infections (Without Systemic Disease)

Yeast or dermatophytic infections.

Yeast skin infections

- Commonly **cutaneous or mucocutaneous candidiasis**

- May disseminate in compromised patients

- Discussed with opportunistic fungi

Dermatophytes (group of fungi)

- **Filamentous** fungi (**monomorphic**)

- **Infect only skin and hair and/or nails** (do not disseminate)

- Three genera:

  Trichophyton—Infects skin, hair and nails
  Microsporum—Infects hair and skin
  Epidermophyton—Infects nails and skin

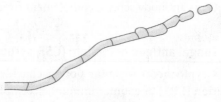

Figure II-5-12. Dermatophyte

Diseases

- Dermatophytic Infections = **Tineas** (Ringworms)
  - Itching is the most common symptom of all tineas.
  - If highly inflammatory, generally from animals (zoophilic)
  - If little inflammation, generally from humans
  - Tinea capitis = ringworm of the scalp
  - The most serious of the tineas capiti is favus (tinea favosa), which causes permanent hair loss and is very contagious.
  - Tinea barbae = ringworm of the bearded region
  - Tinea corporis = dermatophytic infection of the glabrous skin
  - Tinea cruris = jock itch
  - Tinea pedis = athlete's foot
  - Tinea unguium = ringworm of the nails

Diagnosis

- *Microsporum* fluoresces a bright yellow-green (Wood lamp)
- **KOH mount** of nail or skin scrapings should show **arthroconidia and hyphae.**

Treatment

- Topical imidazoles or tolnaftate
- Oral imidazoles or griseofulvin where hairs are infected, or skin contact hurts
- **Keep areas dry.**

ID reaction

(Dermatophytid) = Allergic response to circulating fungal antigens

Key Vignette Clues

Dermatophytes

- Patient with scaly, pruritic ring-like lesions of skin. May involve hair shaft or nails.
- KOH scraping shows arthroconidia and hyphae.

Subcutaneous Mycoses

Sporothrix schenckii

Dimorphic Fungus

- **Environmental form**: on **plant material**, worldwide as **hyphae with rosettes and sleeves of conidia**
- **Traumatic implantation** (rose or plum tree thorns, wire/sphagnum moss)
- **Tissue form: cigar-shaped yeast** in tissue

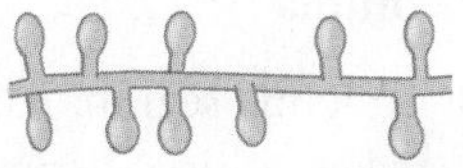

Figure II-5-13. *Sporothrix* Hyphae

Diseases

- **Sporotrichosis (rose gardener disease): subcutaneous or lymphocutaneous lesions.** Treatment: itraconazole or **potassium iodide in milk**
- **Pulmonary** (acute or chronic) **sporotrichosis.** Urban alcoholics, particularly homeless (**alcoholic rose-garden-sleeper disease**)

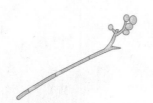

Figure II-5-14. *Sporothrix*

Treatment: Itraconazole or amphotericin B

Key Vignette Clues

Sporothrix schenckii

- Patient with subcutaneous/lymphocutaneous mycetoma
- Gardener, florist, basket weaver
- Cigar-shaped yeasts in pus

DEEP FUNGAL INFECTIONS

Classical Pathogens

Three important classical pathogens in the U.S.:

- *Histoplasma*
- *Coccidioides*
- *Blastomyces*

All 3 pathogens **cause**

- **Acute pulmonary** (asymptomatic or self-resolving in about **95%** of the cases)
- **Chronic** pulmonary, or
- **Disseminated** infections

Diagnosis

(Most people never see a doctor.)

- Sputum cytology (calcofluor white helpful)
- **Sputum cultures** on blood agar and **special fungal media** (inhibitory mold agar, Sabouraud)
- **Peripheral blood cultures are useful for *Histoplasma* since it circulates in RES cells.**

Histoplasma capsulatum

Dimorphic Fungus

- **Environmental form: hyphae** with **microconidia** and **tuberculate macroconidia**
  - Endemic region: Eastern Great Lakes, Ohio, Mississippi, and Missouri River beds

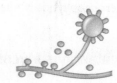

Figure II-5-15. *Histoplasma* Environmental Form

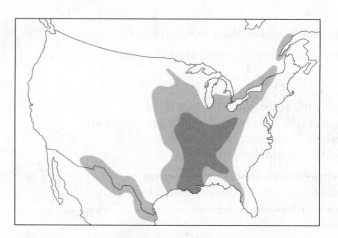

Figure II-5-16. *Histoplasma* Endemic Region

- Found in soil (dust) enriched with bird or bat feces
- Spelunking (cave exploring), cleaning chicken coops, or bulldozing starling roosts
- **Tissue form: small intracellular yeasts** with narrow neck on bud; **no capsule**
- **Facultative intracellular parasite** found in **reticuloendothelial (RES) cells** (tiny; can get 30 or so in a human cell)

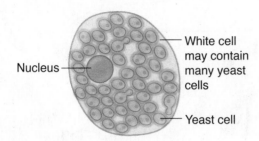

Figure II-5-17. Human RES Cell

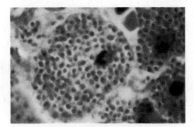

Histoplasma capsulatum
yeast cells within an RES cell

Disease

Fungus flu (a pneumonia)

- Asymptomatic or acute (but self-resolving) pneumonia with flu-like symptomatology
- **Hepatosplenomegaly may be present** even in acute pulmonary infections (facultative intracellular RES)
- Very common in summer in endemic areas: children or newcomers (80% of adults are skin-test positive in some areas)
- Lesions have a tendency to **calcify as they heal**.
- Relapse potential increases with T cell immunosuppression.
- **Disseminated infections**: Mucocutaneous lesions are common; also common **in AIDS** patients in endemic area.

Treatment: Itraconazole for mild, amphotericin B for severe

Coccidioides immitis

Dimorphic Fungus

- **Environmental form: hyphae** breaking up into **arthroconidia** found **in desert sand**

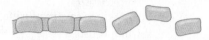

Figure II-5-18.
Coccicioides immitis

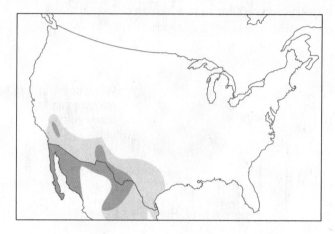

Figure II-5-19. *Coccidioides* Endemic Region

- Endemic region: Southwestern United States—Southern California (especially San Joaquin Valley), Arizona, New Mexico, Texas, Nevada

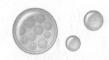

Figure II-5-20.
Coccidioides immitis Spherules

- Arthroconidia are inhaled, round up, and enlarged, becoming spherules inside which the cytoplasm walls off, forming endospores.

- **Tissue form: spherules with endospores**

Disease: **Valley fever** (asymptomatic to **self-resolving pneumonia**)

- **Desert bumps** (erythema nodosum) and arthritis are generally good prognostic signs.

- Very common in endemic region

- **Pulmonary lesions have a tendency to calcify as they heal.**

- **Systemic infections are a problem in AIDS and immunocompromised patients** in endemic region (meningitis, mucocutaneous lesions).

- Tendency to **disseminate in third trimester of pregnancy**.

Treatment: Azoles for mild to moderate (itraconazole, etc.), amphotericin B for severe

Blastomyces dermatitidis

Dimorphic Fungus

- **Environmental form**: **hyphae** with **nondescript conidia** (i.e., no fancy arrangements)

- Association not definitively known, **appears to be associated with rotting wood** such as beaver dams

- Endemic region: Upper Great Lakes, Ohio, Mississippi River beds, plus the southeastern seaboard of the U.S. and northern Minnesota into Canada

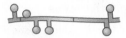

Figure II-5-21. *Blastomyces dermatitidis* Hyphae with Conidia

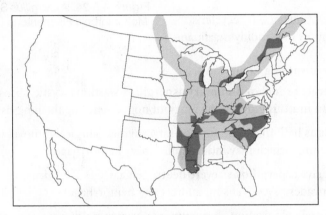

Figure II-5-22. Blastomycosis Endemic Region

- **Tissue form: broad-based budding yeasts** and a double refractile cell wall (not capsule)

Disease: Blastomycosis

- Acute and chronic pulmonary disease

- Considered less likely to self-resolve than *Histoplasma* or *Coccidioides*, so many physicians will treat even acute infections.

Figure II-5-23. *Blastomyces dermatitidis* Broad-Based Budding Yeasts

- Disseminated disease

Treatment: Itraconazole for mild, amphotericin B for severe

Key Vignette Clues

Blastomyces dermatitidis

- Normal patient with acute pulmonary symptoms

- Immunocompromised patient with chronic pulmonary or disseminated infection

- North and South Carolina (otherwise coexists with *Histoplasma*)

- Sputum has broad-based, budding yeasts with double, refractile cell walls

Key Vignette Clues

Aspergillus fumigatus

- Patient with asthma, cystic fibrosis—growing mucous plugs in lung
- Patient with cavitary lung lesions—fungus ball
- Patient with burns—cellulitis, invasion
- Immunocompromised patient—pneumonia, meningitis
- Septate hyphae branch at acute angles

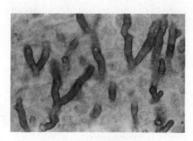

Aspergilus fumigatus

Key Vignette Clues

Candida albicans

- Immunocompromised patient, overuse of antibiotics—thrush, spread down GI tract, septicemia
- IV drug abusers—endocarditis
- Germ tube test demonstrates pseudohyphae and hyphae

Opportunistic Fungi

Aspergillus fumigatus

Monomorphic filamentous fungus

- **Dichotomously branching**
- **Generally acute angles**
- **Frequent septate hyphae with 45° angles**
- One of our **major recyclers**: compost pits, moldy marijuana

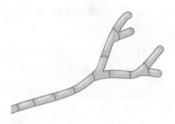

Figure II-5-24. *Aspergillus* Showing Monomorphic Filamentous Fungus

Diseases/Predisposing Conditions

- **Allergic bronchopulmonary aspergillosis**/asthma, cystic fibrosis (growing in mucous plugs in the lung but not penetrating the lung tissue)
- **Fungus ball**: free in preformed lung cavities (surgical removal to reduce coughing, which may induce pulmonary hemorrhage)
- **Invasive aspergillosis**/severe neutropenia, CGD, CF, burns
  - Invades tissues causing infarcts and hemorrhage.
  - Nasal colonization → pneumonia or meningitis
  - Cellulitis/in burn patients; may also disseminate

Treatment: Voriconazole for invasive and aspergilloma, glucocorticoids + itraconazole for ABPA

Candida albicans (and other species of Candida)

- **Yeast** endogenous to our mucous membrane normal flora
- *C. albicans* yeasts form germ tubes at 37°C in serum.
- Forms **pseudohyphae** and **true hyphae** when it invades tissues (nonpathogenic *Candida* do not).

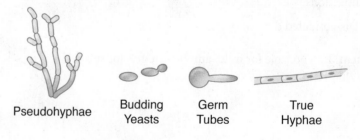

| Pseudohyphae | Budding Yeasts | Germ Tubes | True Hyphae |

Figure II-5-25. *Candida albicans*

Diseases/Predisposing Conditions

- **Perlèche**: crevices of mouth/malnutrition
- **Oral thrush**/prematurity, antibiotic use, immunocompromised (IC) host, AIDS
- **Esophagitis**/antibiotic use, IC host, AIDS
- **Gastritis**/antibiotic use, IC host, AIDS
- **Septicemia** (with endophthalmitis and macronodular skin lesions)/ immunocompromised, cancer and intravenous (IV) patients
- **Endocarditis** (with transient septicemias)/**IV drug abusers**
- **Cutaneous infections**/obesity and infants; patients with rubber gloves
- **Yeast vaginitis**/particularly a problem in diabetic women
- Chronic mucocutaneous candidiasis/endocrine defects; anergy to *Candida*

Diagnosis

- KOH: pseudohyphae, true hyphae, budding yeasts
- Septicemia: culture lab identification: biochemical tests/formation of germ tubes

Treatment

- Topical imidazoles or oral imidazoles; nystatin
- Disseminated: Amphotericin B or fluconazole

Cryptococcus neoformans

Encapsulated Yeast (Monomorphic)

Environmental Source: Soil enriched with pigeon droppings

Diseases/Predisposing Conditions

- **Meningitis/Hodgkin, AIDS (the dominant meningitis)**
- **Acute pulmonary** (usually asymptomatic)/**pigeon breeders**

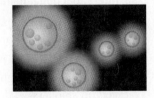

Cryptococcus neoformans

Diagnosis of Meningitis: CSF

- Detect capsular antigen in CSF (by latex particle agglutination or counter immunoelectrophoresis)
- India ink mount (misses 50%) of CSF sediment to find budding yeasts with capsular "halos"
- Cultures (urease positive yeast)

Treatment: AMB+5FC (flucytosine) until afebrile and culture negative (minimum of 10 weeks), then fluconazole

Mucor, Rhizopus, Absidia (Zygomycophyta)

Nonseptate filamentous fungi

Environmental Source: Soil; sporangio-spores are inhaled

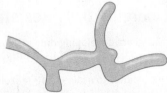

Figure II-5-26. Nonseptate Hyphae with Broad Angles

Disease

- **Rhinocerebral infection** caused by *Mucor* (or other zygomycophyta)
- (Old names: Mucormycosis = Phycomycosis = Zygomycosis)
- Characterized by paranasal swelling, necrotic tissues, hemorrhagic exudates from nose and eyes, and mental lethargy
- Occurs in **ketoacidotic diabetic patients and leukemic patients**
- These fungi penetrate without respect to anatomical barriers, progressing rapidly from sinuses into the brain tissue

Diagnosis: KOH of tissue; broad ribbon-like nonseptate hyphae with about 90° angles on branches.

Treatment

- Debride necrotic tissue and start Amphotericin B fast
- High fatality rate because of rapid growth and invasion

Key Vignette Clues

Pneumocystis jirovecii

- Premature infant or AIDS patient with atypical pneumonia
- Biopsy with honeycomb exudate and silver-staining cysts
- X-ray: ground glass

Pneumocystis jirovecii (formerly P. carinii)

Fungus (based on molecular techniques like **ribotyping**)

- **Obligate extracellular parasite**
- **Silver stained cysts in tissues**

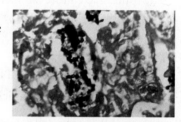

Pneumocystis, silver stain, exudate

Disease: Interstitial pneumonia

- Pneumonia in AIDS patients even with prophylaxis (mean CD4+/mm^3 of 26), malnourished babies, premature neonates, and some other IC adults and kids
- Symptoms: fever, cough, shortness of breath; sputum nonproductive except in smokers
- Serum leaks into alveoli, producing an exudate with a foamy or **honeycomb appearance on H & E stain.** (Silver stain reveals the holes in the exudate are actually the cysts and trophozoites, which do not stain with H & E.)
- X-ray: **patchy infiltrative** (ground glass appearance); the lower lobe periphery may be spared.

Diagnosis: Silver-staining cysts in bronchial alveolar lavage fluids or biopsy

Treatment: Trimethoprim/sulfamethoxazole for mild; dapsone for moderate to severe

Emerging Drug Resistances in Fungi

- Fungi are developing drug resistances by mechanisms analogous to those seen in bacteria.
- Resistance to azoles (clotrimazole, miconazole, ketoconazole, fluconazole) becoming widespread
- *Aspergillus, Candida, Cryptococcus*

Medical Parasitology 6

Learning Objectives

❏ Demonstrate understanding of classification of parasites

❏ Use knowledge of important protozoan parasites

❏ Answer questions about important metazoan parasites

CLASSIFICATION OF PARASITES

Medical parasitology is the study of the invertebrate animals and the diseases they cause. Parasites are classified as protozoans or metazoans.

The most important organisms in the U.S. are identified in the following two tables in boldface type.

Table II-6-1. Protozoans

Common Name	Amebae	Flagellates	Apicomplexa
Important Genera	**Entamoeba** Naegleria Acanthamoeba	LUMINAL (GUT, UG) **Trichomonas** **Giardia** HEMOFLAGELLATES Leishmania Trypanosoma	BLOOD/TISSUE **Plasmodium** **Toxoplasma** Babesia INTESTINAL **Cryptosporidium** Isospora

Pneumocystis, which was formerly classified as a protozoan, has been determined to be a fungus through ribotyping and other molecular biologic techniques.

Table II-6-2. Metazoans: Worms*

Phylum	Flat worms (Platyhelminthes)		Roundworms
Classes: Common name:	Trematodes (flukes)	Cestodes (tapeworms)	Nematodes** (roundworms)
Genera:	*Fasciola* *Fasciolopsis* *Paragonimus* *Clonorchis* *Schistosoma*	*Diphyllobothrium* *Hymenolepis* *Taenia* *Echinococcus*	**_Necator_** **_Enterobius_** (W)uchereria/Brugia **_Ascaris_** and **_Ancylostoma_** *Toxocara, Trichuris &* *Trichinella* *Onchocerca* *Dracunculus* *Eye worm (Loa loa)* *Strongyloides*

* Metazoans also include the Arthropoda, which serve mainly as intermediate hosts (the crustaceans) or as vectors of disease (the Arachnida and Insecta).

**Nematodes mnemonic.

Hosts

The infected host is classified as

- **Intermediate**—host in which **larval or asexual stages develop**.
- **Definitive** —host in which the **adult or sexual stages occur**.

Vectors

Vectors are **living transmitters** (e.g., a fly) of disease and may be

- **Mechanical,** which transport the parasite but there is no development of the parasite in the vector.
- **Biologic,** in which some stages of the life cycle occur.

IMPORTANT PROTOZOAN PARASITES

Table II-6-3. Protozoan Parasites

Species	Disease/Organs Most Affected	Form/Transmission	Diagnosis	Treatment
Entamoeba histolytica	***Amebiasis:*** dysentery **Inverted flask**-shaped lesions in large intestine with extension to peritoneum and liver, lungs, brain, and heart **Blood and pus** in stools **Liver abscesses**	Cysts Fecal-oral transmission—water, fresh fruits, and vegetables	Trophozoites: or cysts in stool: Serology: Nuclei have sharp central karyosome and fine chromatin "spokes".	Metronidazole followed by iodoquinol
Giardia lamblia	Giardiasis: Ventral sucking disk attaches to lining of duodenal wall, causing **a fatty, foul-smelling diarrhea** (diarrhea → *malabsorption* duodenum, jejunum)	Cysts Fecal (human, beaver, muskrat, etc.), oral transmission—water, food, day care, oral-anal sex	Trophozoites or cysts in stool or fecal antigen test (replaces "string" test) "Falling leaf" motility	Metronidazole
***Cryptosporidium* sp.** *C. parvum*	Cryptosporidiosis: transient diarrhea in healthy, severe in immunocompromised hosts	Cysts Undercooked meat, water; not killed by chlorination	**Acid fast oocysts in stool:** Biopsy shows dots (cysts) in intestinal glands	Nothing is 100% effective; nitrazoxanide, puromycin, or azithromycin are the DOCs
Isospora belli	Transient diarrhea in AIDS patients; diarrhea mimics giardiasis malabsorption syndrome	Oocysts Ingestion Fecal-oral	**Acid-fast and elliptical oocysts in stool;** contain 2 sporocysts each with 4 sporozoites	TMP-SMX or pyrimethamine/ sulfadiazine
Cyclospora cayetanensis	Self-limited diarrhea in immunocompetent; prolonged and severe **diarrhea in AIDS** patients	Oocysts, water	Fecal; **acid-fast and spherical oocysts;** contain 2 sporocysts each with 2 sporozoites; UV fluorescence	TMP-SMX

(Continued)

Table II-6-3. Protozoan Parasites (*Cont'd*)

Species	Disease/Organs Most Affected	Form/Transmission	Diagnosis	Treatment
Microsporidia (6 genera)	Microsporidiosis: persistent, debilitating **diarrhea in AIDS** patients; other spp → neurologic, hepatitis, disseminated	Spores ingested	**Gram (+), acid-fast spores** in stool or biopsy material	None proven to be effective
Trichomonas vaginalis (urogenital)	Trichomoniasis: often asymptomatic or **frothy vaginal discharge**	Trophozoites **Sexual**	Motile trophozoites in methylene blue wet mount; **corkscrew motility**	**Metronidazole**

Free Living Amebae

- Occur in water or soil (*Naegleria, Acanthamoeba*)
- Occur in contact lens saline solutions (*Acanthamoeba*): cysts from dust contaminate

Table II-6-4. Free Living Amoebae That Occasionally Infect Humans

Species	Disease / Locale	Form / Transmission	Diagnosis	Treatment
Naegleria	**Primary amebic meningoencephalitis (PAM):** severe **prefrontal headache,** nausea, high fever, **altered sense of smell;** often fatal	Free-living amebae picked up while swimming or **diving in very warm fresh water**	Motile trophozoites in CSF Culture on plates seeded with gram-negative bacteria; amebae will leave trails	Amphotericin B (rarely successful)
Acanthamoeba	**Keratitis; granulomatous amebic encephalitis** (GAE) in immunocompromised patients: insidious onset but progressive to death	Free living amebae in contaminated **contact lens solution (airborne cysts)** Not certain for GAE: inhalation or contact with contaminated soil or water	Star-shaped cysts on biopsy; rarely seen in CSF Culture as above	Keratitis: topical miconazole and propamidine isethionate GAE: ketoconazole, sulfamethazine (rarely successful)

Plasmodium Species

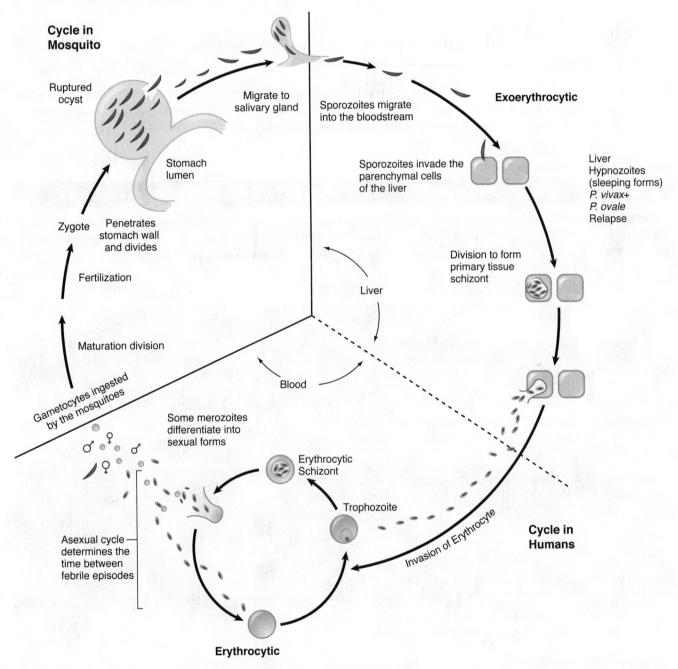

Cycle in Mosquito

Ruptured ocyst

Migrate to salivary gland

Sporozoites migrate into the bloodstream

Exoerythrocytic

Stomach lumen

Sporozoites invade the parenchymal cells of the liver

Liver Hypnozoites (sleeping forms) *P. vivax+* *P. ovale* Relapse

Zygote

Penetrates stomach wall and divides

Fertilization

Liver

Division to form primary tissue schizont

Maturation division

Blood

Gametocytes ingested by the mosquitoes

Some merozoites differentiate into sexual forms

Erythrocytic Schizont

Trophozoite

Cycle in Humans

Asexual cycle determines the time between febrile episodes

Invasion of Erythrocyte

Erythrocytic

Figure II-6-1. *Plasmodium* Life Cycle

Each *Plasmodium* has two distinct hosts.

- A vertebrate such as the human where asexual phase (schizogony) takes place in the liver and red blood cells.

- An arthropod host (*Anopheles* mosquito) where gametogony (sexual phase) and sporogony take place.

Cause disease by a wide variety of mechanisms, including metabolism of hemoglobin and lysis of infected cells leading to anemia and to agglutination of infected RBC.

Cause paroxysms (chills, fever spike, and malarial rigors) when the infected RBC are lysed, liberating a new crop of merozoites.

HbS heterozygote—selective protection against *P. falciparum*. Duffy blood group Ag—receptor for *P. vivax*. Other abnormal hemoglobins (e.g., thalassemia) are indigestible to all *Plasmodium* spp.

Table II-6-5. Plasmodium Species

Species	Disease	Important Features	Blood Smears	Liver Stages	Treatment**
Plasmodium vivax	**Benign tertian**	48-hour fever spikes	Enlarged host cells; ameboid trophozoites 	Persistent **hypnozoites** **Relapse***	Chloroquine PO$_4$ then **primaquine**
Plasmodium ovale	Benign tertian	48-hour fever spikes	Oval, jagged, infected RBCs	Persistent hypnozoites Relapse	Chloroquine PO$_4$ then primaquine
Plasmodium malariae	**Quartan** or malarial	72-hour fever spikes; recrudescence*	Bar and band forms; rosette schizonts	No persistent stage*; Recrudescence*	Chloroquine PO$_4$ (no radical cure necessary)
Plasmodium falciparum	**Malignant tertian**	Irregular fever spikes; causes **cerebral malaria**	**Multiple ring forms crescent-shaped gametes** 	No persistent stage*; recrudescence	Chloroquine resistance a problem***

*Recrudescence is a reoccurrence of symptoms from low levels of organisms remaining in <u>red</u> cells.
Relapse is a return of clinical symptoms from liver stages (hypnozoites).

**Treatment:
1. Suppressive (to avoid infection)
2. Therapeutic (eliminate erythrocytic)
3. Radical cure (eliminate hypnozoites)
4. Gametocidal (destruction of gametocytes)
   Successful treatment is accomplished with chloroquine followed by primaquine. Chloroquine therapy is suppressive, therapeutic, and gametocidal, whereas primaquine eliminates the exoerythrocytic form.

***Use quinine sulfate plus pyrimethamine-sulfadoxine.

Hemoflagellates (Trypanosomes and Leishmanias)

Hemoflagellates infect blood and tissues.

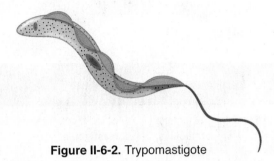

Figure II-6-2. Trypomastigote

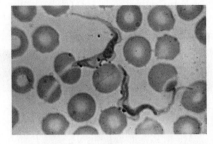

Trypomastigote in blood smear

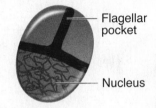

Flagellar pocket

Nucleus

Figure II-6-3. Amastigote

Trypanosomes are found
- In human blood as trypomastigotes with flagellum and undulating membrane
- In tissues as **amastigotes (oval cells having neither the flagellum nor undulating membrane)**

Leishmania found always as amastigotes in macrophages.

Table II-6-6. Hemoflagellates

Species	Disease	Vector/Form/Transmission	Reservoirs	Diagnosis	Treatment
Trypanosoma cruzi*	**Chagas disease** (American trypanoso-miasis) Latin America Swelling around eye: (**Romaña sign**) common early sign Cardiac muscle, liver, brain often involved	**Reduviid bug (kissing or cone bug**; genus *Triatoma*) passes trypomastigote (flagel-lated form) **in feces**; scratching implants in mucosa	Cats, dogs, armadillos, opossums Poverty hous-ing	Blood films, **trypo-mastigotes**	Benzimidazole
Trypanosoma brucei gambiense Trypanosoma b. rhodesiense	**African sleeping sick-ness** (African trypanosomia-sis) **Antigenic variation**	Trypomastigote in saliva of **tsetse fly** contaminates bite	Humans, some wild animals	Trypomastigotes in blood films, CSF High immunoglob-ulin levels in CSF	Acute: suramin Chronic: melar-soprol
Leishmania donovani** complex	**Visceral Leishmaniasis**	**Sandfly** bite	Urban: humans Rural: rodents and wild ani-mals	**Amastigotes in macrophages** in bone marrow, liver, spleen	Stibogluconate sodium (from CDC)
Leishmania (About 15 differ-ent species)	Cutaneous Leishmani-asis (Oriental sore, etc.)	**Sandfly** bite	Urban: humans Rural: rodents and wild ani-mals	**Amastigotes in macrophages** in cutaneous le-sions	Stibogluconate sodium
Leishmania braziliensis complex	Mucocutaneous Leish-maniasis	**Sandfly** bite	Urban: humans Rural: rodents and wild ani-mals	Same	Stibogluconate sodium

**T. cruzi:* An estimated 1/2 million Americans are infected, creating some risk of transfusion transmission in U.S. In babies, acute infections often serious involving CNS.

In older children and adults, mild acute infections but may become chronic with the risk of development of cardiomyopathy and heart failure.

**Leishmania all: Intracellular, sandfly vector, stibogluconate.

Miscellaneous Apicomplexa Infecting Blood or Tissues

Table II-6-7. Miscellaneous Apicomplexa Infecting Blood or Tissues

Species	Disease/Locale of Origin	Transmission	Diagnosis	Treatment
Babesia (primarily a disease of cattle) Humans: *Babesia microti*, WA1, & MO1 strains	Babesiosis (hemolytic, **malaria-like**) Same range as lyme: NE, N Central, California, and NW U.S.	***Ixodes*** **tick** **Co-infections with** *Borrelia*	Giemsa stain of thin smear or hamster inoculation; small rings, maltese cross, tetrad in RBCs	Clindamycin + quinine
Toxoplasma gondii	See below	**Cat** is **essential definitive** host. Many other animals are intermediate host. Mode: 1) Raw meat in U.S. #1 = pork 2) Contact with cat feces	Serology High IgM or rising IgM acute infection	**Pyrimethamine + sulfadiazine**

Toxoplasmosis

Diseases

Healthy individuals

- *Toxoplasma* acquired after birth is most commonly asymptomatic or a mild, non-specific flu-like illness with lymphadenopathy and fever; heterophile-negative mononucleosis
- Once infected, as immunity develops, bradyzoites encyst, but generally remain viable as evidenced by a positive antibody titer.

Pregnant patients

- Women who acquire *Toxoplasma* as a primary infection during pregnancy present with flu-like illness/heterophile-negative mononucleosis.
- If primary maternal infection occurs during pregnancy, the fetus may be infected.
- If *Toxoplasma* crosses the placenta early, severe congenital infections (intracerebral calcifications, chorioretinitis, hydro- or microcephaly or convulsions) may occur.
- If *Toxoplasma* crosses the placenta later, infection may be inapparent, but may lead to progressive blindness in the child later in life (teens).
- Maternal antibodies (secondary infection) protect the fetus during pregnancy, even if the mother is re-exposed during pregnancy.

AIDS patients

- Leading cause of focal CNS disease in AIDS patients
- Brain scan will describe ring-enhancing lesions.
- Unless prophylactic drugs are given, AIDS patients who are seropositive for *Toxoplasma* will have reactivational infections.

IMPORTANT METAZOAN PARASITES

Trematodes

- Are commonly called flukes.

- Are leaf-shaped worms, which are generally flat and fleshy.

- Are hermaphroditic except for *Schistosoma*, which has separate male and female.

- Have complicated life cycles occurring in two or more hosts.

- Have operculated eggs (except for *Schistosoma*), which contaminate water, perpetuating the life cycle, and which are also used to diagnose infections.

- **The first intermediate hosts are snails.**

Table II-6-8. Trematode (Fluke) Diseases

Organism	Common Name	Reservoir Host	Acquisition	Progression in Humans	Important Ova	Treatment
S. mansoni Schistosoma japonicum	**Intestinal schistoso-miasis**	Cats, dogs, cattle, etc.	Contact with water; **skin penetration**	Skin penetration (itching)→ mature in veins of mesentery → eggs cause granulomas in liver (liver enlargement in chronic cases)		Praziquantel
Schistosoma haemato-bium	**Vesicular schistoso-miasis**	Primates	Contact with water; **skin penetration**	Skin penetration (itching) → mature in bladder veins; chronic infection has high association with **bladder carcinoma in Egypt and Africa**		Praziquantel
Non-human schisto-somes	**Swimmer's itch**	Birds (Great Lakes U.S.)	Contact with water; **skin penetration**	Penetrate skin, producing **dermatitis** without further development in humans; itching is most intense at 2 to 3 days		Trimeprazine Calamine Sedatives
Clonorchis sinensis	**Chinese liver fluke**	Dogs, cats, humans	Raw fish ingestion	Serum-like sickness	Operculated eggs	Praziquantel

Cestodes

- Are the tapeworms.

- Consist of 3 basic portions: the head or scolex; a "neck" section, which produces the proglottids; and the segments or proglottids, which mature as they move away from the scolex. (The combination of the neck and proglottids is called the strobila.)

- Are hermaphroditic, with each proglottid developing both male and female reproductive organs, and mature eggs developing in the most distal proglottids.

- Adhere to the mucosa via the scolex, which is knobby looking and has either suckers or a sucking groove.

- Have no gastrointestinal (GI) tract; they absorb nutrients from the host's GI tract.

- Are diagnosed by finding eggs or proglottids in the feces.

- Have for the most part complex life cycles involving extraintestinal larval forms in intermediate hosts. When humans are the intermediate host, these infections are generally more serious than the intestinal infections with adult tapeworms.

Gastrointestinal Cestodes (Tapeworms)

Table II-6-9. Gastrointestinal Cestodes (Tapeworms)

Cestode*	Form/Transmission	Humans Are:	Disease/Organ Involvement/Symptoms (Sx)	Diagnosis	Treatment
Taenia saginata (beef tapeworm) IH: cattle DH: humans	Rare beef containing the **cysticerci** is ingested	DH*	**Intestinal tapeworm/** small intestine Sx: Asymptomatic or vague abdominal pains	**Proglottids** or **eggs** in feces	Praziquantel
Taenia solium (pork tapeworm) IH: swine; Rarely: humans DH: humans; developing and Slavic countries	Water, vegetation, food contaminated with **eggs** **Autoinfection**	IH*	**Cysticercosis**/eggs → larva develop in brain, eye, heart, lung, etc. Adult-onset epilepsy	Biopsy	Praziquantel: surgery in some sites
	Rare/raw pork containing the **cysticerci** is ingested by humans	DH	**Intestinal tapeworm** Sx: as for *Taenia saginata*	**Proglottids** or **eggs** in feces	Praziquantel
Diphyllobothrium latum (fish tapeworm) IH (2): crustaceans → fish; rare: humans DH: humans/mammals; cool lake regions	Drinking pond water w/ → copepods (crustaceans) carrying the **larval** forms or frog/snake poultices	IH	**Sparganosis**/larvae penetrate intestinal wall and encyst	Biopsy	Praziquantel
	Rare, raw pickled fish → containing a **sparganum**	DH	**Intestinal tapeworm** (up to 10 meters)/small intestine **megaloblastic anemia**	Proglottids or eggs in feces	Praziquantel
Echinococcus granulosus IH: herbivores; rare: humans DH: carnivores in sheep-raising areas	Ingestion of eggs	IH	**Hydatid cyst disease/** liver & lung where cysts containing brood capsules develop	Imaging; serology	Surgery; albendazole
Echinococcus multilocularis IH: rodents DH: canines and cats; northern areas	Ingestion of eggs	IH	**Alveolar hydatid cyst disease**	As above	Surgical resection

* Definitive host = adult tapeworm develops in; intermediate host = cysticerci or larvae develop in; cysticerci = encysted larvae found in intermediate host. Common name is in parentheses.

Nematodes

- Are the roundworms
- Cause a wide variety of diseases (pinworms, whipworms, hookworms, trichinosis, threadworms, filariasis, etc.)
- Have round unsegmented bodies
- Are transmitted by:
  - ingestion of eggs (*Enterobius, Ascaris,* or *Trichuris*);
  - direct invasion of skin by larval forms (*Necator, Ancylostoma,* or *Strongyloides*);
  - ingestion of meat containing larvae (*Trichinella*); or
  - infection involving insects transmitting the larvae with bites (*Wuchereria, Loa loa, Mansonella, Onchocerca,* and *Dracunculus*).

Table II-6-10. Round Worms (Nematodes) Transmitted by Eggs

Species	Disease/Organs Most Affected	Form/ Transmission	Diagnosis		Treatment
Enterobius vermicularis Most frequent helminth parasite in U.S.	**Pinworms**, large intestine, perianal itching	**Eggs**/person to person **autoinfection**	Sticky swab of perianal area Ova have flattened side with larvae inside		Pyrantel, **mebendazole** Treat entire family (albendazole)
Trichuris trichiura	**Whipworm** cecum, appendicitis, and rectal prolapse	**Eggs** ingested	**Barrel-shaped eggs with bipolar plugs** in stools		Albendazole
Ascaris lumbricoides Most common helminth worldwide Largest roundworm	**Ascariasis** Ingest egg → larva migrate thru lungs (cough) and mature in small intestine; may obstruct intestine or bile duct	**Eggs** ingested	**Bile stained, knobby eggs** Adults **6–12"** roundworms		Supportive therapy during pneumonitis; surgery for ectopic migrations; mebendazole
Toxocara canis or cati (dog/cat ascarids)	**Visceral Larva Migrans** Larvae wander aimlessly until they die, cause inflammation	**Eggs** ingested/ from handling puppies or from eating dirt in yard (pica)	Clinical findings and serology		Mebendazole; self-limiting in most cases (albendazole)

Table II-6-11. Roundworms (Nematodes) Transmitted By Larvae

Species	Disease/Organs	Form/Transmission	Diagnosis	Treatment
Necator americanus New World hookworm	**Hookworm** infection Lung migration → pneumonitis bloodsucking → anemia	Filariform **larva penetrates intact skin of bare feet**	Fecal larvae (up to 13 mm) and ova: oval, transparent with 2–8 cell-stage visible inside Occult blood fecal may be present	**Mebendazole** and iron therapy (albendazole)
Ancylostoma braziliense Ancylostoma caninum (dog and cat hookworms)	**Cutaneous Larva Migrans**/ intense skin itching	Filariform larva penetrates intact skin but cannot mature in humans	Usually a presumptive diagnosis; exposure	Thiabendazole Topical corticosteroids
Strongyloides stercoralis	**Threadworm** strongyloidiasis: Early: pneumonitis, abdominal pain, diarrhea Later: malabsorption, ulcers, bloody stools	Filariform **larva penetrates intact skin; Autoinfection** leads to indefinite infections unless treated	Larvae in stool, serology	Thiabendazole
Trichinella spiralis	Trichinosis: larvae encyst in muscle → pain	**Viable encysted larvae in meat** are consumed: wild game meat	Muscle biopsy; clinical findings: **fever, myalgia, splinter hemorrhages, eosinophilia**	Steroids for severe symptoms + mebendazole (albendazole)

Table II-6-12. Filarial Nematodes

Species	Disease	Transmission/Vector	Diagnosis	Treatment
Wucheria bancrofti; Brugia malayi	Elephantiasis	Mosquito	Microfilariae in blood, eosinophilia	Surgery, ivermectin and diethylcarbamazine (DEC)
Loa loa (African eye worm)	Pruritus, calabar swellings	*Chrysops*, mango flies	Microfilariae in blood, eosinophilia	Surgical removal of worms; DEC
Onchocerca volvulus	River blindness, itchy "leopard" rash	Blackflies	Skin snips from calabar swellings	Surgical removal of worms; DEC or ivermectin
Dracunculus medinensis (guinea worm, fiery serpent)	Creeping eruptions, ulcerations, rash	Drinking water with infected copepods	Increased IgE; worm eruption from skin	Slow, cautious worm removal with stick; albendazole

Clinical Infectious Disease

7

Learning Objectives

❏ Answer case-based questions related to infectious disease

•••

These charts are designed for self-study after the organisms have all been reviewed in class. They represent the basics used in clinical scenarios on the USMLE.

Cover the last column on each chart and write the causal agent(s) on paper. Then think about how the organism causes disease. Is there a major virulence factor?

Abbreviations Used

→ means progressing on to

~ means about or approximately

HIV+ = patient with known human immunodeficiency virus infection; can be used for anyone who is infected but often used for those who are HIV+ but do not have full blown AIDS (in other words, CD4+ count >200)

AIDS = acquired immunodeficiency syndrome (CD4+ count <200)

abd = abdominal

CF = cystic fibrosis

CMI = cell-mediated immunity

CGD = chronic granulomatous disease

GU = genitourinary

IC = immunocompromised

Infl'd = inflamed

Infl'n = inflammation

IV = intravenous

mo = month(s)

NF = normal flora

occ = occasional

PMNs = polymorphonuclear leukocytes

pt = patient

RBCs = red blood cells

subQ = subcutaneous

If there are multiple causal agents, at the end of the description there may be a # with the abbreviation "CA." This means you should be able to list that number. If it specifically says "species," you should give species.

Table II-7-1. Diseases of Skin, Mucous Membranes, and Underlying Tissues

Type Infection	Case Vignette/Key Clues	Common Causal Agents
Furuncles, carbuncles	Neck, face, axillae, buttocks	*Staphylococcus aureus*
	Inflamed follicles from neck down	*Pseudomonas aeruginosa* (hot tub folliculitis)
Acne vulgaris	Inflammation of follicles and sebaceous glands	*Propionibacterium acnes*
Impetigo	Initially vesicular; skin erosion; **honey-crusted** lesions; catalase negative organism	*Streptococcus pyogenes*
	Initially vesicular but with longer lasting **bullae**; catalase-positive organism	*Staphylococcus aureus*
Vesicular lesions	Sometimes preceded by neurologic pain	Herpes
SubQ granulomas/ulcers/cellulitis	Tropical fish enthusiasts; granulomatous lesion	*Mycobacterium marinum* (fish tank granuloma)
	Cellulitis following contact with saltwater or oysters	*Vibrio vulnificus*
Mycetoma (swelling with pain, sinus tract formation, yellow granules in exudate)	Solitary or lymphocutaneous lesions, rose gardeners or florists, sphagnum moss	*Sporothrix schenckii* (rose gardener disease)
	Subcutaneous swelling (extremities, shoulders) multiple CA	Bacteria: *Actinomyces, Nocardia,* Fungi: *Madurella, Pseudallescheria, Sporothrix*
	Jaw area, associated with carious teeth, dental extraction, or trauma	*Actinomyces israelii* "lumpy jaw"
Malignant pustule	Pustule → dark red fluid-filled, tumor-like lesion → necrosis → black eschar surrounded by red margin	*Bacillus anthracis*
	Ecthyma gangrenosum (as above)	*Pseudomonas* septicemia
Cellulitis	Blue-green pus, grape-like odor, burns	*Pseudomonas aeruginosa*
	Dermal pain, edema, heat and rapid spread. Red, raised butterfly facial rash	*Streptococcus pyogenes* (Erysipelas)
	Hot inflamed tissues. Deeper tissues from extension of skin lesions or wounds including surgical	Variety of bacteria: *S. aureus, S. pyogenes*, gram (−) rods, *Clostridium* and anaerobes

(Continued)

Table II-7-1. Diseases of Skin, Mucous Membranes, and Underlying Tissues (*Cont'd*)

Type Infection	Case Vignette/Key Clues	Common Causal Agents
Wounds	Surgical wounds (clean)	*Staphylococcus aureus*
	Surgical wounds (dirty)—list groups	*S. aureus, Enterobacteriaceae*, anaerobes
	Trauma—list groups	*Clostridium*, Enterobacteriaceae, *Pseudomonas*
	Shallow puncture wound through tennis shoe sole	*Pseudomonas aeruginosa*
Animal bites	Various	*Pasteurella multocida*
	Human bites, fist fights	*Eikenella corrodens*
	Dog bites	*Capnocytophaga canimorsus*
	Rat bites	*Streptobacillus moniliformis and Spirillum minus*
	Cat scratches resulting in lymphadenopathy with stellate granulomas	*Bartonella henselae*

Table II-7-2. Ear, Nose, Throat, Upper Respiratory System Infections

Type Infection	Case Vignette/Key Clues	Common Causal Agents
Acute otitis media	Red, bulging tympanic membrane, fever 102–103; pain goes away if drum ruptures or if ear tubes are patent. 5 CA	*Streptococcus pneumoniae* *H. influenzae* (often nontypeable, recurs) *Moraxella catarrhalis* RSV Rhinovirus
Otitis externa	Ear pain—list of organisms	Normal flora often involved Often mixed infections: *Staph aureus* (from NF)* *Candida albicans* (from NF)* *Proteus* (water organism) *Pseudomonas* (water)
Malignant otitis externa	Severe ear pain in diabetic; life threatening	*Pseudomonas aeruginosa*
Sinusitis	Sinus pain; low-grade fever	As for acute otitis media
Oral cavitary disease	Painful mouth—overgrowth of spirochetes and fusiform bacteria	*Fusobacterium* and treponemes (normal oral spirochetes)
	Sore mouth with thick white coating (painful red base under); increased risk: premature infants, AIDS, IC pts, pts on antibiotics, vitamin C deficiency	*Candida*
Sore throat	Inflamed tonsils/pharynx, which may be purulent and may develop abscesses; cervical lymphadenopathy, fever, stomach upset; sandpaper rash	*Streptococcus pyogenes* (group A strep) Rash indicates presence of erythrogenic exotoxin A
	White papules with red base on posterior palate and pharynx, fever	Coxsackie A
	Throat looking like Strep with severe fatigue, lymphadenopathy, fever, rash; heterophile (+); Downey type II cells	Epstein-Barr virus
	Low-grade fever with a 1–2 day gradual onset of membranous nasopharyngitis and/or obstructive laryngotracheitis; bull neck from lymphadenopathy; elevated BUN; abnormal ECG; little change in WBC (toxin). Exudate bleeds profusely when dislodged	*Corynebacterium diphtheriae* (diphtheria)
Common cold	Rhinitis, sneezing, coughing; list CA with seasonal peaks	Rhinoviruses (summer–fall) Coronaviruses (winter–spring) Human metapneumovirus Adenovirus, many others

*NF = normal flora

Table II-7-3. Eye Infections

Type Infection	Case Vignette/Key Clues	Common Causal Agents
Eyelid	Bilateral eye lid swelling, >10% eosinophilia, fever, muscle pain; earlier GI Sx	*Trichinella*
	Stye; 2 CA	*Staphylococcus aureus* *Propionibacterium acnes*
	Unilateral inflammation at bite site often around eye or mouth; travel to Mexico, Central or South America	*Trypanosoma cruzi*
Conjunctivitis neonate	Red itchy eye(s)/pus; onset 2–5 days Red itchy eye(s)/pus; onset 5–10 days	Bacterial pink eye *Neisseria gonorrhoeae* *Chlamydia trachomatis* (serotypes D–K U.S.)
	Neonate with "sticky eye"	*Staphylococcus aureus*
Conjunctivitis (other age groups)	Red itchy eye(s), thin exudate; pain, photophobia	Viral pink eye: adenovirus (more common than bacterial pink eye)
	Red eye, pus; 4 CA	*S. aureus*, group A Strep, *Strep pneumoniae* (all gram [+]) *Haemophilus influenzae, H. aegyptius*
	Red eye, pus, presence of inclusion bodies in scrapings; CA with serotypes in U.S.	*Chlamydia trachomatis* serotypes D-K (inclusion conjunctivitis)
	Granulomas and inturned eye lashes, corneal scarring, blindness; CA with serotypes	*Chlamydia trachomatis* serotypes A, B, Ba, C (trachoma)
Chorioretinitis	Neonate or AIDS; 2 CA	*Toxoplasma*, CMV
Retinopathy with keratitis in baby	Mom IV drug abuser	*Treponema pallidum* (congenital syphilis)

Table II-7-4. Cardiac Symptoms

Type Infection	Case Vignette/Key Clues	Common Causal Agents
Acute endocarditis: Chills, fever, arthralgia, myalgia, back pain, acutely ill, Janeway lesions; emboli	Developing a heart murmur; IV drug user	*Staphyloccoccus aureus*
	Not IV drug user	*Staphyloccoccus aureus*
Subacute endocarditis: Fever with vague symptoms with insidious onset, fatigue, weakness, weight loss, night sweats, anorexia, myalgias; murmur may have been long present; emboli, splinter hemorrhages	Poor oral hygiene or dental work	*Viridans* streptococci (55% of cases in native hearts)
	Gram neg. endocarditis (normal oral flora)	HACEK organisms (**H**aemophilus aphrophilus **A**ctinobacillus actinomycetemcomitans **C**ardiobacterium hominis **E**ikenella corrodens **K**ingella kingae)
	Bilary or urinary tract infection GU manipulation in elderly men	*Enterococcus faecalis*
	IV drug user	*Staph. epidermidis* *Aspergillus* (branching <45) *Candida* (pseudohyphae) *Pseudomonas* *Viridans* streptococci
Dilated cardiomyopathy	Rural South America	*Trypanosoma cruzi*

Table II-7-5. Middle and Lower Respiratory System Infections

Type Infection	Case Vignette/Key Clues	Most Common Causal Agents
Respiratory difficulty or obstruction	Inflamed epiglottis; patient often 2–3 and unvaccinated	*Haemophilus influenzae* (epigottitis)
	Infant with fever, sharp barking cough, inspiratory stridor, hoarse phonation	Parainfluenza virus (Croup)
Bronchitis	Wheezy; infant or child ≤5 years	RSV
	›5 years	*Haemophilus influenzae, Mycoplasma pneumoniae, Chlamydophila pneumoniae*
	With cough ›2 weeks, afebrile; ›9	*Bordetella pertussis*
Pneumonia **Typical:** high fever, productive cough, diffuse infiltreates	Poorly nourished, unvaccinated baby/child; giant cell pneumonia with hemorrhagic rash	Measles: malnourishment ↑ risk of pneumonia and blindness
	Adults (including alcoholics) #1 CA Rusty sputum, often follows influenza	*Streptococcus pneumoniae*
	Neutropenic pts, burn pts, CGD, CF	*Pseudomonas*
	Foul smelling sputum, aspiration possible	Anaerobes, mixed infection (*Bacteroides, Fusobacterium, Peptococcus*)
	Alcoholic, abscess formation, aspiration, facultative anaerobic, gram-negative bacterium with huge capsule, currant jelly sputum	*Klebsiella pneumoniae*
	Nosocomial, ventilator, post-influenza Abscess formation Gram +, catalase +, coagulase + Salmon-colored sputum	*Staphylococcus aureus*
Atypical: low fever, dry cough, diffuse infiltrates	Pneumonia teens/young adults; bad hacking cough; initially non-productive cough	*Mycoplasma pneumoniae* (most common cause of pneumonia in school age children)
	Atypical with air conditioning exposure especially ›50 yr, heavy smoker, drinker	*Legionella* spp.
	Atypical with bird exposure, hepatitis	*Chlamydophila psittaci*
	AIDS patients with staccato cough; "ground glass" x-ray; biopsy: honeycomb exudate with silver staining cysts, progressive hypoxia	*Pneumocystis jiroveci*
Acute respiratory distress	Travel to Far East, winter, early spring, hypoxia	SARS-CoV
	Spring, 4 corners region, exposure to rodents	Hanta virus
Acute pneumonia or chronic cough with weight loss, night sweats, calcifying lesions	Over 55, HIV+, or immigrant from developing country	*Mycobacterium tuberculosis*
	Dusty environment with bird or bat fecal contamination (Missouri chicken farmers), yeasts packed into phagocytic cells	*Histoplasma capsulatum*
	Desert sand, SW U.S.	*Coccidioides immitis*
	Rotting contaminated wood, North and South Carolina	*Blastomyces dermatitidis*

Table II-7-6. Genitourinary Tract Infections

Type Infection	Case Vignette/Key Clues	Most Common Causal Agents
Urethritis	Gram-negative diplococci in PMNs in urethral exudate	*Neisseria gonorrhoeae*
	Culture negative, inclusion bodies	*Chlamydia trachomatis*
	Urease positive, no cell wall	*Ureaplasma urealyticum*
	Flagellated protozoan with corkscrew motility	*Trichomonas vaginalis*
Cystitis	Frequent and painful urination, hematuria, and fever	#1 *E. coli*, other gram-negative enterics, *Pseudomonas*, *Proteus*
	Young, newly sexually active individual; gram-positive cocci	*Staphylococcus saprophyticus*
Pyelonephritis	As above, with flank pain and prominent fever	*E. coli, Staphylococcus*
Cervicitis	Friable, inflamed cervix with mucopurulent discharge; probes or culture to distinguish	*Neisseria gonorrhoeae* (gram-negative diplococci) *Chlamydia trachomatis* (non-staining obligate intracellular parasite) Herpes simplex (virus)
Vaginal itching, pain, discharge odor	Adherent yellowish discharge, pH >5, fishy amine odor in KOH, clue cells; gram-negative cells dominate	(Bacterial vaginosis) overgrowth of *Gardnerella vaginalis* and anaerobes
	Vulvovaginitis, pruritis, erythema, discharge: consistency of cottage cheese	*Candida* spp.
	Foamy, purulent discharge, many PMNs and motile trophozoites microscopically (corkscrew motility)	*Trichomonas vaginalis*
Pelvic inflammatory disease	Adnexal tenderness, bleeding, deep dyspareunia, vaginal discharge, fever; tenderness from cervical movement, possibly palpable inflammatory mass on bimanual exam, onset often follows menses	*Neisseria gonorrhoeae* or *Chlamydia trachomatis* or both or a variety of other organisms
Genital lesions	Genital warts	Human papilloma virus (most common U.S. STD), *Treponema pallidum*, molluscum contagiosum
	Multiple painful vesicular, coalescing, recurring	Herpes simplex virus
	Nontender, indurated ulcer healing spontaneously 2–10 weeks	*Treponema pallidum*
	Non-indurated, painful papule, suppurative with adenopathy, slow to heal	*Haemophilus ducreyi*
	Soft, painless ulcer, pt from Caribbean or New Guinea, gram negative intracellular bacilli	*Klebsiella granulomatis (granuloma inguinale)*
Genital elephantitis	Initial papule heals; lymph nodes enlarge and develop fistulas; genital elephantiasis may develop Tropics, microfilariae in bloodstream	*Chlamydia trachomatis* L1–L3 *Wuchereria* or *Brugia* (filarial nematodes)

Diarrhea

Dysentery

- Abdominal cramps, tenesmus, and pus and blood in the stool
- Usually associated with invasive bacterial disease in the colon

Diarrhea

- Refers to profuse watery feces
- Most commonly associated with increased secretion of fluid across the mucosal surfaces of the small intestine in response to a toxin or a viral infection
- No inflammatory cells, usually no fever

Table II-7-7. Diarrhea by Intoxication

Most Common Sources	Common Age Group Infected	Incubation Period	Pathogenesis	Symptoms	Duration of Symptoms	Organism
Ham, potato salad, cream pastries	All	**1–6 hours**	**Heat stable entero-toxin is produced in food contaminated** by food handler; food sits at room temperature	**abd cramps, vomiting, diarrhea; sweating and headache may occur; no fever**	‹24 hours	***Staphylococcus aureus***
Rice	All	‹6 hours	**Heat stable toxin causes vomiting**	As above	8–10 hours	***Bacillus cereus:*** emetic form
Meat, vegetables	All	›6 hours	Heat labile toxin causes diarrhea (similar to *E. coli* LT)	Nausea, abd cramps, diarrhea	20–36 hrs	*Bacillus cereus:* diarrheal form

Table II-7-8. Microbial Diarrhea: Organisms Causing NoninflammatoryDiarrhea

Common Age Group Infected	Most Common Sources	Incubation Period	Pathogenesis	Symptoms	Duration of Symptoms	Organism
Infants and toddlers	Day care, water, nosocomial, fecal-oral	1–3 days (fall, winter, spring)	Microvilli of small intestine blunted; mononuclear infiltrate in lamina propria; disaccharidase activity down; glucose coupled transport normal; lactose intolerance may cause build up and osmotic influx creating watery diarrhea	Noninflammatory watery diarrhea, vomiting, fever, and dehydration	**5–7 days**	Rotaviruses
Young kids, IC	Nosocomial	7–8 days	?	Diarrhea, fever, and vomiting	8–12 days	Adenovirus 40/41
Infants in developing countries	Food, water, fecal-oral	2–6 days	**Adherence to enterocytes through pili causes damage** to adjoining microvilli	Watery to profusely watery diarrhea	1–3 weeks	Enteropathogenic *E. coli*
Older kids and adults	Water, food, fecal-oral	18–48 hours	Jejunal biopsy shows blunting of microvilli; cytoplasmic vacuolization is seen along with mononuclear infiltrates of tissue; virus appears to decrease brush border enzymes causing malabsorption	Diarrhea, nausea, and vomiting; fever in some	12–48 hours	Norwalk virus
	Cruise ships					Noro-like virus
All	**Beef, poultry, gravies** Mexican food	8–24 hours	Enterotoxin	Abd cramps and **watery diarrhea**, rarely fever or vomiting	<24 hours	*Clostridium perfringens*
All	Water, food, fecal-oral	9–72 hours	**Toxin stimulates adenylate cyclase and causes increase in cAMP in the small intestine without inflammation or invasion**	**Profuse watery diarrhea with vomiting; fever may be present** (rice water stools)	3–4 days	*Vibrio cholerae*
All	Raw or **undercooked shellfish**	5–92 hours	Self-limited gastroenteritis mimicking cholera; there is a severe, rarer dysentery form, no clear enterotoxin; hemolysins, phospholipase and lysophospholipase; tests for invasiveness are negative	Explosive watery diarrhea along with headache, abdominal cramps, nausea, vomiting, and fever.	Up to 10 days	*Vibrio parahaemolyticus*
All	Water, uncooked fruits and vegetables	12–72 hours	**Heat labile toxin (LT) stimulates adenylate cyclase resulting in efflux of water and ions into the small intestine;** stable toxin guanylate cyclase	Watery diarrhea with some vomiting and sometimes fever	3–5 days	Enterotoxigenic *E. coli*
50% <10 yrs., all	Food, fecal-oral (**hamburger**)	3–5 days	**Verotoxin, which is a cytotoxin, causes bloody diarrhea** with no invasion of the organism	Abdominal cramps, watery diarrhea with blood (**no fever**)	7–10 days	Enterohemorrhagic *E. coli.*
All	Water, day care, **camping**, beavers, dogs, etc.	5–25 days	Cysts ingested; excyst in the duodenum and jejunum; **multiply and attach to intestinal villi by sucking disk**	**Loose, pale, greasy diarrhea; mild to severe malabsorption** syndrome	1–2 weeks to years	*Giardia lamblia*
Children, AIDS patients	Day care, fecal-oral, animals, **homosexuals**	2–4 weeks	Sporozoites attach to the epithelial surface of the intestine and replicate	Mild diarrhea in immunocompetent; severe chronic diarrhea in AIDS **Acid-fast** spores/oocysts in stool	4 days to 3 weeks **in AIDS: indefinite**	*Cryptosporidium parvum Isospora belli, Cyclospora, Microsporidia*

Table II-7-9. Microbial Diarrhea: Organisms Causing Inflammatory Diarrhea/Dysentery

Common Age Group Infected	Most Common Sources*	Incubation Period	Pathogenesis	Symptoms	Duration of Symptoms	Organism
All, esp <1 year and young adults	**Poultry, domestic animals, water,** unpasteurized milk, day care, fecal-oral	3–5 days	**Multiply in the small intestine; invades epithelium** resulting in inflammation and RBC and WBC in stools.	Diarrhea, abd pain, malaise; enteritis with diarrhea, malaise, fever	1–2 days mild; <1 week normal self-limiting	*Campylobacter jejuni*
All, esp infants and kids	**Poultry, domestic animals,** water, day care, fecal-oral	8–48 hours	Adsorb to epithelial cells in terminal small intestine; penetrate to lamina propria of ileocecal region causing **PMN response and PG response, which stimulates** cAMP and watery diarrhea	Diarrhea (occ bloody), abd cramps, abd tenderness, fever, and nausea w/occ vomiting; osteomyelitis in sickle cell anemia	3–5 days; spontaneous resolution	*Salmonella* gastroenteritis
All, esp 6 mo to 10 yr.	Water, day care, no animal reservoirs, fecal-oral	1–7 days	*Shigella* colonize the small intestine producing at first an enterotoxin-induced watery diarrhea; ultimately the *shigellae* penetrate the colon mucosa producing **shallow mucosal ulcerations and dysentery; septicemia rare**	Watery diarrhea at first → lower abdominal cramps, tenesmus and abundant pus and blood in the stools (dysentery)	4–7 days; antibiotics can reduce spread	*Shigella*
All, esp older kids and young adults	Milk, wild **domestic animals** water, fecal-oral	2–7 days	The terminal ileum is infected with enlargement of the mesenteric lymph nodes; produces focal necrosis difficult to distinguish from appendicitis; organism is able to grow in cold; produces heat insensitive enterotoxin. Arthritis may occur.	Fever, diarrhea (frequently with leukocytes & blood in stools), abdominal pain; also a noninflammatory gastroenteritis	1 day – 3 weeks (avg. 9 days)	*Yersinia enterocolitica*
Pt on antibiotics	Associated with **antibiotic use (most common clindamycin)**	NA	Intense inflammatory response creates the friable yellow plaque-like colonic lesions (pseudo-membrane) associated with this disease	Mild diarrhea to severe **colitis;** abd cramps; spiking fever, systemic toxicity; blood, mucus, and pus in stools	Until antibiotic stopped; treat with metronidazole or change antibiotic	*Clostridium difficile*
Adults	Food, water, fecal-oral	2–3 days	Similar to *Shigella* dysentery	Fever and cramps with blood and pus in the stools	1–2 weeks; fluid and electrolyte replacement	Enteroinvasive *E. coli*
All	Food, water, fecal-oral, **tropical** generally	2–4 weeks	Ingested cysts survive (trophozoites die) and multiply in the colon with invasion of the colon wall producing the **characteristic flask-like lesions and extra-intestinal abscesses**	Gen. acute diarrhea with cramping; sometimes dysentery; ulceration of colon may produce peritonitis	Weeks to monthsRx with metronidazole followed by iodoquinol	*Entamoeba histolytica*

*Sources: Water = those listed are the most common diarrhea diseases spread through water
Day care = organisms listed are ones that have caused outbreaks in day care facilities, but note that any organism spread by the oral-fecal route may be a problem in this setting
Milk = unpasteurized milk or dairy products

Table II-7-10. Other Gastrointestinal or Liver Infections

Signs and Symptoms	Case Vignette/Key Clues	Most Common Causal Agents
Hepatitis: Jaundice, anorexia, nausea, right upper quadrant pain on palpation, cigarettes taste foul, elevated liver enzymes*	Food-borne (possibly contaminated raw oysters or clams); 14–45 days; without chronicity; sturdy naked RNA virus	Hepatitis A ("infectious" hepatitis) (picornavirus)
	IV drug abuse, needle stick; chronic carrier state, cirrhosis, primary hepatocellular carcinoma; DNA virus easily inactivated by alcohol	Hepatitis B ("serum" hepatitis) neonatal transmission (Hepadnavirus)
	Transfusion, IV drug abuse, or prison-acquired tatoos; acute illness is less severe than hepatitis B but chronicity is higher, with 60% of those infected having chronic active hepatitis; RNA, enveloped virus	Hepatitis C (Flavivirus)
	Enterically transmitted with high fatality in pregnant women, no chronic form	Hepatitis E (Hepevirus)
Acute abdominal pain	Intestinal blockage	*Ascaris lumbricoides* or *Diphyllobothrium latum*
Bile duct blockage		*Ascaris lumbricoides* (following surgery) *Fasciola hepatica*
Peritonitis		Mixed flora often involving anaerobic normal flora: *Bacteroides fragilis* and facultative anaerobes such as *E. coli*
Cirrhosis	Travel history: Puerto Rico, Peace Corps, etc.; egg granulomas block triads → fibrosis	*Schistosoma mansoni*
	IV drug use	Hepatitis viruses
Pancreatitis	Generally with swelling of salivary glands	Mumps virus

*Hepatitis may also occur with two other viruses: CMV and yellow fever virus or with toxoplasmosis or leptospirosis.

Table II-7-11. Changes in Blood Cells

Symptoms and Signs	Case Vignette/Key Clues	Most Common Causal Agents
Anemia	Megaloblastic	*Diphyllobothrium latum*
	Normocytic	Chronic infections
	Microcytic and hypochromic (iron deficiency anemia)	*Ancylostoma, Necator, Trichuris*
Patient with cyclic or irregular fever, decreased hemoglobin and hematocrit	Often foreign travel to tropics, rings or schizonts in RBCs	*Plasmodium*
Splenectomized patient, New England, hemolytic anemia, no travel history, summer months (tick exposure)	Multiple ring forms inside RBC	*Babesia microti*
Reduced CD4 cell count		HIV
Increases in PMNs		Generally found in many extracellular bacterial infections
Increases in eosinophils		Allergy
		Helminths during migrations
Increases in mononuclear leukocytes (monocytes or lymphocytes)		Viruses and other intracellular organisms: *Listeria, Legionella, Leishmania, Toxoplasma*
	Infectious mononucleosis Heterophile (+)Downey type II cells (reactive T cells) sore throat, lymphadenopathy, young adult	Epstein-Barr virus (EBV)
	Heterophile negative	CMV *Toxoplasma* *Listeria* (Listeriosis)
Lymphocytosis with paroxysmal cough, stridor on inspiration	Unvaccinated child, hypoglycemic	*Bordetella pertussis*

Table II-7-12. Central Nervous System Infections

Signs and Symptoms	Case Vignette/Key Clues	Most Common Causal Agents
Meningitis: Headache, fever, vomiting, sepsis, seizures, irritability, lethargy, bulging fontanelles, nuchal rigidity	Neonate to 2 months	*Streptococcus agalactiae* #1 (gram-positive coccus) *E. coli* (gram-negative rod) More rarely: *Listeria monocytogenes* (motile gram-positive rod)
	3 months to 2 years; unvaccinated child	*Haemophilus influenzae* type B* (gram-negative pleomorphic rod with polyribitol capsule)
	3 mo to young adult. Prodrome may be very rapid; child may be properly vaccinated; rash	*Neisseria meningitidis* (gram-negative diplococcus with capsule; ferments maltose)
	‹2 yrs Young adults to elderly	*Streptococcus pneumoniae* (gram-positive coccus, catalase negative, alpha hemolytic, inhibited by optochin, lysed by bile)
	Renal transplant patient	*Cryptococcus neoformans* (#1); encapsulated, urease (+) yeast *Listeria monocytogenes* (motile gram-positive rod)
	Several month prodrome (except in severely compromised). Usually some underlying condition, endemic area	Fungal, e.g., Cryptococcal, or if in Southwestern U.S., *Coccidioides* If near U.S. great river beds with exposure to bird, bat feces; *Histoplasma capsulatum*
	Patient with low CMI, nerve palsies in a patient with tuberculosis and low CSF glucose	*Mycobacterium tuberculosis* (Tuberculous meningitis)
Meningoencephalitis:	Swimming and often diving in very warm waters (hot springs). Prefrontal headache, high fever, disturbance of smell	*Naegleria*
	Immunocompromised patients	*Acanthamoeba* or *Toxoplasma*

*By 1990, with day care centers and the dramatic increase in *Haemophilus* meningitis, *Haemophilus* meningitis became overall the most common. Since late 1990, when the conjugated vaccine went into use, there has been a dramatic decrease in *Haemophilus* meningitis in **vaccinated kids**.

(Continued)

Table II-7-12. Central Nervous System Infections (*continued*)

Signs and Symptoms	Case Vignette/Key Clues	Most Common Causal Agents
Encephalitis: Headache, and fever → drowsiness, coma, hemiplegia, cranial nerve palsy, hallucinations, behavioral disturbances, and other focal neurological findings	Summer–fall, mosquito-borne from bird reservoirs (except for California encephalitis, which is a rodent reservoir)	Encephalitis with **arboviruses:** **Western equine encephalitis** (midwest and west U.S.) **St. Louis encephalitis** elderly blacks with hypertension, most severe infections **West Nile Virus** (North America) **California encephalitis** (entire U.S.) **Eastern equine encephalitis** all age groups, but most common in young and old; highest morbidity of viral CNS infections; with mental retardation, seizures, personality changes in survivors
	Focal uptake of radionucleotide, RBCs in CSF, high opening pressure, frontal temporal lobe involvement.	**Herpes simplex encephalitis**
Mass lesion	Generally following: sinus, ear, or dental infection, infection at distant site, head trauma, etc. (symptoms dependent on location of mass) and elevated intracranial pressure along with headache, mental changes, nausea, vomiting, fever with chills, and seizure	Don't do lumbar puncture; CT generally shows ring enhancing lesion; 45% mixed infections; Streptococci and *Bacteroides* are the two most commonly identified groups of bacteria
Reye Syndrome	Child following a viral illness with pernicious vomiting, lethargy and irritability, which may lead to brain swelling, indication of aspirin usage.	Influenza or varicella infection (Reye syndrome)
Epilepsy	Mexico, immigrant, onset after age 20	*Taenia solium* (neurocysticercosis)
Bell palsy (acute facial nerve paralysis)	Systemic disease following bull's-eye rash	*Borrelia burgdorferi*
Guillain-Barré (acute inflammatory demyelinating polyneuropathy with ascending paralysis)	With GI tract problems	*Campylobacter jejuni*
	With respiratory problems	*Influenza*

Table II-7-13. Cerebrospinal Fluid Finding in Meningitis

Pressure	CSF Appearance	Cell Count (cells/mm)³	Dominant Cell Type	Glucose mg/dL	Protein mg/dL	Condition
‹100 mm H2O	Clear	0–5	Lymphocytes	40–70	‹40	Normal
Normal or +	Clear	0–500	Early: PMNs Late: lymphocytes	Normal or –	Normal or +	Viral infection
++	Opaque	1–60,000	PMNs	–	++	Bacterial infection
+	Clear	10–500	Early: PMNs Late: lymphocytes	–	+ to ++	Fungal infection

– Below normal range, + above normal range

Table II-7-14. Selected Rashes

Type Rash	Progression	Other Symptoms	Disease	Causal Agent/Toxin
Erythematous maculopapular rash (sandpaper-like rash)	Trunk and neck → extremities	Sore throat, fever, nausea	Scarlet fever	*Strep. pyogenes* Exotoxin A-C
Diffuse erythematous, macular, sunburn-like rash	Trunk and neck → extremities with desquamation on palms and soles	Acute onset, fever >102°F, myalgia, pharyngitis, vomiting, diarrhea; hypotension leading to multi-organ failure	Toxic shock syndrome	*Staph. aureus* TSST-1
Perioral erythema, bullae, vesicles, desquamation	Trunk and neck → extremities, except tongue and palate; large bullae and vesicles precede defoliation	Abscess or some site of infection	Staphylococcal skin disease: scalded skin disease & scarletina	*Staph. aureus* Exfoliatin
Petechiae → purpura	Trunk → extremities; spares palms, soles, and face	Fever, rash, headache, myalgias, and respiratory symptoms	Epidemic typhus	*Rickettsia prowazekii* ? Endotoxin
	Ankles and wrists → generalized with palms and soles	Fever, rash, headache, myalgias, and respiratory symptoms	Rocky Mountain spotted fever (most common on East Coast)	*Rickettsia rickettsii* ? Endotoxin
	Generalized	Abrupt onset, fever, chills, malaise, prostration, exanthem → shock	Early meningococcemia	*N. meningitidis* Endotoxin
Skin: maculopapular; mucous membrane: condyloma	Generalized involving the palms and soles, bronze or copper colored	Fever, lymphadenopathy, malaise, sore throat, splenomegaly, headache, arthralgias	Secondary syphilis	*Trep. pallidum* Endotoxin
Confluent erythematous maculopapular rash	Head → entire body	Cough coryza, conjunctivitis, and fever (prodrome), oral lesions (Koplik spots), exanthem, bronchopneumonia, and ear infections	Measles	Rubeola virus Rash from T cell destruction of virus-infected cells in capillaries
Erythematous concentric rings (Bull's eye)	Outward from site of tick bite	Fever, headaches, myalgias, Bell's palsy	Lyme disease	*Borrelia burgdorferi*

Table II-7-15. Osteomyelitis

Type Infection	Case Vignette/Key Clues	Most Common Causal Agents
Fever, bone pain with erythema and swelling, some patients (diabetic particularly) may have associated cellulitis	Adults, children, and infants without major trauma or special conditions	*Staphylococcus aureus*
	Neonates (<1 mo)	*Staphylococcus aureus* Group B Streptococcus, Gram-negative rods (*E. coli, Klebsiella, Proteus, Pseudomonas*)
	Sickle cell anemia*	*Salmonella*
	Trauma	*Pseudomonas*

* Sickle cell anemia patients are functionally asplenic and may have defective opsonic and alternate complement pathway activities. The most common bacterial infections include

- Encapsulated organisms
  Streptococcus pneumoniae
  Haemophilus influenzae
  Neisseria meningitidis
  Salmonella enterica subsp.
- Osteomyelitis due to *Salmonella enterica* subsp.
- Pneumonia, bacteremia, and meningitis are all a problem.

Table II-7-16. Arthritis Related to Infections

Type Infection	Case Vignette/Key Clues	Most Common Causal Agents
Pain, redness, low-grade fever, tenderness, swelling, reduced joint mobility	#1 overall except in the 15–40 age group where gonococcal is more prevalent	*Staphylococcus aureus*
	Multiple joints	From septicemia, e.g., staphylococci, gonococci
	15–40 years; mono- or polyarticular	*Neisseria gonorrhoeae*
	Prosthetic joint	Coagulase negative staphylococci
	Viral	Rubella, hepatitis B, and parvovirus
	Chronic onset, monoarticular	*M. tuberculosis* or fungal
	Large joint resembling Reiter following tick bite or erythema migrans	*Borrelia burgdorferi*
Postinfectious (reactive arthritis)	Following gastrointestinal infection	*Salmonella, Shigella, Campylobacter,* or *Yersinia enterocolitica*
	Following sexual contact	*Chlamydia trachomatis*

Comparative Microbiology   8

Learning Objectives

❏ Differentiate infectious organism that have clinically relevant and distinctive morphology, physiology, pathogenicity, epidemiology, transmission, pathology, lab diagnosis, treatment, or prevention

MORPHOLOGY/TAXONOMY

Spore-Forming Bacteria (Have Calcium Dipicolinate)
Bacillus
Clostridium

Non-motile Gram-Positive Rods
Corynebacterium diphtheriae
Nocardia
Clostridium perfringens (rest of the pathogenic *Clostridia* are motile)
Bacillus anthracis (most other *Bacillus* species are motile)

Acid Fast Organisms
Mycobacterium
Nocardia (partially acid fast)
Cryptosporidium oocysts
Isospora oocysts

Bacteria and Fungi That Characteristically Have Capsules
The "biggies" can be remembered by the mnemonic: Some Killers Have Pretty Nice Capsules!

Streptococcus pneumoniae
Klebsiella pneumoniae
Haemophilus influenzae
Pseudomonas aeruginosa—slime producer especially in cystic fibrosis patients' lungs
Neisseria meningitidis
Cryptococcus neoformans (only encapsulated fungal pathogen)
Bordetella pertussis

Other Important Capsule Producers

E. coli meningeal strains have capsule, mostly K_1

Bacillus anthracis—poly D-glutamate capsule

Salmonella enterica subsp. *typhi*—(virulence; Vi) capsular antigen

Streptococcus pyogenes when first isolated; non-immunogenic (but anti-phagocytic) hyaluronic acid capsule

Biofilm Producers

Staphylococcus epidermidis (catheter-related infections)

Streptococcus mutans (dental plaque)

Pigment Production

***Pseudomonas aeruginosa* (blue-green)—pyocyanin, fluorescein**

Serratia—red pigment

Staphylococcus aureus—yellow pigment

Photochromogenic and scotochromogenic *Mycobacteria*—Carotenoid pigments (yellow and orange)

Corynebacterium diphtheriae—black to gray

Unique Morphology/Staining

Metachromatic staining—*Corynebacterium*

Lancet-shaped diplococci—*Pneumococcus*

Kidney bean-shaped diplococci—*Neisseriae*

Bipolar staining—***Yersinia pestis***

Gulls wings—*Campylobacter*

Table II-8-1. Viral Cytopathogenesis

Inclusion Bodies	Virus
Intracytoplasmic (Negri bodies)	Rabies
Intracytoplasmic acidophilic (Guarnieri)	Poxviruses
Intranuclear (Owl eye)	Cytomegalovirus
Intranuclear (Cowdry)	Herpes simplex virus Subacute sclerosing panencephalitis (measles) virus
Syncytia formation	**Virus** Herpes viruses Varicella-zoster Paramyxoviruses (measles, mumps, rubella and respiratory syncytial virus) HIV

PHYSIOLOGY

Table II-8-2. Metabolism*

Aerobes	Anaerobes	Microaerophilic
Mycobacterium	*Actinomyces*	*Campylobacter*
Pseudomonas	*Bacteroides*	*Helicobacter*
Bacillus	*Clostridium*	
Nocardia	Fusobacterium	
Corynebacterium diphtheriae	Prevotella	
	Propionibacterium (aerotolerant)	
	Eubacterium	
	Lactobacillus (aerotolerant)	

*Most others are considered facultative anaerobes.

Enzymes

Oxidase

- **All Enterobacteriaceae are oxidase negative.**
- **All *Neisseria* are oxidase positive** (as are most other Gram-negative bacteria).

Urease Positive (mnemonic: PUNCH)

- All **Proteus** species produce urease; this leads to alkaline urine and may be associated with renal calculi.
- *Ureaplasma* (renal calculi)
- *Nocardia*
- *Cryptococcus* (the fungus)
- **Helicobacter**

Catalase

$$H_2O_2 \xrightarrow{\text{catalase}} H_2O + 1/2\ O_2$$

Staphylococci have catalase, *Streptococci* do not.

Most anaerobes lack catalase.

Catalase positive organisms are major problems in chronic granulomatous disease (CGD):

- All staphylococci
- *Pseudomonas aeruginosa*
- *Candida*
- *Aspergillus*
- Enterobacteriaceae

Coagulase positive

- ***Staph. aureus***
- ***Yersinia pestis***

DETERMINANTS OF PATHOGENICITY

Genetics

Genes encoding pathogenic factors reside on:

- The bacterial **chromosome**

  Endotoxin

- A **plasmid**

  Most toxins and multiple drug resistances

- A **bacteriophage genome** stably integrated into the host DNA as a prophage. Virulence modified by the stable presence of phage DNA in bacterial cell = lysogenic conversion.

  ### Examples:

  C = cholera toxin

  O = *Salmonella* O antigen

  B = Botulinum toxin (phage CEβ and DEβ)

  E = Erythrogenic toxin of *Streptococcus pyogenes*

  D = Diphtheria toxin (Corynephage β)

  S = Shiga toxin

  Mnemonic: **COBEDS** (when 2 people share a bed somebody gets a little pregnant [with phage])

Antigenic variation

Neisseria gonorrhoeae (pili)

Borrelia recurrentis

Trypanosoma brucei

HIV

Toxins

Table II-8-3. Disease Due to Toxin Production

Bacterium	Disease	Activity of Toxin
Corynebacterium diphtheriae	**Diphtheria**	ADP ribosylation of eEF-2 results in inhibition of protein synthesis
Clostridium tetani	**Tetanus**	Binds to SV2 ganglioside protein receptor. SV2 enables internalization and cellular intoxication.
Clostridium botulinum	**Botulism**	Prevents release of acetylcholine
Vibrio cholerae	**Cholera**	Choleragen stimulates adenylate cyclase
E. coli (ETEC)	**Travelers' diarrhea**	LT stimulates adenylate cyclase
Clostridium difficile	Diarrhea	Toxin A and B inhibit protein synthesis and cause loss of intracellular K$^+$
Bordetella pertussis	Whooping cough	Hypoglycemia due to activation of islets Edema due to inhibition Gi Lymphocytosis due to inhibition of chemokine receptors Sensitivity to histamine

eEF-2 = eukaryotic elongation factor-2

Heat stable toxins

60°C

- *Staphylococcus aureus* enterotoxin
- ST toxin of *E. coli*
- *Yersinia enterocolitica* toxin

100°C

- Endotoxin

Toxins with ADP-ribosylating activity

Table II-8-4. Toxins with A-B ADP-Ribosyl Transferase Activity

Toxin	ADP-Ribosylated Host Protein	Effect on Host Cell
Pseudomonas Exotoxin A Exotoxin S	eEF-2 unknown	Inhibits translocation during protein synthesis
Diphtheria toxin	eEF-2	Inhibits translocation during protein synthesis
E. coli heat-labile toxin (LT)	G-protein (G_S)	Increases cAMP in instestinal epithelium causing diarrhea
Cholera toxin	G-protein (G_S)	Increases cAMP in intestinal epithelium causing diarrhea
Pertussis toxin	G-protein (G_i)	Increases cAMP causing edema, lympho-cytosis and increased insulin secretion

A is the ADP-ribosyl transferase.
B binds to cell receptor and translocates the A subunit into the cell.

Invasive factors

Table II-8-5. Invasive Factors

Invasive Factor	Function	Bacteria
All capsules	Antiphagocytic	See earlier list with morphology
Slime layer (capsule or glycocalyx)	Antiphagocytic	*Pseudomonas*
M protein	Antiphagocytic	Group A Streptococci
A protein	Inhibits opsonization	*Staph. aureus*
Lipoteichoic acid	Attachment to host cells	All gram-positive bacteria
N. gonorrhoeae pili	Antiphagocytic	*N. gonorrhoeae*

Table II-8-6. Extracellular Enzymes

Enzyme	Function	Bacteria
Hyaluronidase	Hydrolysis of ground substance	Group A Streptococci
Collagenase	Hydrolysis of collagen	*Clostridium perfringens* *Prevotella melanino-genica*
Kinases	Hydrolysis of fibrin	*Streptococcus* *Staphylococcus*
Lecithinase (alpha toxin)	Damage to membrane	*Clostridium perfringens*
Heparinase	May contribute to thrombophlebitis	*Bacteroides fragilis* *Prevotella melanino-genica*
IgA Proteases	Colonizing factor	*Neisseria* *Haemophilus* *Strep. pneumoniae*

Ability to Survive and Grow in Host Cell

Obligate Intracellular Parasites

Cannot be cultured on inert media. Virulence is due to the ability to survive and grow intracellularly where the organism is protected from many B-cell host defenses.

- Bacteria

    All Rickettsiae

    All Chlamydiaceae

    Mycobacterium leprae

- Viruses

    All are obligate intracellular parasites.

- Protozoa

    Plasmodium

    Toxoplasma gondii

    Babesia

    Leishmania

    Trypanosoma cruzi (amastigotes in cardiac muscle)

- Fungi

    None

Facultative intracellular parasites of humans

- Bacteria

  Francisella tularensis

  Listeria monocytogenes

  Mycobacterium tuberculosis

  Brucella species

  Non-tuberculous *mycobacteria*

  Salmonella enterica subsp. *typhi*

  Legionella pneumophila

  Yersinia pestis

  Nocardia species

- Fungi

  Histoplasma capsulatum

Obligate Parasites That Are Not Intracellular

(e.g., cannot be cultured on inert media but are found extracellularly in the body)

- *Treponema pallidum*
- *Pneumocystis jirovecii*

EPIDEMIOLOGY/TRANSMISSION

Bacteria That Have Humans as the Only Known Reservoir

Mycobacterium tuberculosis

M. leprae (armadillos in Texas)

Shigella species

Salmonella enterica subspecies **typhi**

Rickettsia prowazekii (epidemic typhus)

Group A β-hemolytic streptococcus

Neisseria meningitidis and *N. gonorrhoeae*

Corynebacterium diphtheriae

Streptococcus pneumoniae

Treponema pallidum

Chlamydia trachomatis

Zoonotic Organisms

(Diseases of animals transmissible to humans)

Bacillus anthracis

Salmonella enterica all subspecies except *typhi*

Leptospira

Borrelia

Listeria monocytogenes

Brucella species

Francisella tularensis

Pasteurella multocida (cat bites)

Vibrio parahaemolyticus (from fish)

Capnocytophaga canimorsus (dog bites)

Bartonella henselae (cat scratches)

Streptobacillus moniliformis (rat bite fever)

Mycobacterium marinum (fish tank granuloma)

Vibrio vulnificus (oysters)

Yersinia pestis, Y. enterocolitica, Y. pseudotuberculosis

Campylobacter fetus, C. jejuni

Most Rickettsia

Chlamydophila psittaci (birds)

Rabies virus

Arthropod Vectors in Human Disease: Insects

- Lice

   Epidemic or louse-borne typhus (*Pediculus h. humanus*)

   Epidemic relapsing fever

   Trench fever

- **True bugs**

   Chagas' disease (American trypanosomiasis)—kissing bugs (Reduviidae)

- Mosquitoes

   Malaria (*Anopheles* mosquito)

   Dengue (*Aedes*)

   Mosquito-borne encephalitides: WEE, EEE, VEE, SLE, WNV

   Yellow Fever (*Aedes*)

   Filariasis

- **Sandflies**

   Leishmaniasis

   Bartonellosis

- Midges

   Filariasis

- Blackflies

   Onchocerciasis

- Deerflies (*Chrysops*) and horse flies

   Loaloasis

   Tularemia

- Tsetse flies

  African trypanosomiasis

- Fleas

  Plague

  Endemic typhus

Arthropod Vectors That Are Not Insects

- Ticks

  Rocky Mountain spotted fever (*Dermacentor*)

  Colorado tick fever (*Dermacentor*)

  Lyme disease (*Ixodes*)

  Ehrlichia (Ixodes, Amblyomma)

  Babesiosis (*Ixodes*)

  Tularemia (*Dermacentor*)

  Recurrent fever or tick-borne relapsing fever (*Ornithodoros*, a soft tick)

- Mites

  Scrub typhus (*Leptotrombium*) (transovarial transmission in vector)

  Rickettsialpox

Parasitic Infections Transmitted by Ova

Enterobius vermicularis (pinworm)

Ascaris lumbricoides (roundworm)

Toxocara canis (visceral larva migrans)

Trichuris trichiura (whipworm)

Echinococcus granulosus/multilocularis

Taenia solium (cysticercosis)

All others are transmitted in larval stage.

Bacterial and Fungal Infections That Are Not Considered Contagious

(i.e., no human-to-human transmission)

Nontuberculous mycobacterial infections, e.g., ***Mycobacterium avium-intracellulare***

Non-spore forming anaerobes

Legionella pneumophila

All fungal infections except the dermatophytes

Infections That Cross the Placenta

(Mnemonic: TORCH)

Toxoplasma

Other (Syphilis)

Rubella

CMV

Herpes and **H**IV

<5% perinatal hepatitis B could possibly have been acquired by crossing placenta.

- Viruses

    Cytomegalovirus

    Rubella

    HSV 2 (in primary infection)

    Coxsackie B

    Polio

    HIV

    B19

- Parasites

    Toxoplasma gondii

- Bacteria

    Treponema pallidum

    Listeria monocytogenes

Spread by Respiratory Droplet

Streptococcus pyogenes (Group A)

Streptococcus pneumoniae

Neisseria meningitidis

Mycobacterium tuberculosis

Bordetella pertussis

Haemophilus influenzae

Corynebacterium diphtheriae

Mycoplasma pneumoniae

Influenza

Rubella

Measles

Chickenpox

Pneumocystis jirovecii

Spread by Inhalation of Organisms from the Environment

Histoplasma

Coccidioides

Blastomyces

Nontuberculous mycobacteria, e.g., M. avium-intracellulare (MAC)

Legionella

Chlamydophila psittaci

Pseudomonas (also spread by ingestion and contact)

Spread by Oral/Fecal Route
(Infections may be spread by oral sex.)

Salmonella

Shigella

Campylobacter

Vibrio

Yersinia enterocolitica

Yersinia pseudotuberculosis

Bacillus cereus

Clostridium

Staphylococcus (also other routes commonly)

Enteroviruses, including poliovirus

Rotavirus

Norwalk agent

Hepatitis A

Toxoplasma—cat feces

Entamoeba

Giardia

All nematodes except filaria and *Trichinella*

All cestodes

Contact: (Person-to-Person) Nonsexual
Impetigo (*Strep* and *Staph*)

Staphylococcus

Herpes I

Epstein-Barr (kissing)

Hepatitis B (all body fluids)

Molluscum contagiosum (wrestling teams)

Contact: Sexual

Chlamydia	HPV	HBV
Neisseria	HIV	HCV
Treponema	HSV 2	
Trichomonas	CMV	

PATHOLOGY

Organisms that Produce Granulomas
(most are intracellular, others have persistent antigen)

Fran Likes My Pal Bruce And His Blasted Cockerspaniel (in) Salt Lake City. (Mnemonic by M. Free.)

(ic) = intracellular organism

Francisella (ic)

Listeria (ic)

Mycobacterium (ic)

Treponema **p**allidum

Brucella (ic)

Actinomyces

Histoplasma (ic)

Blastomyces

Coccidioides

Schistosoma species

Lymphogranuloma venereum (ic)

Cat scratch fever

Infections Causing Intracerebral Calcifications

Toxoplasma

CMV

Cysticercosis

Cryptococcus neoformans

Tuberculous meningitis

LABORATORY DIAGNOSIS

Special Stains

- Silver stains

   Dieterle—*Legionella*

   Gomori methenamine—*Pneumocystis*, fungi

- Acid fast (Ziehl-Neelsen or Kinyoun)

   Mycobacterium, *Nocardia* (partially AF), *Cryptosporidium*, *Isospora*, *Cyclospora*, and *Microsporidia* (oocysts in feces)

- India ink—*Cryptococcus* (if negative not a reliable diagnostic method)

- Calcofluor white—fungi

- Giemsa

   Blood protozoa (*Plasmodium*, *Babesia*, *Trypanosoma*, *Leishmania*)

   Histoplasma capsulatum in RES cells

Name Tests

Tests	Disease
PPD or Tuberculin (Mantoux)	TB
Lepromin	Leprosy
Fungal skin tests	Clinically valuable only to demonstrate exposure or anergy
CAMP test	*Strept agalactiae* carriers
Elek test	Toxin producing *C. diphtheriae* strains
Weil-Felix	Rickettsia (with *Proteus* strain OX antigens)

Unusual Growth Requirements

Haemophilus (most species require one or both)

- **X factor** = protoporphyrin IX, the precursor of **hemin**

- **V factor** = NAD (nicotinamide dinucleotide) or NADP

Mycoplasma

- **Cholesterol**

Salt (halophilic organisms)

- *Staph aureus* will grow on high salt media.

- Group D enterococci will grow on 6.5% NaCl.

- *Vibrio* species requires NaCl to grow and grows at 6.5%.

Cysteine requirement for growth

- Four Sisters Ella of the Cysteine Chapel (mnemonic by M. Free) *Francisella*, *Legionella*, *Brucella*, and *Pasteurella*

Cultures that must be observed for a long time

- *Mycobacterium tuberculosis* and all non-tuberculous mycobacteria except rapid growers

- *Mycoplasma pneumoniae*

- Systemic fungal pathogens (*Blastomyces*, *Histoplasma*, and *Coccidioides* in U.S.)

TREATMENT/PREVENTION

Treat Prophylactically

- *Neisseria meningitidis* (household and day care contacts—vaccination also used in outbreaks)

- *Mycobacterium tuberculosis* with a recent skin test conversion or known household (i.e., significant) exposure; or persons under 35 with a positive skin test who have never been treated

- *Haemophilus influenzae* B (unvaccinated household contacts <6 years old)—also vaccinate

- *Neisseria gonorrhoeae* (sexual contacts)

- *Treponema pallidum* (sexual contacts)

- *Yersinia pestis*
- Neonatal eyes (*Neisseria gonorrhoeae, Chlamydia trachomatis, Treponema pallidum*)

Vaccines Available in the U.S.

Inactivated vaccines (RIP-A; Rest In Peace Always)

- Rabies
- Influenza virus
- Salk polio (killed)—all primary vaccinations in U.S., including IC patients
- Hepatitis A
- Japanese encephalitis and several other encephalitis vaccines
- *Vibrio cholerae*

Live, attenuated vaccines

- *Francisella tularensis*
- Measles (rubeola)
- Rubella
- Mumps (killed vaccine available for IC patients)
- Sabin polio (oral)
- Smallpox
- Yellow fever
- Varicella-Zoster
- Rotavirus

Live, Pathogenic Virus (in enteric-coated capsules)

- Adenovirus

Toxoid: Chemically Modified Toxin—-Vaccines

- Tetanus
- Diphtheria
- Pertussis toxoid (in DTaP)

Subunit Vaccines

- *Haemophilus*—purified capsular polysaccharide conjugated to protein
- *Neisseria meningitidis*—capsular polysaccharides, pediatric version is conjugated to protein
- Pneumococcal—capsular polysaccharide (7 and 23 serotypes) (pediatric version is conjugated to protein)

Recombinant Vaccines

- Hepatitis B—HBsAg (produced in yeast)
- Human papilloma virus vaccine, 4 capsid proteins

Reference Charts and Tables

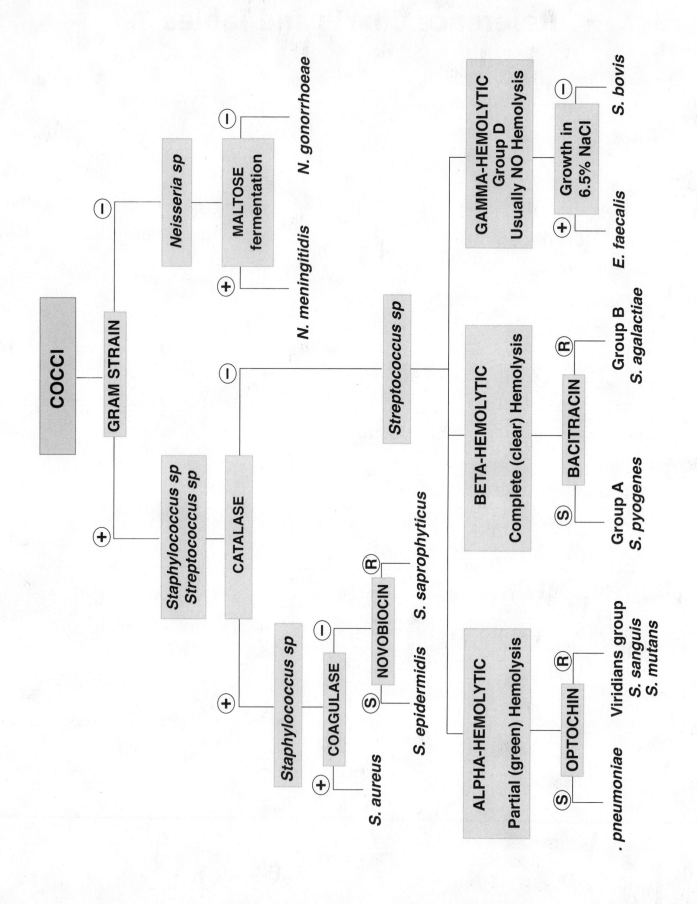

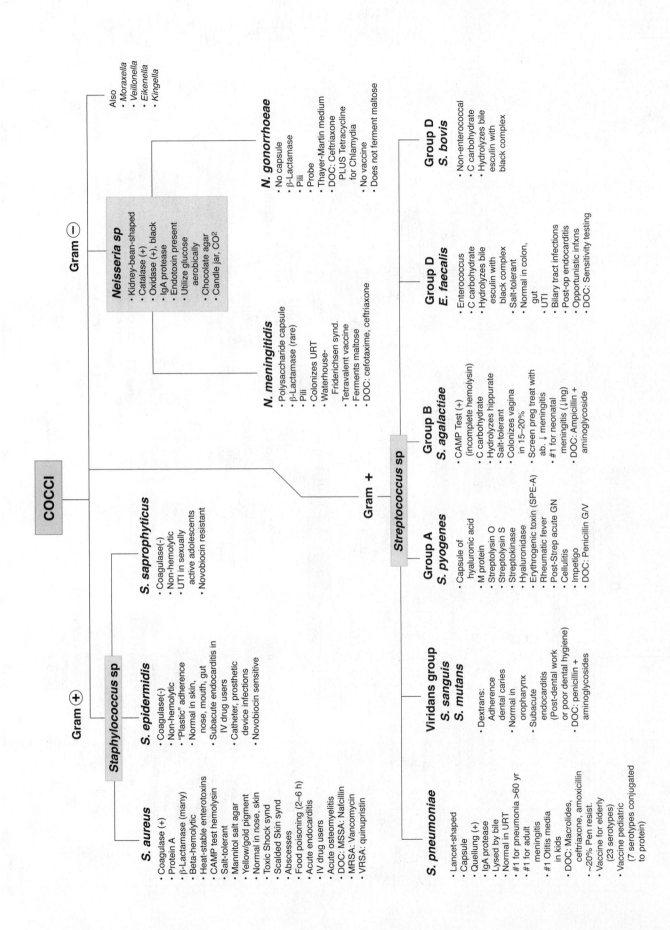

COCCI

Gram (+)

Staphylococcus sp

S. aureus
- Coagulase (+)
- Protein A
- β-Lactamase (many)
- Beta-hemolytic
- Heat-stable enterotoxins
- CAMP test hemolysin
- Salt-tolerant
- Mannitol salt agar
- Yellow/gold pigment
- Normal in nose, skin
- Toxic Shock synd
- Scalded Skin synd
- Abscesses
- Food poisoning (2–6 h)
- Acute endocarditis
- IV drug users
- Acute osteomyelitis
- DOC: MSSA: Nafcillin
- MRSA: Vancomycin
- VRSA: quinupristin

S. epidermidis
- Coagulase(-)
- Non-hemolytic
- "Plastic" adherence
- Normal in skin, nose, mouth, gut
- Subacute endocarditis in IV drug users
- Catheter, prosthetic device infections
- Novobiocin sensitive

S. saprophyticus
- Coagulase(-)
- Non-hemolytic
- UTI in sexually active adolescents
- Novobiocin resistant

Streptococcus sp

S. pneumoniae
- Lancet-shaped
- Capsule
- Quellung (+)
- IgA protease
- Lysed by bile
- Normal in URT
- #1 for pneumonia >60 yr
- #1 for adult meningitis
- #1 Otitis media in kids
- DOC: Macrolides, ceftriaxone, amoxicillin
- ~20% Pen resist.
- Vaccine for elderly (23 serotypes)
- Vaccine pediatric (7 serotypes conjugated to protein)

Viridans group
S. sanguis
S. mutans
- Dextrans:
  Adherence
  dental caries
- Normal in oropharynx
- Subacute endocarditis (Post-dental work or poor dental hygiene)
- DOC: penicillin + aminoglycosides

Group A
S. pyogenes
- Capsule of hyaluronic acid
- M protein
- Streptolysin O
- Streptolysin S
- Streptokinase
- Hyaluronidase
- Erythrogenic toxin (SPE-A)
- Rheumatic fever
- Post-Strep acute GN
- Cellulitis
- Impetigo
- DOC: Penicillin G/V

Group B
S. agalactiae
- CAMP Test (+) (incomplete hemolysin)
- C carbohydrate
- Hydrolyzes hippurate
- Salt-tolerant
- Colonizes vagina in 15–20%
- Screen preg treat with ab. ↓ meningitis
- #1 for neonatal meningitis (↓ing)
- DOC: Ampicillin + aminoglycoside

Group D
E. faecalis
- Enterococcus
- C carbohydrate
- Hydrolyzes bile esculin with black complex
- Salt-tolerant
- Normal in colon, gut
- UTI
- Biliary tract infections
- Post-op endocarditis
- Opportunistic infxns
- DOC: Sensitivity testing

Group D
S. bovis
- Non-enterococcal
- C carbohydrate
- Hydrolyzes bile esculin with black complex

Gram (−)

Neisseria sp
- Kidney-bean-shaped
- Catalase (+)
- Oxidase (+), black
- IgA protease
- Endotoxin present
- Utilize glucose aerobically
- Chocolate agar
- Candle jar, CO_2

N. meningitidis
- Polysaccharide capsule
- β-Lactamase (rare)
- Pili
- Colonizes URT
- Waterhouse-Friderichsen synd.
- Tetravalent vaccine
- Ferments maltose
- DOC: cefotaxime, ceftriaxone

N. gonorrhoeae
- No capsule
- β-Lactamase
- Pili
- Probe
- Thayer-Martin medium
- DOC: Ceftriaxone PLUS Tetracycline for Chlamydia
- No vaccine
- Does not ferment maltose

Also
- *Moraxella*
- *Veillonella*
- *Eikenella*
- *Kingella*

GRAM (+) RODS

NON-SPORE-FORMING

Aerobic

Motile

L. monocytogenes
- Tumbling motility
- "Jets" from cell to cell
- Fac intracellular organism
- Beta-hemolytic
- Cold enrichment
- Sepsis
- Crosses placenta
- Meningitis
  - Renal transplant
  - Neonatal
  - Cancer
- DOC: Ampicillin and Gentamicin for IC

Non-Motile

C. diphtheriae
- Club-shaped
- "Chinese Characters"
- Exotoxin (ADP-R of eEF-2) Heart, Nerves, epithelium
- Volutin granules on Loeffler's medium
- Tellurite: black colonies
- ELEK test
- Gray pseudomembrane
- Myocarditis
- Recrnt larngl nerve palsy
- DOC: Antitoxin PLUS Erythromycin
- Toxoid vaccine

N. asteroides
- Filaments to rods
- Urease (+)
- Partially acid-fast
- Cavitary bronchopulmonary
- Multiple brain abscesses
- Mycetoma (granules)
- DOC: Sulfonamides

Anaerobic

A. israelii
- Rods with branching
- Non-motile
- Not restricted by anatomical boundaries
- Sulfur "granules" in exudates from sinus tract
- Normal in mouth and female genitourinary tract
- Cervicofacial (lumpy jaw)
- IUD-associated infections
- Solitary brain abscess
- Mycetoma
- Rx: Penicillin plus drainage

SPORE-FORMING

Aerobic

Motile

B. cereus
- Heat-stable exotoxin: vomiting increase cAMP
- Heat-labile toxin: diarrhea
- Fried rice
- Food poisoning (2–18 h)
- Symptomatic Rx

Non-Motile

B. anthracis
- Poly-D-glutamate capsule
- Spores
- In R-E cells
- Toxin:
  - Protective Ag
  - Lethal factor
  - Edema factor (an adenylate cyclase)
- Painless skin ulcer 95%
- Black eschar
- Striking local edema
- Woolsorter's disease Pneumonia
- DOC: Ciprofloxacin or doxycycline

Anaerobic

Motile

C. tetani
- Terminal spores
- Exotoxin Tetanospasmin Inhibits GABA Glycine
- Tetanus
  - Spastic paralysis
- DOC: hyperimmune globulin, Penicillin PLUS spasmolytic
- Toxoid vaccine

C. botulinum
- Neurotoxin heat-labile
- Blocks ACh release
- Flaccid paralysis
- Canned-food poisoning
- Trivalent antitoxin
- DOC: antitoxin PLUS Penicillin
- Infant botulism human hyperimmune serum, no drugs

Non-Motile

C. difficile
- Nosocomial
- Diarrhea to pseudomembranous colitis
- Antibiotic (Clindamycin) usage
- Yellow plaques
- Colon
- Toxins A + B
- DOC: Change or stop antibiotic

C. perfringens
- Subterminal spore
- Alpha lecithinase= Phospholipase C
- Enterotoxin
- Stormy fermentation
- Double-zone hemolysis
- Egg yolk agar
- Normal in colon
- Food poisoning
- Gas gangrene
- Myonecrosis
- High mortality
- DOC: Penicillin G ± Clindamycin PLUS debridement

GRAM (-) RODS & SPIROCHETES

AEROBES

Facultative Anaerobes →

B. pertussis
- Adhesion to cell via hemagglutinin and pertussis toxin
- Adenylate cyclase txn (local edema)
- Tracheal toxin
- Dermanecrosis toxin
- Endotoxin - Lipid X, A
  - ADP-R of GNBP
- Bordet-Gengou agar
- Regan-Lowe agar
- Whooping cough
- DOC: Erythromycin
- Vaccine toxoid and filamentous hemagglutinin

Brucella sp
- In R-E cells
- Endotoxin
- Requires CYS, CO_2
- Unpasteurized milk
- Undulant Fever
  - Bang's disease
  - Malta fever
- *B. abortus* cattle, mild
- *B. suis* pigs suppurative, chronic
- *B. melitensis* goats severe, acute
- DOC: rifampin and doxycycline

F. tularensis
- In R-E cells
- Requires CYS
- *Dermacentor* tick bite Transovarian trans.
- Aerosol
- Rabbits, rodents
- Granulomatous rxn
- Tularemia - AR, MO, TX
- Live, attntd vaccine
- DOC: Streptomycin

L. pneumophila
- Water-loving air conditioning
- Requires CYS & Fe
- Buffered Charcoal Yeast agar
- Dieterle silver stain
- Stains poorly Gram (-)
- Atypical pneumonia
- Mental confusion
- Diarrhea
- DOC: Erythromycin
- Not contagious

P. aeruginosa
- Slime-layer
- Grape-like odor
- Exotoxin A: ADP-R of eEF-2 Liver
- Oxidase (+)
- Pigments pyocyanin, pyoverdin
- Transient colonization In 10% of normal pop
- Osteomyelitis in drug abusers
- Pneumonia in cystic fibrosis
- Nosocomial infections Burn patients Neutropenic patients
- Ecthyma gangrenosum
- DOC: Penicillin PLUS Aminoglycoside

ANAEROBES

Bacteroides sp
- *B. fragilis* - obligate
- Modified LPS, capsules
- Predominant colonic flora
- Normal in oropharynx, vagina
- Predisposing factors: surgery, trauma chronic disease (cancer)
- Septicemia, peritonitis aspiration pneumonia
- *Prevotella melaninogenica* Human oropharynx
- *Fusobacterium* (combined w/ *Treponema microdentium*) Vincent's angina Trench mouth
- DOC: Metronidazole OR Clindamycin OR Cefoxitin

SPIROCHETES
- Thin-Walled
- Spiral-Shaped
- Axial Filaments
- Jarisch-Herxheimer Rxn

Treponema sp
- *T. pallidum* - Syphilis Obligate parasite
- 1° PAINLESS chancre, infectious
- 2° Rash infectious
- 3° - Gummas, CVS, CNS
- Congenital: stillbirths, malformed
- VDRL & RPR - Screening tests
- Reagin ab - xrxn with Cardiolipin
- FTA-ABS (immunofluorescence) specific test
- Dark-field microscopy
- DOC: Benzathine Penicillin

Borrelia sp
- Microaerophillic
- Giemsa stain
- *B. burgdorferi* Lyme disease (*I. scapularis*), *I. pacificus* Reservoirs: mice, deer CT, WI, CA Erythema Migrans Target lesions
- *B. recurrentis* Relapsing fever Vector: body louse Antigenic variation
- DOC: Penicillin or azithromycin

Leptospira sp
- Dark-field microscopy
- Contaminated water Animal urine
- Fever, jaundice, uremia
- Non-icteric Leptospirosis Meningitis - No PMN in CSF uveitis, rash
- Icteric Leptospirosis Weil's disease Renal failure, myocarditis
- DOC: Penicillin G or doxycycline

FACULTATIVE ANAEROBES

Other Gram (–) RODS →

P. multocida
- Requires CYS
- Animal bites (cats & dogs)
- Cellulitis with Lymphadenitis
- DOC: Amoxicillin/Clav (prophylaxis)

H. influenzae
- Polyribitol capsule
- Quellung (+)
- IgA protease
- Requires X (Hemin), V (NAD) and
- Normal in nasopharynx and conjunctiva
- Pathogenic in kids: type B
- Meningitis in 1–2 yr
- Otitis media, pneumonia
- Acute epiglottitis
- DOC: Cefotaxime/Ceftriaxone
- Prev: HIB vaccine, Rifampin

Vibrio sp
- Polar flagella, comma-shaped
- Enterotoxin (Choleragen) ADP-R, increase cAMP
- Catalase (+), Oxidase (+)
- Alkaline culture (TCBS)
- Classic cholera O_1
- Biotypes: El Tor, Cholerae
- Rice-water stools
- Most severe dehydration
- Rx: fluid & electrolytes tetracycline for contacts
- *V. parahaemolyticus*
  Catalase (–), salt-tolerant
  Raw seafood
- *V. vulnificus*
  Brackish water • Oysters
  Cellulitis, Septicemia
  DOC: tetracycline

Campylobacter sp
Helicobacter sp
- Microaerophilic
- Polar flagella
- Comma or S-shaped
- Oxidase (+), Catalase (+)
- Skirrow's agar CO_2
- Invasive
- **H. pylori**
  37°C, urease(+)
  gastritis, ulcers
  carcinoma
- DOC: omeprazole + amoxicillin + clarithromycin
- **C. jejuni**
  42°C enterocolitis
  #1 bacterial diarrhea U.S.A.
- "Gull-Wings"
- *C. fetus* escapes GIT
- DOC: Erythromycin, fluoroquinolones

Also:
- *Gardnerella*
- *Capnocytophaga*
- *Actinobacillus*
- *Cardiobacterium*

ENTEROBACTERIACEAE
- Ferment Glucose
- Oxidase (–), Catalase (+)
- Reduce Nitrates to Nitrites

Lactose-Fermenting

E. coli
- Normal in colon
- #1 for UTI
- P-pili, X-Adhesins
- Nosocomial infections
- Neonatal meningitis (K_1)
- ETEC • Traveler's Drha
  Toxins: LT, ST
- EIEC • Invasive
- EHEC • VTEC 0157:H7
  Hemorrhagic colitis
  Hemolytic uremic S
  Does not ferment Sorbitol
- EPEC
  Plasmid-coded EAF
- EAEC
  Fimbriae/biofilm
- DAEC
  Infants
  Bacteria in microvilli
- DOC: Ampicillin or
  Sulfonamides
  Cephalosporins

K. pneumoniae
- Capsule
- Quellung (+)
- Pneumonia
  Currant jelly septum
  Chronic lung disease
  Alcoholism
  Aspiration
- UTI
  Nosocomial
  Catheterization
- DOC: Cephalosporin
  +/– aminoglycoside

Non-Lactose-Fermenting

Motile and H₂S-Producing

Proteus sp.
- Swarming motility
- Indole (+), Urease (+)
- UTI, Septicemia
  Staghorn calculi
- DOC: Fluoroquinolones

Salmonella enterica subsp.
- Antigens: Vi, O, H
- EMB/MacConkey
- Predisposing factors
  High gastric pH
  Gastrectomy
- Widal test (O, H ag)
- Osteomyelitis in Sickle
  Cell disease
- *S. enterica* subsp. *typhi*
  No animal res.
  No H₂S produced
  Invasive (R-E) cells
  Rose spots
  - DOC: fluoroquinolones
    or cephalosporins
- *S. enterica* subsp. *enteritidis*
  Poultry, reptiles
  Rx: Symptomatic
  - DOC for invasive:
    ampicillin, cephalosporins

Non-Motile and Non-H₂S-Producing

Shigella sp
- No H Antigens
- Invasive
  Shigatoxin
  Nicks 60S SU
  Neurotoxin
  Cytotoxin
  Enterotoxin
- Enterocolitis
- Bloody diarrhea
- DOC: fluid and electrolytes
  FQ, Azithro

Y. pestis
- Coagulase (+)
- V&W antigens
- Safety-pin appearance
  (bipolar staining
  Wayson's stain)
- Wild rodents
- Flea bite
- Southwest U.S. (Sylvatic)
- Bubonic plague
  fever, buboes,
  conjunctivitis
- Pneumonic plague
- DOC: Aminoglycosides
  PLUS Quarantine (72 h)
- *Y. enterocolitica*
  Cold growth
  Heat-stable toxins

Poorly Gram-Staining Organisms*

ACID FAST

Mycobacteria

M. tuberculosis
- Gram (+) wall but doesn't stain due to waxy CW
- Acid fast, obligate aerobe
- Respiratory transmission
- Pathogen, contagious
- Cord factor-trehalose mycolate-inhib. WBC migration
- Sulfatides-inhib. resp./ oxid. phosphor mitoch.
- Sulfatides-inhib. phagosome-lysosome fusion
- Niacin (+), catalase (+) at 37°C, (–) at 68°C
- Slow growing
- Drug resistance
- Lowenstein-Jensen medium
- DOC: isoniazid + rifampin + pyrazinimide (2 mo) then isoniazid + rifampin (4 mo)

M. avium-intracellulare
- Gram (+) wall but doesn't stain due to waxy CW
- Acid fast
- Obligate aerobe
- Soil organism
- Opportunist, non-contagious
- Pulmonary → diss infections CA pts, late AIDS pts

M. leprae
- Obligate intracellular bacterium
- Tuberculoid (CMI damage)
- Lepromatous leprosy (poor CMI)
- DOC: dapsone + rifampin + clofazimine

M. marinum
- Cutaneous lesions (fish tank granuloma)
- DOC: isoniazid, rifampin, ethambutol

SOME ATP

Rickettsias

R. rickettsii
- Obligate intracellular bacteria
- Gram-negative envelope but stain poorly
- Rocky MT Spt'd Fever-rash on wrists/ankles → trunk, palms, soles
- Vector: *Dermacentor* tick
- Reservoirs: ticks, wild rodents
- Dx: serol: 4x incr indir Fl. Ab + Weil-Felix
- DOC: Doxycycline

R. prowazekii
- Obligate intracellular bacteria
- Epidemic typhus
- Vector: *Pediculus* louse
- Reservoir: humans, squirrel fleas, flying squirrels

Bartonella henselae
- Cat scratch fever
- Bacillary angiomatosis in AIDS

Ehrlichia
- Ehrlichiosis
- Morulae in WBC
- DOC: doxycycline
- *E. chafeensis*-monocytes + macrophages
- *E. phagocytophila* - PMNs
- *Ixodes* tick

NO ATP, mod. peptidoglycan

Chlamydiaceae

Chlamydia trachomatis
- Obligate intracellular bacteria
- Gram-negative envelope but stain poorly; lack muramic acid
- Elementary body-transmitted
- Reticulate body-intracellular
- Dx: serology or tissue culture growth confirmed by inclusion bodies (Fl Ab, Giemsa, iodine)
- **Serotypes D-K**
- U.S.-Most common bacterial STD (HPV and HSV2 more common)
- Neonatal/adult inclus. conjunct, neonatal. pneumo; urethritis cervicitis, PID, infertility
- **Serotypes L1, 2, 3**
- Lymphogranuloma venereum
- STD in Africa, Asia, S. America
- **Serotypes A, B, Ba, C**
- Trachoma-folic conjunctivitis → conj. scarring, entropion → corneal scarring
- Leading infectious cause blindness
- DOC: Doxycycline or azithromycin

Chlamydophila pneumoniae
- TWAR agent
- Respiratory infections
- Probably very common
- Potential association with atherosclerosis
- DOC: macrolides and tetracycline

Chlamydophila psittaci
- Atypical pneumonia
- Birds (parrots)
- DOC: tetracycline

NO CELL WALL

Mycoplasmas

M. pneumoniae
- Lack cell wall peptidoglycan → non-Gram-staining
- Cholesterol (req'd) in membr.
- Atypical pneumonia in youth and young adults
- Free living (culturable, extracell.)
- Slow growth, special media: Myco-plasma, Eaton's or Hayflick's media-sterols+pur/pyrimidines: mulberry colonies
- Cold aggulutinins in 65% cases
- No Penicillins nor Cephalosporins
- DOC: erythromycin, azithromycin

Ureaplasma urealyticum
- Urethritis, prostatitis
- Urease positive
- No cell wall
- DOC: erythromycin or tetracycline

*Also note that *Legionella* and the spirochetes (*Treponema*, *Leptospira*, and *Borrelia*)—all Gram-negative—do not show up reliably with Gram stain.

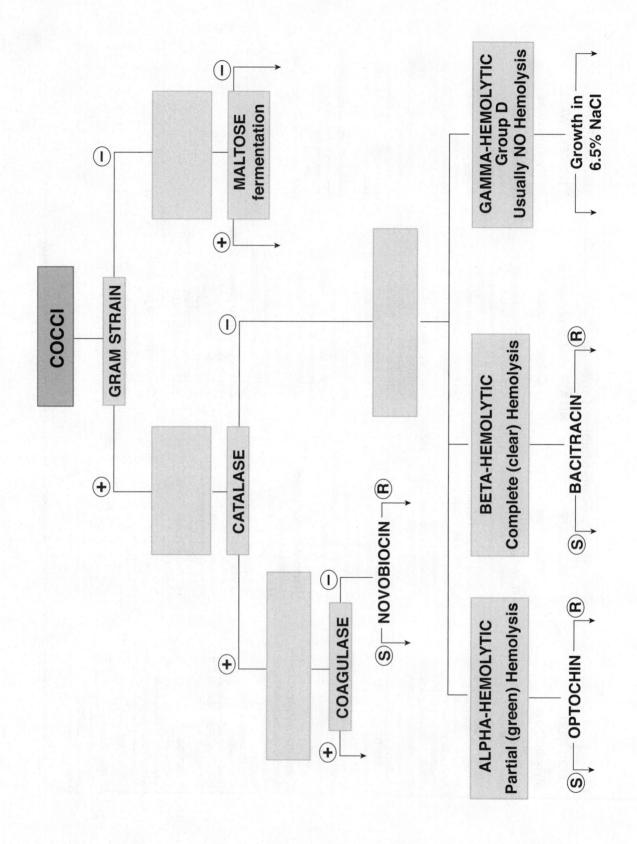

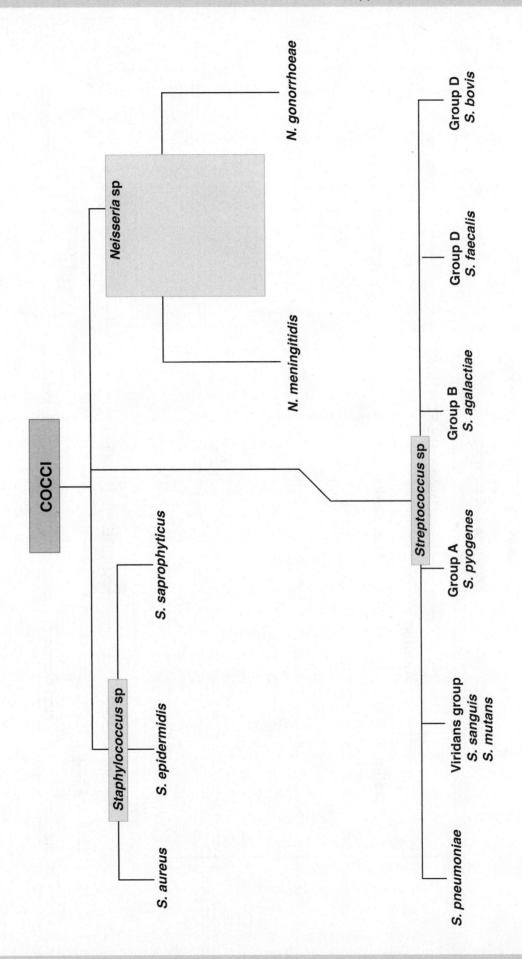

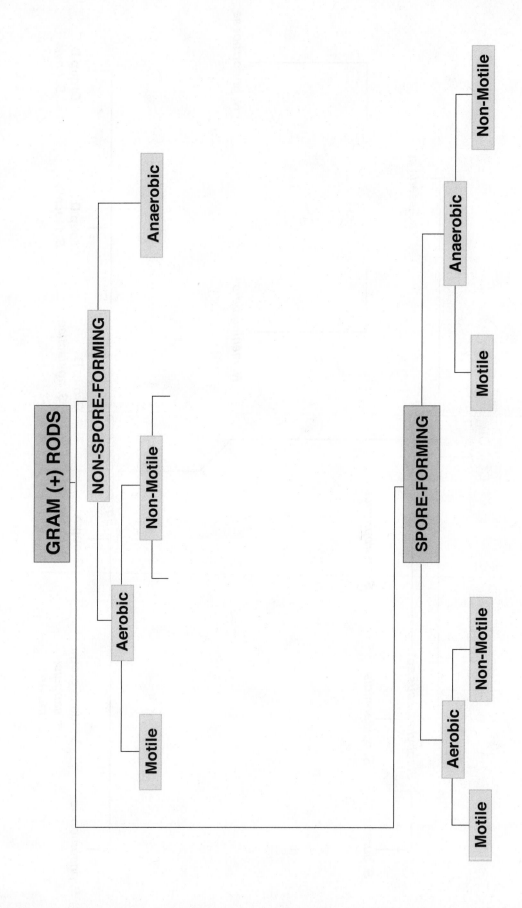

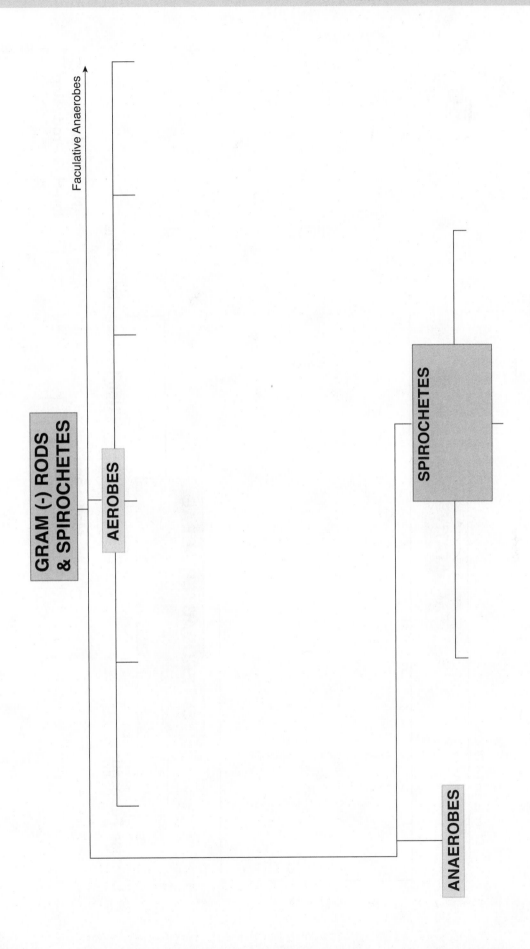

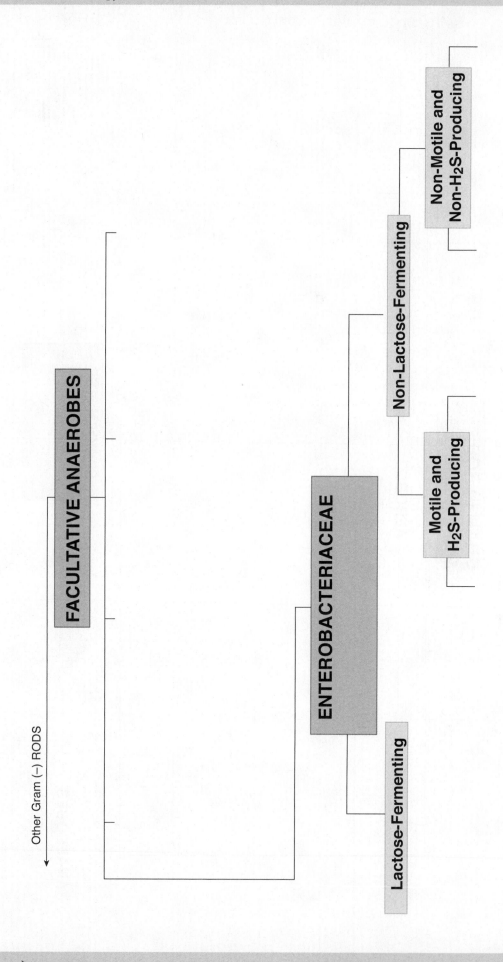

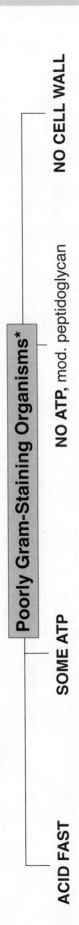

Poorly Gram-Staining Organisms*

ACID FAST

SOME ATP

NO ATP, mod. peptidoglycan

NO CELL WALL

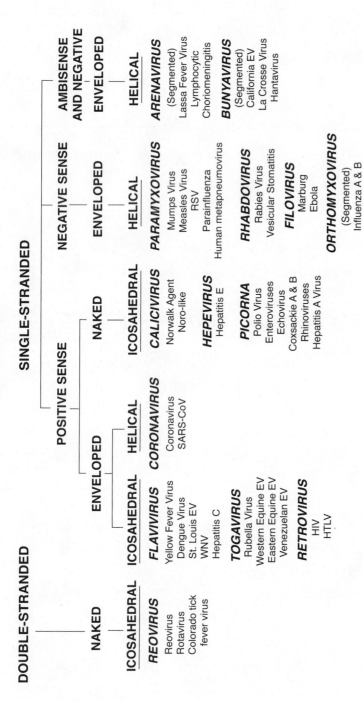

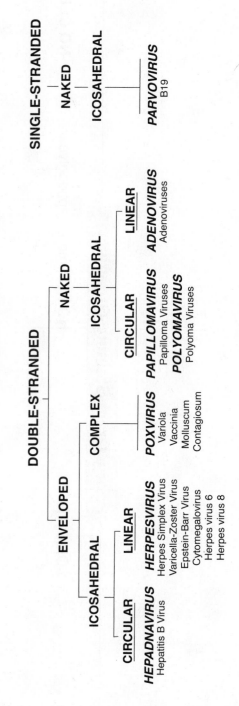

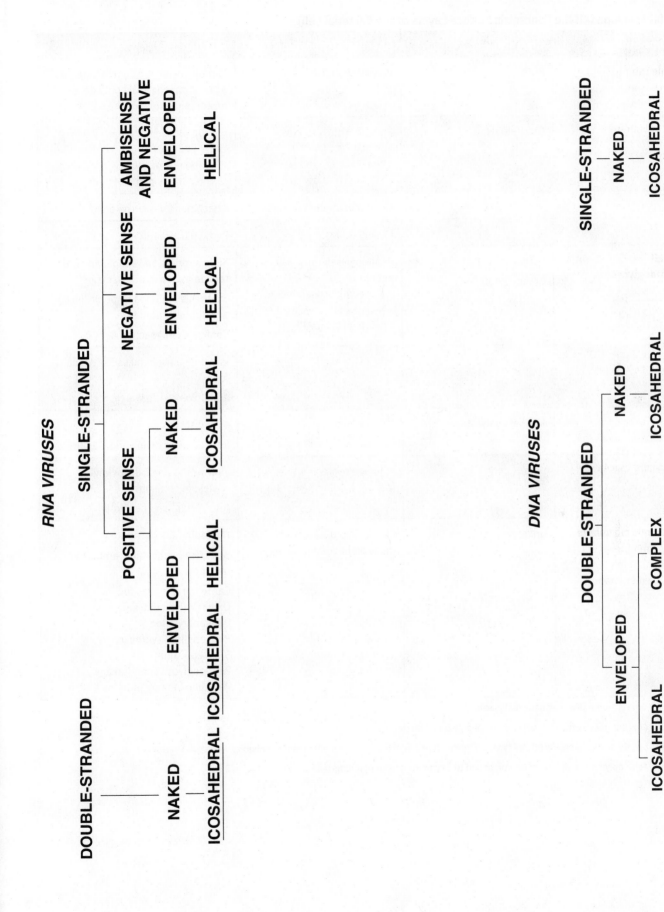

Bacterial Envelope (All the Concentric Surface Layers of the Bacterial Cell)

Envelope Structure	Gram + or −	Chemical Composition	Function
Capsule (Non-essential) = Slime layer = Glycocalyx	Both	Polysaccharide gel*	Pathogenicity factor protecting against phagocytosis until opsonized; immunogenic**
Outer membrane	Gram − only	Phospholipid/proteins: Lipopolysaccharide Lipid A Polysacccharide	Hydrophobic membrane: LPS = endotoxin Lipid A = toxic moiety PS = immunogenic portion
		Outer membrane proteins	Attachment, virulence, etc.
		Protein porins	Passive transport
Cell wall = peptidoglycan	Gram + (thick) Gram − (thin)	Peptidoglycan-open 3-D net of: N-acetyl-glucosamine N-acetyl-muramic acid amino acids (DAP)	Rigid support, cell shape, and protection from osmotic damage Synthesis inhibited by penicillins and cephalosporins Confers Gram reaction
	Gram + only	Teichoic acids***	Immunogenic, induces TNF-alpha, IL-1 Attachment
	Acid-fast only	Mycolic acids	Acid-fastness Resistance to drying and chemicals
Periplasmic space	Gram − only	"Storage space" between the inner and outer membranes	Enzymes to break down large molecules, (β-lactamases) Aids regulation of osmolarity
Cytoplasmic membrane = inner membrane = cell membrane = plasma membrane	Gram + Gram −	Phospholipid bilayer with many embedded proteins	Hydrophobic cell "sack" Selective permeability and active transport Carrier for enzymes for: Oxidative metabolism Phosphorylation Phospholipid synthesis DNA replication Peptidoglycan cross linkage Penicillin binding proteins (PBPs)

Definition of abbreviation: DAP, diaminopimelic acid.

* Except *Bacillus anthracis*, which is a polypeptide of poly D-glutamate.

** Except *S. pyogenes* (hyaluronic acid) and type B *N. meningitidis* (sialic acid), which are nonimmunogenic.

*** Teichoic acid: polymers of ribitol or glycerol, bound to cell membrane or peptidoglycan.

Outer Surface Structures of the Bacterial Cell

Pilus or fimbria 1. Common 2. Sex 3. Virulence	Primarily Gram −*	Glycoprotein (pilin)	Adherence to cell surfaces, including attachment to other bacteria during conjugation
Flagellum	+ and −	Protein (flagellin)	Motility
Axial filaments (internal flagellum)	Spirochetes gram −	Protein	Motility

*M-protein of group A strep described as diffuse fimbriate layer or fimbriae.

Internal Bacterial Structures*

Structure	Cell Type	Chemical Composition	Function
Nucleoid region No membrane No histones No introns	Gram + and gram −	DNA RNA Proteins	Genetic material (all essential genes) Primers, mRNA Linker proteins, polymerases
Plasmids	Gram + and gram −	DNA	Non-essential genetic material Roles in conjugation, drug resistance, toxin production
Ribosomes	Gram + and gram −	70S (protein/RNA) 30S (16S RNA) 50S (23 and 5S)	Protein synthesis
Granules (various types)	Gram + and gram −	Glycogen, lipids, polyphosphate, etc.	Storage: polymerization of molecules present in high numbers in cells reduces osmotic pressure. Volutin granules of *Corynebacterium diphtheriae* are used in clinical identification.
Endospores	Gram + *only*	Keratin coat, calcium dipicolinate	Resistance to heat, chemicals, and dehydration

*Note that there are no mitochondria or membrane-bound structures, such as chloroplasts.

Microbiology Practice Questions

GENERAL MICROBIOLOGY

1. A 21-year-old student was seen by his family physician with complaints of pharyngitis. Examination of the pharynx revealed patchy erythema and exudates on the tonsillar pillars. Throat smear showed gram-positive cocci in chains and gram-negative diplococci. He admitted to having been sexually active. What is the significance of the Gram stain smear in this case?

   (A) It provides a rapid means of diagnosing the infection
   (B) It indicates laboratory contamination
   (C) It is not useful as it is not possible to make a diagnosis this way
   (D) It strongly suggests gonococcal pharyngitis
   (E) It is evidence of infection with hemolytic streptococci and *Neisseriae*

2. Your laboratory isolates an entirely new and unknown pathogen from one of your patients, which has all the characteristics of an aerobic filamentous fungus except that the ribosomes are prokaryotic. Unfortunately, your patient with this pathogen is very ill. Which agent would most likely be successful in treating your patient?

   (A) Third generation of cephalosporins
   (B) Isoniazid
   (C) Metronidazole
   (D) Careful limited usage of Shiga toxin
   (E) Tetracycline

3. Mitochondria are missing in

   (A) Filamentous fungi
   (B) Protozoan parasites
   (C) Viruses
   (D) Yeasts
   (E) Cestodes

4. A culture isolate from a patient with subacute endocarditis is reported to be gram positive and possess a complex carbohydrate cell wall. What is the most likely taxonomic group of the causal agent?

   (A) Fungus
   (B) Parasite
   (C) Prion
   (D) Prokaryot
   (E) Virus

5. A patient with a non-healing skin lesion has that lesion biopsied to determine its cause. The pathology lab reports back that the lesion has the characteristics of a stellate granuloma. Which of the following is most likely to be true of the causal agent?

    (A) It has lipopolysaccharide.

    (B) It has pili.

    (C) It is an exotoxin producer.

    (D) It is a superantigen.

    (E) It is intracellular.

6. A cancer chemotherapy patient has to have her intravenous port revised after it becomes blocked and the catheter is found to contain bacterial contaminants. Which of the following attributes is most likely to be a factor in this pathogenesis?

    (A) Biofilm production

    (B) Ergosterol containing membrane

    (C) Peptidoglycan layer

    (D) Possession of IgA protease

    (E) Possession of pili

7. A 45-year-old female executive goes to a cosmetic surgeon with the complaint of frown lines on her forehead which she feels are negatively affecting her appearance. Rather than undergoing surgery, she opts to try injection of BOTOX. What is the mechanism of action of this toxin?

    (A) It blocks release of acetylcholine.

    (B) It inhibits glycine and GABA.

    (C) It is a lecithinase.

    (D) It is a superantigen.

    (E) It ribosylates eukaryotic elongation factor-2.

    (F) It ribosylates Gs.

MEDICALLY IMPORTANT BACTERIA

8. A 4-year-old boy develops several honey-crusted lesions behind his ears and on his face. The simplest test for the physician to determine the genus of bacteria responsible for this child's illness is the

    (A) catalase test

    (B) coagulase test

    (C) growth of the organism in 6.5% sodium chloride

    (D) hemolysis pattern on blood agar

    (E) polymerase chain reaction

9. An atherosclerotic 80-year-old man develops a pelvic abscess following a ruptured appendix. What is/are the most likely causal agent(s)?

    (A) *Bacteroides* species and microaerophilic streptococci

    (B) *Candida albicans*

    (C) *Enterobacter aerogenes*

    (D) *Haemophilus influenzae* group B

    (E) *Streptococcus viridans*

10. A homeless, malnourished chronic alcoholic presents with severe headache and dyspnea. Physical examination reveals a disheveled male with poor hygiene. His temperature is 41°C, blood pressure is 110/78 mm Hg, and his pulse is 96/minute and regular. Auscultation of the chest reveals absence of breath sounds over the left middle lung fields. A chest x-ray confirms left lobar pneumonia. Sputum stain reveals partially acid-fast bacilli with branching rods. Which of the following agents is the most likely cause?

    (A) *Mycobacterium avium-intracellulare*

    (B) *Mycobacterium kansasii*

    (C) *Mycobacterium leprae*

    (D) *Mycobacterium tuberculosis*

    (E) *Nocardia asteroides*

11. A 70-year-old man presents to the emergency department with a fever of 103.5°F, a dry cough, tachypnea, and chest pain. History reveals he has been smoking since he was a teen. He mentions that several people at the assisted living community where he resides have had similar symptoms. A sputum sample isolated organisms that grew on buffered charcoal yeast extract agar and stained weakly gram-negative. Which of the following properties is consistent with the above organism?

    (A) Capsule

    (B) No cell wall

    (C) Optochin sensitive

    (D) Requires iron and cysteine for growth

    (E) Serpentine growth in vitro

12. A 33-year-old man presents to the emergency department with a fever of 102.5°F, facial palsy, headache, and malaise. A circular maculopapular rash was identified on the patients left shoulder; the patient was unaware of the rash. The patient likely acquired the above infection via which of the following routes?

    (A) Consumption of contaminated food

    (B) Direct contact with fomite

    (C) Arthropod vector

    (D) Respiratory route

    (E) Sexual contact

13. A 25-year-old man develops a high fever and swelling in the armpits and groin. Aspirates from the lymph nodes reveal gram-negative rods with bipolar staining. The patient is most likely

   (A) a farmer
   (B) from the southwestern U.S.
   (C) in the military
   (D) living in a dormitory
   (E) sexually promiscuous

14. A previously healthy 5-month-old infant presents with apparent upper body weakness including droopy eyes, head lag, drooling, and inability to sit unassisted. The most likely infectious form is

   (A) elementary body
   (B) endospore
   (C) exotoxin
   (D) reticulate body
   (E) vegetative cell

15. Sixteen residents in a retirement home have fever, malaise, and anorexia. These residents have taken their meals prepared by the same kitchen. Blood cultures from 11 of these residents grow *Salmonella enterica* subsp. *typhi*. The primary reservoir of this organism is

   (A) hen's egg
   (B) dogs and cats
   (C) turkeys
   (D) people
   (E) water

16. If a culture is inoculated to a density of 5×10^2 cells/mL at time 0 and has both a generation time and lag time of 10 minutes, how many cells/mL will there be at 40 minutes?

   (A) 1.5×10^3
   (B) 2×10^3
   (C) 4×10^3
   (D) 6×10^3
   (E) 4×10^6

17. A 6-year-old girl had crashed on a toboggan ride and complained of pain in the perineal area. Exam showed only bruising of the area. Two days later, she develops fever, prostration, discoloration of the buttock, and blebs of the skin in the area. After admission to the hospital, she develops progressive involvement of the leg, thigh, and buttock with extension to the lower abdomen. She goes into shock and dies before surgery could be performed. At autopsy, a 1-inch piece of wood is found in the perineum, which had perforated the anus. The most likely causal agent

    (A) requires an elevated oxidation reduction potential
    (B) is a gram-negative coccobacillus
    (C) is a marked lecithinase producer
    (D) is nonhemolytic on blood agar
    (E) is nonfermentative

18. A 71-year-old man is admitted from his extended care facility (nursing home) because of recent aggravation of an exfoliative skin condition that has plagued him for several years. He had been receiving a variety of topical antibiotic regimens over the last year or two. He now has a temperature of 38.9°C (102°F). The skin of upper chest, extremities, and neck shows erythema with diffuse epidermal peeling and many pustular lesions. Cultures obtained from these lesions were reported back from the laboratory as yielding a gram-positive organism that is highly salt (NaCl) tolerant. What lab result is used to confirm the species of the causal agent?

    (A) Bacitracin sensitivity
    (B) Bile solubility
    (C) Catalase production
    (D) Coagulase production
    (E) Optochin sensitivity

19. Eight of 10 family practice residents who had a potluck 4 days ago now have diarrhea with abdominal cramps, general malaise, and fever ranging from 37.5° to 38.7°C. Stools from 3 residents are blood tinged. Laboratory studies revealed the causal agent was a microaerophilic gram-negative, curved rod with polar flagella often in pairs to give a "seagull" appearance. It grew on special media at 42°C. The original contamination probably was found in

    (A) poultry
    (B) improperly canned food
    (C) fried rice
    (D) fish
    (E) vegetables

20. A 19-year-old man was brought to the emergency department by his dorm mate with a petechial rash, headache, nuchal rigidity, and vomiting. Which of the following describes the most likely causal agent?

    (A) Gram-negative coccus, capsule, ferments maltose

    (B) Gram-negative coccus, ferments glucose only

    (C) Gram-negative coccobacillus, capsular serotype b

    (D) Gram-positive coccus, alpha hemolytic, optochin sensitive

    (E) Gram-positive rods, growth at 4°C

21. A 70-year-old woman is brought to the emergency department by her spouse with complaints of shortness of breath and fever. Physical examination revealed a fever of 103°F, hypotension, and a diastolic murmur. History revealed a cardiac valve replacement 5 years earlier. Three consecutive blood cultures taken during febrile periods revealed gram-positive cocci that were catalase-positive and coagulase-negative. Which of the following organisms is the most likely cause?

    (A) *Enterococcus faecalis*

    (B) *Kingella kingae*

    (C) *Staphylococcus aureus*

    (D) *Staphylococcus epidermidis*

    (E) *Staphylococcus saprophyticus*

22. What is the structure that is found in gram-negative but not in gram-positive bacteria?

    (A) Capsule

    (B) Cell wall

    (C) Cytoplasmic membrane

    (D) Endospore

    (E) Outer membrane

23. A tourist who recently returned from a trip to Peru goes to her physician complaining of persistent high fever, malaise, and constipation that persisted over a week. She recalls that the fever began slowly and climbed to 41°C. A physical exam reveals an enlarged spleen and tender abdomen with rose-colored spots. Laboratory isolation of a bacterium that produces H_2S and is motile is revealed. Which organism is the most likely cause of her condition?

    (A) EHEC

    (B) ETEC

    (C) *Salmonella enterica* subsp. *enteritidis*

    (D) *Salmonella enterica* subsp. *typhi*

    (E) *Shigella dysenteriae*

24. A 5-year-old child of an Eastern European immigrant family is brought to your pediatric clinic. The child is afebrile, but weak and exhausted from a week of paroxysmal coughing with inspiratory whoops, frequently associated with vomiting. The parents profess religious objections to childhood vaccinations, but permit withdrawal of a blood sample, which reveals a lymphocytosis of 44,000/mm^3. Production of lymphocytosis, insulin secretion, and histamine sensitization are all results of which attribute of this organism?

    (A) Motility

    (B) Adenylate cyclase toxin

    (C) Beta-hemolysin

    (D) Anaerobic growth

    (E) Pertussis toxin

    (F) Filamentous hemagglutinin

25. The clinical laboratory reports the presence of 0157:H7 strains of *E. coli* in the bloody stools of 6 children ages 3–5 who attended a local petting zoo. These young children would be at an increased risk for developing

    (A) buboes

    (B) hemolytic uremic syndrome

    (C) infant botulism

    (D) renal stones

    (E) rice water stools

26. A 65-year-old man develops pneumonia. The organisms isolated from the sputum are gram-positive cocci that are alpha hemolytic on blood agar and sensitive to optochin. Which structure of the causal agent provides protection against phagocytosis?

    (A) Capsule

    (B) Catalase

    (C) Coagulase

    (D) M protein

    (E) Teichoic acid

27. A 68-year-old woman on chemotherapy for leukemia has developed sepsis due to an infection with *Escherichia coli*. The following day the patient develops septic shock and dies. The structure on the bacterium most likely responsible for causing septic shock in this patient is

    (A) capsule

    (B) lipopolysaccharide

    (C) pili

    (D) spore

    (E) teichoic acid

28. A 12-year-old boy from North Carolina presents to the emergency department with rash, fever, and severe headache that began 3 days ago. The rash began on his arms and legs and then spread to the trunk. The pediatrician notes conjunctival redness, and lab tests reveal proteinuria. Which of the following events likely led to the child's illness?

    (A) Cutting himself while butchering rabbits

    (B) Eating undercooked meat

    (C) Hiking in the woods

    (D) Kissing

    (E) Not washing his hands

29. A 10-year-old child develops glomerulonephritis a week after he was treated for a sore throat. The causal agent is identified by serotyping of the

    (A) capsule

    (B) M proteins

    (C) outer membrane proteins

    (D) pili

    (E) teichoic acids

30. An 8-year-old boy presents to the emergency department with vomiting and a severe cough in which he can't catch his breath. His vaccination history is incomplete. Physical exam reveals fever and conjunctival injection. A nasopharyngeal aspirate grew gram-negative coccobacilli on Bordet-Gengou media. What is the mechanism of action of the toxin involved?

    (A) ADP ribosylation of eukaryotic elongation factor 2 (eEF-2)

    (B) ADP ribosylation of G_i

    (C) ADP ribosylation of GTP-binding protein

    (D) Blocks release of acetylcholine

    (E) Blocks release of inhibitory transmitters GABA and glycine

31. What is the typical means of transmission of a toxin that blocks the release of inhibitory transmitters GABA and glycine?

    (A) Eating home-canned foods

    (B) Fecal-oral, travel to foreign country

    (C) Infant given honey during the first year of life

    (D) Puncture wound

    (E) Respiratory, with incomplete vaccination history

32. An infant presents to the emergency department due to difficulty breathing, constipation, and anorexia. Upon examination, the physician notes flaccid paralysis. A toxin screen of the stool identified the agent. What is the mechanism of action of the toxin?

    (A) ADP ribosylation of eukaryotic elongation factor 2 (eEF-2)

    (B) ADP ribosylation of G_i

    (C) ADP ribosylation of GTP-binding protein

    (D) Blocks release of acetylcholine

    (E) Blocks release of inhibitory transmitters GABA and glycine

33. A 10-year-old girl with an incomplete vaccination history presents to her pediatrician with a fever of 101.5°F, sore throat, malaise, and difficulty breathing. Physical examination reveals cervical lymphadenopathy and a gray, leathery exudate in the rear of the oropharynx. The area bleeds profusely when disturbed with a tongue depressor. Which of the following correctly describes the causal agent?

    (A) Gram-negative rod; toxin that inhibits protein synthesis

    (B) Gram-negative rod; toxin that increases cAMP

    (C) Gram-positive aerobic rod; toxin that inhibits protein synthesis

    (D) Gram-positive anaerobic rod; toxin that inhibits protein synthesis

    (E) Gram-positive aerobic rod; toxin that increases cAMP

34. A 38-year-old man who recently visited India on business presents to the emergency department with profuse watery diarrhea flecked with mucus, and severe dehydration. Which of the following correctly describes the causal agent?

    (A) Gram-negative curved rod; toxin that increases cAMP

    (B) Gram-negative curved rod; toxin that inhibits protein synthesis

    (C) Gram-negative rod; toxin that increases cAMP

    (D) Gram-negative rod; toxin that inhibits protein synthesis

    (E) Intoxication with a heat labile toxin that blocks the release of acetylcholine

35. A 30-year-old man presents to his physician with complaints of midepigastric pain. He describes the pain as moderate, occasionally waking him at night, and improving immediately following meals. A urease breath test was positive. Which of the following correctly describes the causal agent?

    (A) Gram-negative curved rod; microaerophilic

    (B) Gram-negative rod; aerobic

    (C) Gram-negative rod; facultative anaerobe

    (D) Gram-positive rod; aerobic

    (E) Gram-positive rod; microaerophilic

36. A 13-year-old girl presents to her pediatrician with fever, malaise, and a sore throat. Physical examination reveals a fever of 103°F, cervical lymph-adenopathy, and pharyngeal erythema. A swab is taken from some of the tonsillar exudate and cultured on blood agar. Culture reveals beta hemolytic, gram-positive cocci, and a rapid antigen test is positive. What is the major component that protects the causal agent from osmotic damage?

    (A) Lipopolysaccharide
    (B) Peptidoglycan
    (C) Phospholipids
    (D) Polysaccharide
    (E) Teichoic acid

37. A 27-year-old woman, after returning home from her honeymoon, has developed urinary frequency, dysuria, and urgency. Her urine is grossly bloody. Which lab data are most likely to define the causal agent?

    (A) A gram-negative diplococcus, which is oxidase positive but does not ferment maltose
    (B) A gram-positive coccus, which is catalase positive and coagulase negative
    (C) An optochin-resistant, catalase-negative, gram-positive coccus
    (D) A gram-positive bacillus grown on a low oxidation-reduction medium
    (E) A gram-negative bacterium capable of reducing nitrates to nitrites

38. Two days after eating a meal that included home-canned green beans, 3 people developed various degrees of visual problems, including double vision and difficulties focusing. Describe the Gram reaction of the organism most likely to be isolated from the leftover beans and lab findings which would be used in its identification.

    (A) A gram-positive coccus which is catalase-positive and grows in a high salt environment
    (B) A gram-positive aerobic bacillus which sporulates
    (C) A gram-positive coccus which is catalase-negative and optochin-resistant
    (D) A gram-positive bacillus grown on a low oxidation-reduction medium
    (E) A gram-negative bacillus capable of reducing nitrates to nitrites

39. A 16-year-old has pneumonia with a dry, hacking cough. The x-ray pattern shows a light, diffuse infiltrative pattern. The most likely organism producing these symptoms is

    (A) A non-Gram–staining bacterium requiring sterols
    (B) A bacillus showing granules when stained with methylene blue
    (C) A bacitracin-sensitive, catalase-negative gram-positive coccus
    (D) A coagulase positive, gram-positive, catalase positive coccus in clusters
    (E) A gram-positive bacillus grown on a low oxidation-reduction medium

40. A 7-day-old infant presents to the emergency department with a fever, poor feeding, and a bulging fontanelle. During her physical examination, she begins to convulse. A Gram stain of the CSF reveals gram-positive rods. Which of the following organisms is the most likely causal agent?

    (A) *Escherichia coli*

    (B) *Haemophilus influenzae*

    (C) *Listeria monocytogenes*

    (D) *Neisseria meningitidis*

    (E) *Streptococcus agalactiae*

41. A 55-year-old woman had her rheumatic heart valve replaced with a pros-thetic valve. Six blood cultures became positive after 3 days of incubation. An optochin-resistant, catalase-negative gram-positive coccus that was alpha-hemolytic was isolated. What was the most likely causal agent?

    (A) *Streptococcus viridans*

    (B) *Pseudomonas aeruginosa*

    (C) *Serratia marcescens*

    (D) *Staphylococcus aureus*

    (E) *Streptococcus pneumoniae*

42. A surgical patient develops an abdominal abscess. The abscess was drained, and culture reveals a polymicrobial infection. The predominant organism identified is a gram-negative anaerobic rod. Which of the following is the most likely causal agent?

    (A) *Bacteroides fragilis*

    (B) *Escherichia coli*

    (C) *Pseudomonas aeruginosa*

    (D) *Staphylococcus aureus*

    (E) *Staphylococcus epidermidis*

43. A 40-year-old homeless man presents to the emergency department with fever and night sweats, coughing up blood. Acid-fast bacilli are identified in his sputum. Which of the following virulence factors allows the causal agent to inhibit phagosome-lysosome fusion to survive intracellularly?

    (A) Cord factor

    (B) Calcium dipicolinate

    (C) Peptidoglycan

    (D) Sulfatides

    (E) Tuberculin

44. A 28-year-old woman presents to her gynecologist with complaints of a malodorous vaginal discharge. Upon examination the physician notes a thin, gray vaginal discharge with no vaginal redness. A whiff test was positive for an amine odor. Which of the following is consistent with this case?

    (A) Clue cells

    (B) Gram-negative diplococci in PMNs

    (C) Koilocytic cells

    (D) Owl-eye inclusions

    (E) Tzanck smear

45. Several postal workers come down with symptoms of dyspnea, cyanosis, hemoptysis, and chest pain. Chest x-ray reveals mediastinal widening. Sputum cultures are negative for all routine respiratory pathogens. Serology correctly identifies the causal agent. Which of the following structures is possessed by the causal agent?

    (A) Elementary body

    (B) Endotoxin

    (C) Periplasmic space

    (D) Reticulate body

    (E) Spore

46. A 25-year-old man gets into a fight at the local bar and punches another patron in the mouth. The following day his fist becomes infected and he visits a local urgent care center. Exudate from the wound is cultured on blood and chocolate agar and reveals gram-negative rods that have a bleach-like odor. Which of the following agents is the most likely cause?

    (A) *Actinobacillus actinomycetemcomitans*

    (B) *Cardiobacterium hominis*

    (C) *Eikenella corrodens*

    (D) *Pseudomonas aeruginosa*

    (E) *Kingella kingae*

47. A 45-year-old woman presents to the emergency department with intense pain in her lower back and a burning sensation upon urination. A urine culture was taken and plated on MacConkey agar. Gram-negative rods that did not ferment lactose were identified. Which virulence factor of the causal agent is most important to pathogenesis?

    (A) Capsule

    (B) Catalase

    (C) Coagulase

    (D) Exotoxin

    (E) Urease

48. A 70-year-old man is hospitalized for an infection and treated with clindamycin. The patient improves and returns to his nursing home. Two weeks later he is rushed to the emergency room with fever and loose, mucoid green stools. The diarrhea is voluminous, and he is having severe abdominal pain. Sigmoidoscopy of his colon reveals yellow-white plaques. What is the single most likely event/factor that contributed to this patient's current illness?

    (A) Administration of antibiotics

    (B) Advanced age

    (C) Drinking unpasteurized milk

    (D) Eating contaminated cold cuts

    (E) Living in nursing home

49. A 15-day-old boy presents with conjunctivitis. Iodine staining bodies are seen in conjunctival scrapings. The most likely infectious form is a(n)

    (A) elementary body

    (B) reticulate body

    (C) endospore

    (D) exotoxin

    (E) vegetative cell

50. A 45-year-old man presents to the emergency department with shortness of breath and a productive cough. His sputum was gelatinous and bloody. Gram stain of the sputum revealed numerous PMNs and gram-negative rods. Which of the following descriptions is most likely to fit the patient?

    (A) Alcoholic

    (B) Homeless

    (C) Hiker

    (D) IV drug user

    (E) Veterinarian

51. An infant presents with fever, convulsions, and nuchal rigidity during the first month of life. Which of the following agents is the most likely cause?

    (A) *Escherichia coli*

    (B) *Haemophilus influenzae*

    (C) *Listeria monocytogenes*

    (D) *Streptococcus agalactiae*

    (E) *Streptococcus pneumoniae*

52. A 60-year-old woman is hospitalized following a stroke and develops a high-grade fever with chills. She is catheterized due to urinary incontinence and receives cephalosporin for treatment of pneumonia. Blood cultures and Gram stain are performed by the laboratory. The organisms isolated are gram-positive cocci that are catalase-negative and capable of growth in 6.5% sodium chloride. Which of the following is the most likely causal agent?

    (A) *Enterococcus faecalis*

    (B) *Staphylococcus aureus*

    (C) *Staphylococcus epidermidis*

    (D) *Streptococcus pyogenes*

    (E) Viridans streptococci

53. A 35-year-old man who is positive for HIV develops sepsis with the subsequent development of a necrotic lesion on the buttock that has a black center and an erythematous margin. Which of the following is the most likely causal agent?

    (A) *Bacillus anthracis*

    (B) *Clostridium perfringens*

    (C) *Enterococcus faecalis*

    (D) *Pseudomonas aeruginosa*

    (E) *Staphylococcus aureus*

54. A 15-year-old girl develops a sore throat, fever, and earache of approximately 1 week duration. Upon examination by her physician, an erythematous rash is noted covering most of her body and her tongue appears bright red. Which of the following is the description of the causal agent?

    (A) Gram-positive coccus, alpha hemolytic, catalase negative

    (B) Gram-positive coccus, beta hemolytic, catalase negative

    (C) Gram-positive coccus, alpha hemolytic, catalase positive

    (D) Gram-positive coccus, beta hemolytic, catalase positive

    (E) Gram-positive coccus, gamma hemolytic, catalase negative

55. A patient is admitted to the hospital because of a bleeding duodenal ulcer. Culture at 37°C reveals a urease-positive, gram-negative, curved rod. Which of the following is a likely complication due to infection with the causal agent?

    (A) Diarrhea

    (B) Kidney stones

    (C) Pseudomembranous colitis

    (D) Stomach cancer

    (E) Vomiting

56. Roommates of a 19-year-old college student become alarmed when he does not get up to go to swim practice in the morning and they are unable to wake him for his 11 AM class (he had complained of a headache and not feeling well the night before). The rescue squad finds a febrile, comatose young man with a petechial rash. In the emergency room, Kernig and Brudzinski signs are present. No papilledema is seen, so a spinal tap is done. Protein is high, glucose low. CSF WBC count is 9,000 (mainly PMNs) with few RBCs. The characteristics of the most likely causal agent are

    (A) An enveloped dsDNA virus

    (B) A naked (+)ssRNA virus

    (C) A Gram-negative bacillus with a polyribitol capsule

    (D) A Gram-negative, oxidase-positive diplococcus

    (E) A Gram-positive, lancet-shaped, alpha-hemolytic diplococcus

MICROBIAL GENETICS/DRUG RESISTANCE

57. What type of genetic material is created by repeated transpositional recombination events?

    (A) Chromosomal drug resistance genes

    (B) Genetic operon

    (C) Hfr chromosome

    (D) Insertion sequences

    (E) Multiple drug resistance plasmids

58. Which genetic material is found in pathogenic *Corynebacterium diphtheriae* but not in nonpathogenic normal flora diphtheroids?

    (A) A diphthamide on eEF-2

    (B) An episome

    (C) An F factor

    (D) An integrated temperate phage

    (E) Highly repetitive bacterial DNA

59. How is a prophage created?

    (A) Through activation of the *recA* gene product of an exogenote

    (B) Through infection of a bacterial cell with a virulent bacteriophage

    (C) Through site-specific recombination of a temperate phage and bacterial DNA

    (D) Through infection of a bacterial cell with lambda phage, lacking the lambda repressor

    (E) Through excision of bacterial DNA and active lytic replication of a bacteriophage

60. If one cell of type one (figure below) is mixed into a culture of 100 cells of type two (below), and culture conditions are optimized for conjugation BUT NOT for cell division, the cellular genotype that would predominate after overnight incubation would be that of

   (A) Cell #1

   (B) Cell #1 with new a, b, c, and d alleles

   (C) Cell #2 with new A, B, C, and D alleles

   (D) Cell #1 with a new a allele

   (E) Cell #2 with a new A allele

   (F) Cell #1 with new a and b alleles

   (G) Cell #1 with new A and B alleles

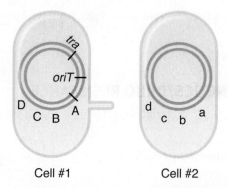

Cell #1   Cell #2

61. Assume the following cells have no plasmids other than those mentioned. Which cell type would contain two molecules of DNA?

   (A) F⁺

   (B) F⁻

   (C) Hfr

62. Assume the cells whose genotype is listed below have no other plasmids than those indicated by the indicated genotype. Which bacterial cell is most likely to transfer chromosomal genes in linear order?

   (A) F⁺

   (B) F⁻

   (C) Hfr

63. What bacterial gene transfer process is most sensitive to extracellular nucleases?

   (A) Conjugation

   (B) Generalized transduction

   (C) Homologous recombination

   (D) Site-specific recombination

   (E) Specialized transduction

   (F) Transformation

64. Following specialized transduction, if any of the bacterial genes transferred in are to be stabilized, what process must occur?

(A) Conjugation

(B) Generalized transduction

(C) Homologous recombination

(D) Site-specific recombination

(E) Specialized transduction

(F) Transformation

65. The ability of a cell to bind DNA to its surface and import it is required for which genetic process?

(A) Conjugation

(B) Generalized transduction

(C) Homologous recombination

(D) Site-specific recombination

(E) Specialized transduction

(F) Transformation

66. The process by which bacterial or plasmid DNA may be mistakenly incorporated (during assembly) into one phage being produced by the lytic life cycle and then that DNA-transferred to another bacterial cell which may acquire some new genetic traits is called

(A) Conjugation

(B) Generalized transduction

(C) Homologous recombination

(D) Site-specific recombination

(E) Specialized transduction

(F) Transformation

67. Recombination is required for stabilization of genetic material newly transferred by all of the following processes EXCEPT

(A) Movement of a transposon

(B) Integration of a temperate bacteriophage

(C) Transduction of a chromosomal gene

(D) Conjugal transfer of an R factor

(E) Transformation of a chromosomal gene

68. Lysogenic conversion

    (A) is a change in pathogenicity due to the presence of a prophage.

    (B) is the induction of a prophage to its virulent state.

    (C) is the conversion of a virulent phage into a temperate phage.

    (D) refers to the incorporation of a prophage into the chromosome.

    (E) is the immunity that a prophage confers on a bacterium.

69. Which of the following events is most likely due to bacterial transformation?

    (A) A formerly non-toxigenic strain of *Corynebacterium diphtheriae* becomes toxigenic.

    (B) A non-encapsulated strain of *Streptococcus pneumoniae* acquires a gene for capsule formation from the extract of an encapsulated strain.

    (C) A strain of *Neisseria gonorrhoeae* starts producing a plasmid-encoded β-lactamase similar to that another Gram-negative strain.

    (D) A gene for gentamicin resistance from an *Escherichia coli* chromosome appears in the genome of a bacteriophage that has infected it.

70. Which of the following mechanisms is most likely to be involved in multiple drug resistance transfer from one cell to another?

    (A) Specialized transduction of a chromosomal gene for drug resistance

    (B) Transformation of chromosomal genes

    (C) Transposition

    (D) Conjugation with a cell with a free plasmid carrying drug resistance

    (E) Conjugation with a cell with chromosomal drug resistance

71. Which of the following agents, if introduced into a growing culture of bacteria, would halt growth but, if then removed, would allow growth to resume?

    (A) Antiseptic

    (B) Bacteriocide

    (C) Bacteriostat

    (D) Disinfectant

    (E) Sterilizing Agent

72. A burn patient develops a purulent infection at the site of a skin graft. Culture of the pus is positive for *Pseudomonas aeruginosa*. The patient is started on anti-pseudomonal penicillin while a Kirby-Bauer agar disc diffusion test is requested for the isolate. The results are shown.

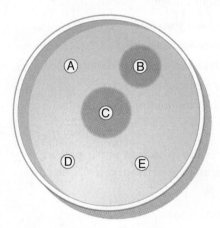

What is the correct interpretation of these lab results?

(A) The isolate is most sensitive to antibiotic B

(B) The isolate is most sensitive to antibiotic C

(C) The isolate is most sensitive to antibiotic E

(D) The isolate is resistant to antibiotic B

(E) Results cannot be analyzed without a key

73. A bacterial isolate from a patient with chronic sinusitis is shown to be sensitive to amoxicillin on a Kirby-Bauer agar disk diffusion test. A follow-up determination of the MIC of the drug is reported back from the laboratory at 2 µg/ml with an MBC of 1 µg/ml. What is the correct interpretation of this data?

(A) The drug is bacteriocidal.

(B) The drug is bacteriostatic.

(C) The drug should be administered to the patient at 1 µg/ml.

(D) The drug should be administered to the patient at 2 µg/ml.

(E) There has been a laboratory error.

MEDICALLY IMPORTANT VIRUSES

74. A 5-year-old presents to the pediatrician with complaints of a sore throat. Her mother also noticed that both of her eyes were slightly red. Examination reveals rhinopharyngitis with bilateral conjunctivitis. What activity likely led to the above illness?

    (A) Hiking in a heavily wooded area

    (B) Eating undercooked shellfish

    (C) Playing with toys in a day care center

    (D) Traveling to a developing country

    (E) Swimming in a community pool

75. Serologic test results from a hepatitis patient reveal: anti-HBc positive, HBsAg positive, and anti-HBs negative. The correct interpretation of the patient's status is

    (A) No longer contagious

    (B) Immune to hepatitis B virus

    (C) Evidence of receiving hepatitis B vaccination

    (D) Hepatitis B virus chronic carrier state

    (E) Impossible to have both surface antigen and core antibody positive

76. A 6-year-old girl presents to the emergency department with a fever and a lacy body rash. Her mother says that yesterday the rash was only on her face, but by this morning, had spread to her trunk and extremities. Which of the following agents is most likely?

    (A) B19

    (B) HHV-6

    (C) Measles

    (D) Rubella

    (E) Varicella zoster virus

77. The best prospects for treatment and cure of microbial diseases are always those unique factors of a pathogen's life cycle that can be altered without affecting the survival of the host's own cells. In HIV, one such therapeutic target would be the products of the *pol* gene, which codes for the reverse transcriptase unique to the retroviral life cycle. If it were possible to ablate expression of the HIV *pol* gene, what other aspect of the virus's life cycle would be directly altered?

    (A) Transcription from proviral DNA

    (B) Production of viral mRNA

    (C) Integration of proviral DNA

    (D) Nucleocapsid

    (E) Viral maturation

78. A 28-year-old male ER resident was accidentally stuck with a needle from a hepatitis B virus-positive patient. He was too embarrassed to tell his attending of his mistake. Two months later, he began to feel fatigued and lost his appetite. When he ordered a hepatitis B serologic panel, he received the results as follows:

    HBsAg   +

    HBsAb   −

    HBcAb   +

    HBeAg   +

    HBeAb   −

    What is the status of the resident?

    (A) Acute infection

    (B) Chronic infection

    (C) Fulminant infection

    (D) Immune

    (E) Uninfected

79. A prison inmate who was diagnosed with hepatitis 6 months ago is tested for his progress with the folllowing results:

    HBsAg   −

    HBsAb   +

    HBcAb   +

    HBeAg   −

    HBeAb   +

    What is the status of the patient?

    (A) Acute infection

    (B) Chronic infection

    (C) Fulminant infection

    (D) Immune

    (E) Uninfected

80. A 10-year-old boy is brought to the emergency department with a high fever, chills, headache, and nausea. He vomits at admission, where his temperature is 104.2°F, and he begins to hallucinate. A CT scan reveals encephalitis in one temporal lobe. Which of the following causal agents is most likely?

    (A) California encephalitis

    (B) Herpes simplex virus 1

    (C) Polio virus

    (D) St. Louis encephalitis

    (E) West Nile virus

81. A 60-year-old woman who recently received a liver transplant develops a high fever and severe dyspnea with a dry hacking cough. Chest x-ray reveals bilateral interstitial infiltrates that are diffuse. Which of the following agents is most likely responsible for her condition?

    (A) Adenovirus

    (B) Cytomegalovirus

    (C) Influenza virus

    (D) Respiratory syncytial virus

    (E) Rhinovirus

82. An 8-year-old boy from India was brought to the emergency department while visiting the U.S. because of a flaccid paralysis in his lower extremities. His mother explains that the child had a flu-like illness a couple of weeks earlier. How was the agent in the above case likely acquired?

    (A) Fecal-oral

    (B) Mosquito

    (C) Respiratory

    (D) Sexual

    (E) Tick

83. A 5-year-old girl presents with a fever and a generalized macular rash that is most dense on the scalp and trunk of the body. Several waves of lesions appear, one after another, and evolve rapidly into vesicles and then pustules over several days. The most likely disease and causal agent is

    (A) Exanthem subitum due to cytomegalovirus

    (B) Chickenpox due to the varicella-zoster virus

    (C) Whitlow infection due to herpes simplex virus type 1

    (D) Herpetic gingivostomatitis due to the varicella-zoster virus

    (E) Infectious mononucleosis due to the Epstein-Barr virus

84. Infection of appropriate cells with a composite virus made up of Coxsackie virus capsid components and poliovirus RNA would yield progeny which would

    (A) Have the host cell range of Coxsackie virus

    (B) Also be composite viruses

    (C) Show phenotypic mixing

    (D) Have a recombinant genome consisting of both Coxsackie and poliovirus

    (E) React with Sabin-vaccine–induced antibodies

85. An epidemic of nausea, vomiting, and watery diarrhea breaks out on shipboard during a cruise to the Virgin Islands. Which of the following accurately describes the most likely causal agent?

    (A) Acid-fast oocysts

    (B) Enveloped DNA virus

    (C) Enveloped RNA virus

    (D) Nonenveloped DNA virus

    (E) Nonenveloped RNA virus

86. To design a vaccine against HIV infection, a logical goal would be to alter some native molecule or product of the virion in order to make it highly immunogenic. If you wished to prevent the attachment of the virus to helper T lymphocytes, which molecule or family of molecules might best be targeted?

    (A) gp41

    (B) gp120

    (C) nucleocapsid protein

    (D) p17

    (E) p24

87. A woman in her late twenties presents to the emergency department disoriented and confused. She is unable to remember where she lived or even her phone number. She is admitted for observation and testing and begins to hallucinate and salivate excessively. On the east coast of the United States, what is the most common reservoir of this disease?

    (A) Bat

    (B) Cat

    (C) Dog

    (D) Fox

    (E) Raccoon

88. An 11-month-old infant was brought to the emergency department with difficulty breathing and wheezing. History and physical examination reveal a slight fever, cough, and rhinorrhea that began about 2 days before. Analysis of the sputum reveals normal flora with the presence of giant multinucleated cells. Which of the following is the most likely cause?

    (A) B19

    (B) Influenza

    (C) Parainfluenza

    (D) Measles

    (E) Respiratory syncytial virus

89. A 37-year-old executive for a local Health Maintenance Organization comes to your office because he has developed multiple blister-like lesions on his penis over the last 1–2 days. They are somewhat painful, and he is worried that he has AIDS. He denies homosexuality and intravenous drug abuse and had an HIV test prior to his marriage 3 years ago. He reports several similar episodes several years ago when he worked as a photographer in Nepal. He was never told what they were, and they resolved over several days without any treatment. His physical examination is remarkable only for the presence of 6–8 vesicular lesions 3–4 mm in diameter on the glans of the penis. There is no crusting, drainage, or bleeding. The lesions are moderately tender and there is mild inguinal adenopathy bilaterally. How does the causal agent produce its messenger RNA?

    (A) By producing a positive sense intermediate
    (B) By direct translation from the genome
    (C) By transcription from proviral DNA
    (D) By producing a negative sense intermediate
    (E) By transcribing from the genomic DNA
    (F) By reverse transcription from the genome
    (G) By semi-conservative replication

90. Several individuals in the central United States from the ages of 5 to 25 have come down with symptoms of nausea, vomiting, and swelling of the parotid glands. Which of the following can be a complication of the above disease?

    (A) Guillain-Barré Syndrome
    (B) Glomerulonephritis
    (C) Orchitis
    (D) Multiple sclerosis
    (E) Reye syndrome

91. In the U.S., a baby has the greatest chance of acquiring which virus in utero?

    (A) Cytomegalovirus
    (B) Hepatitis B virus
    (C) Herpes simplex virus
    (D) Respiratory syncytial virus
    (E) Rubella virus

92. Which of these viruses has RNA for both its genome and replicative intermediate?

    (A) Cytomegalovirus
    (B) Hepadnavirus
    (C) Retroviruses
    (D) Togaviruses
    (E) Poxvirus

93. What is the most common lab testing method for diagnosing infectious mononucleosis?

    (A) The Monospot test to detect EBV-specific antibody

    (B) An assay for Epstein-Barr nuclear antigen

    (C) The presence of atypical lymphocytes in the blood establishes the etiology

    (D) A test for heterophile antibody, which cross-reacts with antigens found on a variety of animal red blood cells

    (E) A simple procedure is done to isolate EBV from saliva, blood, or lymphoid tissue

94. What virus is noted for genetic reassortment, which leads to major pandemics about once every 10 to 11 years?

    (A) Adenovirus

    (B) Herpes virus

    (C) Human immunodeficiency virus (HIV)

    (D) Influenza virus

    (E) Poliovirus

95. What virus is noted for such a high incidence of genetic drift that more than one antigenic variant can be isolated from most infected individuals who have high viral titers?

    (A) Adenovirus

    (B) Herpes virus

    (C) Human immunodeficiency virus (HIV)

    (D) Influenza virus

    (E) Poliovirus

96. A 19-year-old male college student reports sore throat and extreme fatigue following even normal non-taxing tasks like getting dressed and going down to breakfast. He tells you that he has been sick for several weeks, that he has been feverish, and that his girlfriend now appears to be getting the same thing. His tonsils are inflamed with a white exudate adhering; cervical lymphadenopathy is prominent, as is splenomegaly. The most likely causal agent is

    (A) ssDNA, naked icosahedral virus

    (B) dsDNA, naked icosahedral virus

    (C) dsDNA, enveloped complex virus

    (D) dsDNA, enveloped icosahedral virus

    (E) dsRNA, naked segmented virus

    (F) −ssRNA, segmented, enveloped and helical virus

    (G) −ssRNA, bullet-shaped, helical virus

    (H) −ssRNA, naked, helical virus

    (I) +ssRNA, naked, icosahedral virus

    (J) +ssRNA, enveloped, icosahedral virus

    (K) +ssRNA, enveloped, diploid virus

97. Cataracts and patent ductus arteriosus in a newborn suggest in utero infection with what viral family?

    (A) Adenovirus

    (B) Paramyxovirus

    (C) Parvovirus

    (D) Picornavirus

    (E) Reovirus

    (F) Togavirus

98. What is the primary means of spread for measles?

    (A) Animal bite

    (B) Fecal-oral

    (C) Fomite spread

    (D) Respiratory droplet spread

    (E) Sexual contact

    (F) Transfusion or intravenous drug abuse

    (G) Tick bite

99. How are human papilloma virus type 4 warts spread?

    (A) Animal bite

    (B) Fecal-oral

    (C) Fomite spread

    (D) Respiratory droplet spread

    (E) Sexual contact

100. A 15-year-old member of the high school swim team notices painless, umbilicated cutaneous lesions on the toes. Large eosinophilic cytoplasmic inclusions are present in the affected epithelia. What is the most likely causal agent?

    (A) Adenovirus

    (B) B19 virus

    (C) Molluscum contagiosum virus

    (D) Herpes simplex virus

    (E) Human papilloma virus

101. A bone marrow transplant recipient becomes febrile and hypoxic and chest films demonstrate diffuse interstitial pneumonia. What is the most likely causal agent?

    (A) BK virus

    (B) Cytomegalovirus

    (C) Herpes simplex virus

    (D) Molluscum contagiosum virus

    (E) Paramyxovirus

    (F) Varicella-zoster virus

102. A 6-month-old infant presents with painless verrucous growths on the laryngeal folds. What is the most likely causal agent?

    (A) B19 virus

    (B) Cytomegalovirus

    (C) Herpes simplex virus

    (D) Human papilloma virus

    (E) Molluscum contagiosum virus

MEDICALLY IMPORTANT FUNGI

103. An obese 32-year-old diabetic woman presents with complaint of red and painful skin in her abdominal skin folds. Examination reveals a creamy white material at the base of the fold. It is erythematous underneath and extends beyond the creamy material. Microscopic examination of the exudate reveals oval budding structures (3 × 6 μm) mixed with more budding elongated forms. The most likely causal agent is

    (A) *Aspergillus fumigatus*

    (B) *Candida albicans*

    (C) *Epidermophyton floccosum*

    (D) *Microsporum canis*

    (E) *Sporothrix schenckii*

104. A 19-year-old migrant worker from the southwestern U.S. is brought to the family doctor complaining of cough, pleuritic chest pain, fever, and malaise. He also complains of a backache and headache. He is found to have an erythematous skin rash on his lower limbs. A chest radiograph reveals several calcifying lesions. Which of the following structures is most likely to be found?

    (A) Broad-based budding yeast

    (B) Monomorphic encapsulated yeast

    (C) Nonseptate hyphae with broad angles

    (D) Septate hyphae branching dichotomously at acute angles

    (E) Spherules with endospores

105. An 18-year-old high school student in rural north Mississippi develops fever, cough, and chest pain. The cough, associated with weight loss, persisted. Because of poor performance at football practice, he was advised to see a physician. Lymph node biopsies stained with H and E reveal granulomatous inflammation and macrophages engorged with oval structures measuring 2–4 μm. Cultures incubated at room temperature grow powdery white colonies, which on microscopic study have tuberculate spores. The high school student most likely acquired the infection from which of the following?

    (A) Desert sand

    (B) Cat feces

    (C) Soil enriched with bird excrement

    (D) Another human via respiratory secretions

    (E) Contaminated drinking water

106. A 32-year-old man from the southeastern U.S. is referred to a tertiary care center with chronic pneumonia. He also complains of malaise, weight loss, night sweats, chest pain, breathlessness, and hoarseness. Sputum smear revealed thick-walled, refractile, double-contoured yeast cells. What is the most common site of dissemination for the causal organism?

    (A) Heart

    (B) Liver

    (C) Mucocutaneous

    (D) Skin

    (E) Spleen

107. A 55-year-old man who recently recovered uneventfully from a heart valve transplant presents to the emergency room with pleuritic chest pain, hemoptysis, fever, and chills. While he is being examined, he has a myocardial infarction and the medical team is unable to revive him. An autopsy revealed septate, acutely branching hyphae in many tissues. Which of the following organisms is most likely to be identified?

    (A) *Aspergillus fumigatus*

    (B) *Blastomyces dermatitidis*

    (C) *Cryptococcus neoformans*

    (D) *Histoplasma capsulatum*

    (E) *Mucor* species

108. A 33-year-old HIV-positive man complains of headache and blurred vision. Physical examination reveals papilledema and ataxia. A head CT scan is normal, but CSF obtained by lumbar puncture reveals encapsulated organisms visible by India ink. Which of the following is true concerning this organism?

    (A) It can also be seen as "spaghetti and meatballs" on KOH stain

    (B) It consists of branching septate hyphae

    (C) It exists as a mycelial form at room temperature and a yeast at 37°C

    (D) It is an encapsulated nondimorphic yeast found worldwide

    (E) It is a nonencapsulated dimorphic yeast that reproduces by budding

109. A 32-year-old man who has AIDS presents to his physician with progressively increasing dyspnea over the past 3 weeks. He also complains of a dry, painful cough, fatigue, and low-grade fever. A chest x-ray reveals bilateral symmetrical interstitial and alveolar infiltration. Which of the following agents is the most likely cause of the above?

    (A) *Cryptococcus neoformans*

    (B) *Cryptosporidium parvum*

    (C) *Histoplasma capsulatum*

    (D) *Pneumocystis jiroveci*

    (E) *Toxoplasma gondii*

MEDICAL PARASITOLOGY

110. A 44-year-old woman returns home to New York after a 2-week camera safari to East Africa. She started chloroquine antimalarial prophylaxis 2 weeks prior to her departure for Kenya and continued throughout her foreign travel. She stopped taking the pills on her arrival home because they made her nauseated. Two weeks after her return, she develops paroxysmal fever and diaphoresis and is quickly hospitalized with febrile convulsions, jaundice, and anemia. Blood smears reveal red blood cells multiply infected with delicate ring-like trophozoites and rare sausage-shaped gametocytes. The stage of the parasite life cycle that is responsible for the appearance of the parasites 2 weeks after departure from the malarious area is the

    (A) hypnozoite

    (B) sporozoite

    (C) exoerythrocytic schizont

    (D) erythrocytic schizont

    (E) merozoite

111. At a school nurse's request, a clinic in rural South Carolina sees a 9-year-old girl who appears listless and inattentive, although hearing and visual testing has been within normal limits. The physician finds the child thin, with the "potbelly" of malnutrition, and orders a fecal exam and CBC. The CBC reveals a microcytic, hypochromic anemia, and the fecal exam detects brown, oval nematode eggs approximately 65 microns in size, too numerous to count. What was the most likely means by which this child was infected?

    (A) Ingestion of ova

    (B) Ingestion of larvae

    (C) Ingestion of cysts in muscle

    (D) Skin penetration by larvae

    (E) Mosquito transmission of sporozoites

112. An HIV-positive patient with a CD4+ count of 47 presents with diarrhea. Acid-fast structures are found in the stool. From this finding, which of the following is true?

(A) Infection is short lasting and self-resolving and requires no treatment

(B) If treated with antibiotics, the infection should resolve in 3–6 days

(C) Infection will resolve only with a combination of antituberculous drugs, and then it may take weeks

(D) Infection could have been prevented by avoiding cat feces and under-cooked or raw meat

(E) Even with the best treatment, the infection may be unrelenting

113. A 24-year-old primiparous woman in her eighth month of gestation develops a positive IgM titer to *Toxoplasma gondii* for the first time. She should be advised by her physician that

(A) this child and all future fetuses are likely to be infected

(B) a newborn with a positive anti-*Toxoplasma* IgG response should be treated with anti-parasitics

(C) future infections can be avoided by proper vaccination and worming of cats

(D) retinochoroiditis can be prevented by drug treatment of an infant with a positive IgM response

(E) major organ damage can be reversed by prompt treatment of the newborn

114. A 35-year-old captain in the army reserves has been plagued by a painful, erosive lesion near his ear lobe since his return from Operation Desert Storm several years ago. He denies exposure to the toxic by-products of burning oil fields. Punch biopsy of the leading edge of the erosion reveals macrophages distended with oval amastigotes. How was this infection acquired?

(A) Contact with contaminated drinking water

(B) Bite of *Anopheles* mosquito

(C) Bite of reduviid bug

(D) Fecal contamination of food

(E) Direct human contact in barracks

(F) Bite of sandfly

(G) Bite of tsetse fly

115. A group of 6 college students undertake to climb Mt. Rainier outside Seattle on their spring break. They pack food and camping provisions except for water, which they obtain from the many fresh water mountain streams that arise at the summit. The adventure takes a little over a week to accomplish, and all return safely in good spirits to their classes the following week. Within the first week after their return, 5 of the 6 students report to the infirmary with profuse diarrhea and tenesmus. Each affected student experiences weakness and weight loss, and stool samples submitted to the lab are yellow, greasy, and foul smelling. What attribute of this parasite imparts its pathogenicity?

    (A) Lytic enzymes
    (B) Flagella
    (C) Ventral sucking disc
    (D) Encystment
    (E) Toxic metabolites

116. After one week vacationing in Mexico, a 14-year-old girl presents with abdominal pain, nausea, bloody diarrhea, and fever. Stool specimens are collected and sent to the laboratory for bacteriologic and parasitologic examination. Bacterial cultures are negative for intestinal pathogens. The laboratory report reveals organisms with red blood cells inside them. The most likely causal agent is

    (A) *Cryptosporidium parvum*
    (B) *Entamoeba histolytica*
    (C) *Giardia lamblia*
    (D) *Toxoplasma gondii*
    (E) *Shigella dysenteriae*

117. Four weeks after his arrival from Egypt, a 24-year-old graduate student presents with blood in his urine. Microscopic examination of his urine reveals the presence of eggs with terminal spines. In the interview he admits that he has been working on his family's rice field occasionally since his early childhood. The most likely etiologic agent of his complaint is

    (A) *Entamoeba histolytica*
    (B) *Fasciolopsis buski*
    (C) *Schistosoma haematobium*
    (D) *Schistosoma japonicum*
    (E) *Schistosoma mansoni*

118. A 30-year-old woman presents to her gynecologist with complaints of vaginal itching and a frothy, yellow discharge. She also complains of painful urination. She admits to being sexually active with several men in the past two weeks. Cultures are negative for bacterial growth, but organisms are visible via a wet prep on low power. The most likely causal agent is

    (A) *Candida albicans*
    (B) *Trichophyton rubrum*
    (C) *Chlamydia trachomatis*
    (D) *Trichomonas vaginalis*
    (E) *Giardia lamblia*

119. A 30-year-old missionary comes to the emergency department complaining of high fever, chills, severe headache, and confusion. He has recently returned from Africa. A peripheral blood smear reveals multiple ring structures and crescent-shaped gametes. Which of the following organisms is the most likely cause?

    (A) *Leishmania* species

    (B) *Plasmodium falciparum*

    (C) *Plasmodium malariae*

    (D) *Plasmodium ovale*

    (E) *Plasmodium vivax*

120. A 3-year-old girl presents to her pediatrician with intense perianal itching. Her mother explains that the child has also been extremely irritable during the day and has not been sleeping well at night. Eggs with a flattened side were identified by the laboratory technician from a piece of scotch tape brought in by the parent. Infection with which of the following organisms is most likely?

    (A) *Ascaris lumbricoides*

    (B) *Echinococcus granulosus*

    (C) *Entamoeba histolytica*

    (D) *Enterobius vermicularis*

    (E) *Trichuris trichiura*

121. A 12-year-old girl from Guatemala was brought to the emergency room with a prolapsed rectum. Examination of the rectum reveals small worms that resemble whips attached to the mucosa. A stool sample reveals eggs that are barrel shaped, with bipolar plugs. Which of the following is the most likely cause?

    (A) *Ascaris lumbricoides*

    (B) *Echinococcus granulosus*

    (C) *Entamoeba histolytica*

    (D) *Enterobius vermicularis*

    (E) *Trichuris trichiura*

CLINICAL INFECTIOUS DISEASE

Case Histories

Case A: A 28-year-old known alcoholic man presents with fever and productive cough. He was basically well until 3 days ago when he noticed perspiration, cough, shaking chills, and headache. His cough has been associated with the production of a yellowish-green sputum, which occasionally was tinged with brownish streaks, but was not foul smelling. A Gram stain shows Gram-positive cocci in pairs and short chains.

    A. What laboratory tests could you use to identify the genus?

    Answer: Catalase test (negative) to genus.

    B. When plated on blood agar, what other bacterium might you isolate and confuse the causal agent with, and why? What test(s) could distinguish the two?

    Answer: Viridans strep; optochin and bile.

    C. What procedure would you perform to type the isolate?

    Answer: Quellung reaction with known antibodies to capsule (not antibodies to cell-wall antigens).

Case B: The patient in Case A developed meningitis and died.

    A. What would be the expected CSF cell count?

    Answer: High.

    B. What would be the expected CSF protein and sugar values?

    Answer: Protein high, sugar low.

Case C: A 46-year-old, HIV-positive male complains of malaise, weight loss, fever, and night sweats of 6 weeks duration. More recently, he has developed a cough productive of bloody sputum. Physical exam reveals bronchial breath sounds with crepitant rales over the right upper chest. His CD4 cell count is 560 cells/mm^3. Auramine-rhodamine stain of the sputum is positive, and a chest radiograph reveals hilar lymphadenopathy with a small cavity and streaky infiltrates in the upper lobe.

    A. What attribute of the most likely causal agent promotes its survival in reticuloendothelial cells?

    Answer: Sulfatides are sulfolipids which hydrolyze to make sulfuric acid. They impede the fusion of lysosomes with the phagosome.

    B. What attribute of the causal agent is injected in order to elicit a positive skin test?

    Answer: Tuberculin (outermost protein) plus mycolic acids (long-chain fatty acids in the envelope)

    C. What immune cells are most important in the response to this agent?

    Answer: Th1 cells and macrophages (granuloma formation)

Case D: A patient presents with multiple, crusted and oozing, honey-colored lesions.

    A. What is the skin infection?

      Answer: Impetigo.

    B. What two bacteria would you expect to isolate on culture?

      Answer: Streptococcus pyogenes *(often honey-colored crusted) and/or* Staphylococcus aureus *(often longer-lasting vesicular or with bullae).*

    C. How would you separate the two?

      Answer: Catalase test positive for Staphylococcus, *negative for* Strep-tococcus.

Case E: A patient had intermittent bouts of general malaise, fever with weight loss, and progressive anemia. She presents also with a heart murmur.

    A. What additional physical sign might occur and what causes it?

      Answer: Splinter hemorrhages are caused as septic emboli are thrown from heart valves. They are also seen in trichinosis and trauma.

    B. What is her underlying condition and what are the most commonly involved bacteria?

      Answer: Damaged heart valve;
         Viridans streptococci (associated with bad oral hygiene or dental work) or
         Enterococcus faecalis *or* E. faecium *if she has had bowel surgery.*

    C. How would you distinguish the colony on blood agar?

      Answer: Alpha hemolytic not inhibited by optochin; a viridans strepto-coccus.

Case F: A family of Christian Scientists brings their youngest child to the emergency room because of fever and a stiff neck. The 18-month-old child is acutely ill with a temperature of 104°F. CSF is Gram stained, examined in a rapid test, and also cultured. A Gram stain shows pleomorphic, gram-negative rods.

A. What laboratory test could confirm the identity of the isolate?

Answer: Meningitis screen, a series of immunologic rapid identification tests (usually EIAs using known antibodies), followed by growth of CSF sediment or filtrate on special media and drug susceptibilities.

B. What growth factors are required to grow the isolate on blood agar?

Answer: X = hemin and V = NAD.
Chocolate agar provides both X and V.

C. What is the drug of choice?

Answer: Cefotaxime or ceftriaxone.

D. What is the mechanism of action of the vaccine which would have prevented this condition?

Answer: It is a conjugated vaccine containing the polyribitol phosphate capsular material of the most important serotype (the hapten) covalently coupled to the diphtheria toxoid (protein carrier). The hapten stimulates the B lymphocyte, the carrier stimulates the Th cell, and together, isotype switching becomes possible so that something other than IgM is made.

Case G: A 23-year-old woman presents with lower back pain, fever, and dysuria of 3 days' duration. Urinalysis reveals many white blood cells (WBC) and WBC casts. Gram stain of the uncentrifuged urine reveals numerous Gram-negative bacilli per oil immersion field. On culture, extremely motile bacteria form waves of confluent growth.

A. What is the most important biochemical characteristic of this organism? Why?

Answer: Proteus, *urease-producing Enterobacteriaceae; kidney stones induced.*

Case H: A child developed a unilateral mucopurulent conjunctivitis 10 days after birth. A conjunctival specimen was sent to the laboratory and inoculated into tissue culture cells. Iodine-staining inclusion bodies were produced.

A. What is unusual about the chemical makeup of the organism?

Answer: ATP defective mutant, also muramic acid missing from peptidoglycan.

B. What are the two forms of the organism?

Answer: Elementary bodies (extracellular) and reticulate bodies = replicating forms.

C. What would you see on Gram stain?

Answer: Nothing in the cells—poorly Gram staining.

D. What serologic type caused the child's problem?

Answer: If U.S. kid, serotypes D-K.

Case I: A 27-year-old attorney is hospitalized. He was in excellent health until two days earlier when he noted malaise, fatigability, and profound anorexia. He remembers approximately 6–8 weeks ago receiving a tattoo while vacationing in the Caribbean.

A. How would you confirm your clinical diagnosis?

Answer: HBsAg and IgM to HbcAg.

B. What is meant by the "window"?

Answer: A time period between the end of the detectable presence of HBsAg and the beginning of the production of HBsAb. HBcAb and HBeAb are present.

C. What antigen's persistence beyond 6 months post-infection is indicative that the patient is entering a carrier state?

Answer: HBsAg past 6 months.

D. What antigen correlates with viral production?

Answer: HBeAg.

E. Does the virus carry a virion associated polymerase? If so, what kind?

Answer: Yes, RNA-dependent DNA polymerase (Hepatitis B replicates through an RNA intermediate).

Case J: A young man became ill with a sore throat and swollen tonsils, marked fatigue, cervical adenopathy, a palpable spleen, and a pruritic erythematous rash that started after self-administration of ampicillin.

A. What is the most likely disease? What are the most common laboratory diagnostic tests? What does the antibody test measure?

Answer: Infectious mononucleosis; monospot test (measures heterophile antibody which is not specific to EBV antigen) plus CBC.

B. What type of cells are the Downey type II cells?

Answer: T lymphocytes. (Reactive cells, not infected.)

C. What cells does the virus infect? Through what receptor does the lymphocytic infection begin?

Answer: EBV infects epithelial cells and B lymphocytes, whose receptor is CD21 = CR2.

Case K: A 35-year-old woman presents with a unilateral vesicular rash.

A. The most likely diagnosis is

Answer: Shingles.

B. Describe the virion's nucleic acid.

Answer: Linear dsDNA.

C. Patient had a previous history of what other disease?

Answer: Chickenpox.

Case L: A 27-year-old man presents to the hospital emergency room with a cough, chest pain, and fever. Two days before admission he developed a nonproductive cough. Rales are heard. Gram stain of sputum was negative. Sputum cultures on blood agar were also negative. Culture on a special medium containing cholesterol, purines, and pyrimidines produced colonies in 10 days. Serology 3 weeks later (when he returned because of persistent cough but feeling better) showed cold agglutinins.

A. What is the probable causal agent?

Answer: Mycoplasma pneumoniae.

B. Why did the organism not show up on the Gram stain?

Answer: Organism does not have a cell wall and does not stain with either the primary or counterstain in the Gram stain.

C. What antibiotics do you NOT use?

Answer: Penicillin/cephalosporin.

Case M: A 65-year-old retired male police officer reports to an emergent care facility complaining of fever, sore throat, shortness of breath, dry cough, and generalized muscle aches and pains. On examination the patient is pale, tachycardic, and tachypneic. His conjunctivae are congested and rales and wheezes are heard over both lung fields. A chest radiograph shows diffuse bilateral infiltrates and a hemagglutination inhibition antibody test is positive at high titer.

A. What is your diagnosis?

Answer: Influenza

B. What drugs are available to treat this disease?

Answer: Amantidine/rimantidine (inhibit uncoating)
Zanamivir/ostelamivir (inhibit neuraminidase)

C. To what viral family does it belong?

Answer: Orthomyxovirus

D. Where in the cell does it replicate?

Answer: Cytoplasm and nucleus

E. What vaccine might have prevented this?

Answer: Killed, H3N2, H1N1 plus one strain of Influenza B

F. What attribute of the agent causes pandemics?

Answer: Segmented genome can be reassorted, causing genetic shift.

Case N: A 4-year-old male is brought to the pediatrician by his mother, who is concerned by his lack of appetite and loss of weight. He has had diarrhea fairly constantly over the preceding two-week period, which occasionally has been associated with vomiting. On examination, the child is in the 60% percentile of weight for his age, and has mild epigastric tenderness. A fresh stool sample, collected rectally, is yellow, greasy and malodorous and contains motile organisms.

A. To what taxonomic group does this causal agent belong?

Answer: (Giardia lamblia) Flagellated protozoan

B. How was this child infected?

Answer: Fecal/oral contamination with cysts

C. What is the mechanism of pathogenesis?

Answer: Organism adheres in the upper duodenum using a ventral sucking disk. This blocks common bile ducts, causes fat malabsorption and steattorhea

Case O: A 35-year-old worker at a plant nursery seeks his physician for a suppurative lesion on one of his fingers. A smear is taken of the drainage and stained. Cigar-shaped yeasts are detected.

A. What is the causal agent?

Answer: Sporothrix schenckii.

B. Is the fungus dimorphic or monomorphic?

Answer: This is DIMORPHIC FUNGUS consistent with Sporothrix. You can tell from cigar-shaped yeast (in tissues generally tough to visualize) and hyphae with sleeve and rosettes arrangement of conidia in culture.

C. Treatment

Answer: Itraconazole but oral KI given in milk will also clear up.

Case P: A Christian missionary returns to the United States from Central America with high fever, chills, headache, and confusion. On examination his temperature is 39°C and he is pale and tachycardic. Both liver and spleen are enlarged and tender to palpation. Laboratory tests reveal microcytic anemia, thrombocytopenia, hyperbilirubinemia, and hypoglycemia, and a blood film is examined.

A. What is the diagnosis?

Answer: Plasmodium vivax *malaria*

B. What is the treatment?

Answer: Chloroquine, quinine, amodiaquine, fansidar, halofantrine etc. (Lots of drug resistance is now occurring)

C. Is primaquine required? Why or why not?

Answer: Yes, to prevent relapse and kill hypnozoites. This is called "radical cure" and it is necessary for P. vivax *and* P. ovale *malarias.*

D. How did the patient acquire this disease?

Answer: Bite of female Anopheles *mosquito injects sporozoites.*

Case Q: A 50-year-old Missouri farmer was referred to the hospital because of malaise, weakness, weight loss, fever, and a palpable spleen. Examination of the mouth reveals a painless ulcerated lesion. A punch biopsy of the lesion is obtained and submitted for laboratory study. Histologic study revealed oval structures measuring 2–5 μm, packing the macrophages.

A. What is the most likely causal agent, and what are the distinctive forms?

> *Answer:* Histoplasma capsulatum *with the intracellular oval yeasts and the tuberculate macroconidia (and microconidia) in the hyphal state.*

B. Where in nature will you find the fungus in large numbers?

> *Answer: Great central riverbed plains. Chicken coops in Missouri 100% infected. Indianapolis has had an ongoing outbreak and has major problems with it disseminating in their AIDS patients; NY City also high.*

Case R: A 75-year-old woman who has suffered chronic otitis media, is brought to the hospital by the staff of her long-term care facility. She has complained of dizziness and drowsiness, and preliminary examination reveals signs of meningismus. A CT scan is negative for parenchymal lesions of the brain, although the mastoid cavities are inflamed. A lumbar puncture reveals 2130 leukocytes/μl, 1.55 mm glucose/L (concomitant blood sugar 2.6 mmol/L), and 1582 mg protein/L. Gram staining organisms are absent, but filamentous forms are cultured.

A. What is your diagnosis?

> *Answer:* Aspergillus fumigatus *meningitis*

B. How would you describe this organism?

> *Answer: it is a monomorphic, dematiaceous fungus*

C. What is the treatment of choice?

> *Answer: Amphotericin B or itraconazole*

Case S: A 34-year-old accountant presents to the emergency room because of headache and fever of 3 days' duration. The day before admission his wife noted mild confusion and irritability. Lumbar puncture revealed an opening pressure of 300 mm, 200 red blood cells, 90% of the WBCs which are lymphocytes, sugar of 85 mg/dL (concomitant blood sugar of 110 mg/dL), and protein of 65 mg/dL. Bacteriologic smears (and ultimately also the bacterial cultures) were negative, as were India ink preparations. All latex particle agglutination tests for fungal and bacterial capsules done on the patient's CSF were also negative. The patient's condition did not improve despite appropriate therapy, and he died 10 days after hospitalization.

A. What is the most likely diagnosis?

Answer: Herpes simplex encephalitis

B. What is the virus's shape?

Answer: Icosahedral with nuclear membrane envelope.

C. Where within the cell does the virus replicate?

Answer: Nucleus for both DNA synthesis and assembly.

D. What other members belong to the same family?

Answers: EBV, Varicella-Zoster, Cytomegalovirus.

Case T: A 20-year-old male presents to the emergency department complaining of profuse bloody diarrhea of two days duration. On examination he has a purpuric rash over a large portion of his body, although his temperature is normal. The patient is dehydrated and weak, and lab values reveal an elevated blood urea nitrogen and creatinine, with thrombocytopenia. PT and PTT are within normal limits. Culture of the feces grew organisms which produced both colorless and colored colonies on sorbitol MacConkey medium.

A. What is your diagnosis?

Answer: Enterohemorrhagic Escherichia coli, (EHEC)

B. What is the most likely source of his infection?

Answer: Hamburger, fecal contamination from bovine feces

C. What is the most likely serotype in the United States?

Answer: O157:H7

D. What is the mechanism of pathogenesis?

Answer: Toxin (verotoxin) is Shiga-like and inhibits the 60S ribosomal subunit, thereby stopping eukaryotic protein synthesis.

Case U: A patient presents with anogenital warts.

 A. What is the virus that probably caused the tumors?

 Answer: Human papilloma virus.

 B. What serotypes are most commonly associated with this clinical presentation?

 Answer: 6 and 11

 C. Are they premalignant?

 Answer: Rarely.

 D. What serotypes are most commonly associated with cervical intraepithelial neoplasia?

 Answer: 16, 18, and 31. These are sexually transmitted.

 E. What type of vaccine is now available that could have prevented this infection?

 Answer: 4 serotypes of capsid protein created by recombinant DNA technology.

Case V: A girl received a bone marrow transplant for the treatment of leukemia. Nine weeks after the transplant her temperature rose, she became dyspneic, and died. Impression smears were taken from the cut surface of the lower lobe of the left lung. The smears were stained with H&E. Intranuclear inclusions with perinuclear clearing were found.

 A. Why did the patient develop the pneumonia?

 Answer: Immunocompromised—No T cells.

 B. How would you describe what you would see (using only two words)?

 Answer: Owl's eyes: cells with prominent basophilic intranuclear inclusion bodies.

 C. What is the virion's nucleic acid type? To what viral family does it belong?

 Answer: dsDNA; Herpes viruses.

Case W: A young woman developed a feverish illness with painful swelling of her knee, elbow, and wrist joints. She has a sparse rash on the distal parts of her limbs, consisting of small hemorrhagic pustules with an erythematous base. A smear was obtained from the exudate of the exanthem and Gram stained. The stain showed intracellular gram-negative diplococci.

 A. What disease does she have?

 Answer: Disseminated gonococcal infection.

 B. What is the major mechanism of pathogenesis?

 Answer: Pili, for attachment to epithelial surfaces—colonizing factor along with outer membrane proteins. Also exhibit antigenic variation and protect from phagocytosis.

ANSWERS AND EXPLANATIONS

1. **Answer: C.** Gram-positive cocci (alpha hemolytic streptococci) and gram-negative cocci (*Neisseriae*) are normally present in the throat. There is no way to differentiate pathogens from non-pathogens by the Gram stain.

2. **Answer: E.** The cephalosporin that inhibits prokaryotic cell peptidoglycan cross linkage will not likely be effective against the complex carbohydrate cell wall. Isoniazid, which appears to inhibit mycolic acid synthesis, also would not likely work. Metronidazole would not work on an aerobic organism. Shiga toxin is only effective against eukaryotic ribosomes. Tetracycline (the correct answer) would have the greatest chance of success. However, it may not be taken up by the cell, or the cell could have an effective pump mechanism to get rid of it quickly.

3. **Answer: C.** Mitochondria are found only in eukaryotic organisms so both viruses and bacteria lack them.

4. **Answer: A.** The clue of a complex carbohydrate cell wall (chitin, glucan or mannan) defines the organism as a fungus. The mention that the organism was gram positive was a tricky clue, because of course, the gram stain is used diagnostically to differentiate between the two major categories of bacteria (prokaryots; **choice D**). The student should remember that some fungi will stain gram positive, however, because their thick cell wall makes them retain the gram stain just as a gram positive bacterium would. Parasites (**choice B**) do not possess a cell wall, prions (**choice C**) are infectious proteins, prokaryots (**choice D**) have a peptidoglycan cell wall, and viruses (**choice E**) are acellular.

5. **Answer: E.** The attribute of microorganisms which associates most strongly with the causation of granulomas is the fact that they live intracellularly. This causes stimulation of the Th1 arm of the immune response, and the production of the cytokines of cell-mediated immunity, with the net result of the formation of granulomas in the infected tissues. Some organisms which are extracellular will also produce granulomas, but in those cases it is generally the chronic persistence and indigestibility of the pathogen which cause that result. Lipopolysaccharide (**choice A**) is a synonym for endotoxin, which causes gram negative shock, but not granuloma formation. Pili (**choice B**) are surface structures of some bacteria which mediate attachment to cellular surfaces. Exotoxins (**choice C**) are secreted toxins which may cause cell damage in a number of ways, and superantigens (**choice D**) cause stimulation of large numbers of clones of T lymphocytes and macrophages to cause symptoms similar to endotoxin shock.

6. **Answer: A.** Catheters, shunts and prosthetic devices which are left in the body long-term, are almost always coated with Teflon which is extremely slippery. Organisms which are capable of adherence to Teflon (or the enamel of teeth), do so by creation of a biofilm, which allows them to change the surface tension of the liquid around them and thereby "glue" themselves to the material. Ergosterol (**choice B**) is the major sterol in the cell wall of fungi, and is important in membrane integrity, but not adherence. Peptidoglycan (**choice C**) is the cell wall material of bacteria, and is responsible for the shape of bacteria, but not their adherence. IgA proteases (**choice D**) can

assist in the adherence of bacteria to mucosal surfaces, but would not be important in adherence to an intravenous catheter, and although pili (**choice E**) mediate attachment of bacteria to human cells, they would not be important in adherence to Teflon.

7. **Answer: A.** Botulinum toxin (in BOTOX) inhibits release of acetylcholine and results in a flaccid paralysis. Inhibition of glycine and GABA (**choice B**) describes the action of Tetanus toxin which causes a rigid paralysis. The toxin of *Clostridium perfringens* is a lecithinase (**choice C**) which directly disrupts cell membranes. Toxic shock syndrome toxin-1 and the pyrogenic exotoxins of *Streptococcus pyogenes* act as superantigens (**choice D**) which cause systemic inflammatory response syndrome. Ribosylation of eukaryotic elongation factor-2 (**choice E**) is the mechanism of action of the diphtheria toxin and *Pseudomonas* exotoxin A. Ribosylation of Gs (**choice F**) is the mechanism of action of the cholera toxin and the labile toxin of Enterotoxigenic *Escherichia coli*.

8. **Answer: A.** The easiest way to differentiate between *Staphylococcus* and *Streptococcus* is the catalase test (**choice A**). This is important because they can have similar presentations. Coagulase (**choice B**) differentiates between members of the genus *Staphylococcus*. Hemolysis pattern (**choice D**) is inconclusive. Growth of organism in sodium chloride (**choice C**) can be useful for *Enterococcus*. PCR (**choice E**) is currently used to identify organisms that are difficult to culture.

9. **Answer: A.** Atherosclerosis leads to poor circulation to the lower extremities, which in turn lowers the oxidation-reduction potential of the tissues. All this predisposes to infections caused by anaerobic microorganisms, in this case, *Bacteroides* and streptococci. The patient is suffering from anaerobic cellulitis or possibly myonecrosis.

10. **Answer: E.** Partially acid-fast branching rods in a patient with lobar pneumonia suggests *Nocardia*. All the other agents listed are acid-fast bacilli, not branching rods.

11. **Answer: D.** The causal agent is *Legionella pneumophila*. The clues are dry cough, smoking, weakly gram-negative, and growth on buffered charcoal yeast agar. Remember that *Legionella* is one of the 4 sisters **ELLA** that worship in the **cysteine** chapel. Other sisters include *Francisella*, *Brucella*, and *Pasteurella*. A capsule (**choice A**) would identify agents such as *Streptococcus pneumoniae*. No cell wall (**choice B**) describes *Mycoplasma*. Optochin-sensitive (**choice C**) also describes *Streptococcus pneumoniae*. Serpentine growth in vitro (**choice E**) describes *Mycobacterium tuberculosis*.

12. **Answer: C.** The causal agent is *Borrelia burgdorferi*, and the disease is known as Lyme disease. The clues are facial palsy, rash, fever and malaise. *Borrelia* is spread by ticks.

13. **Answer: B.** The causal agent is *Yersinia pestis*. The clues are high fever, swelling in the armpits and groin, and gram-negative rods with bipolar staining. *Yersinia pestis* is endemic in the U.S. in the desert southwest.

14. **Answer: B.** Infant botulism is an infection started by the ingestion of *Clostridium botulinum* endospores from the environment. The spores germinate in the alkaline pH of the immature gastrointestinal tract and the toxin is produced *in vivo*. In adult botulism, the preformed toxin is ingested.

15. **Answer: D.** The reservoir for *S. enterica* subsp. *typhi* is humans. Other subspecies of *Salmonella* have animals as their reservoirs.

16. **Answer: C.** Each cell divides into two at each generation following the single lag phase. So at the end of the first 10 minutes there are still 5×10^2, and then at the end of the first 20 minutes (total) there are 10×10^2. At the end of 30 minutes total time there will be 20×10^2, and at the end of the total time, 40×10^2, which is written 4×10^3 in proper scientific notation.

17. **Answer: C.** The description strongly suggests that she has myonecrosis. Therefore, the causal agent (at least one) is *C. perfringens*. *C. perfringens* is an anaerobe; therefore **choice A** is wrong. *Clostridia* are all gram-positive; therefore, **choice B** is wrong. *C. perfringens* produces concentric areas of hemolysis; therefore, **choice D** is wrong. *C. perfringens* is a marked lecithinase producer; therefore, **choice C** is correct.

18. **Answer: D.** The patient has "scalded skin" syndrome caused by *S. aureus*. The <u>genus</u> *Staphylococcus* would be distinguished from *Streptococcus* by staphylococcal production of catalase. But the <u>species</u> (*S. aureus*) would be distinguished from *S. epidermidis* on the basis of *S. aureus* production of coagulase. Bacitracin sensitivity is characteristic of *Streptococcus pyogenes*, and bile solubility is characteristic of *Streptococcus pneumoniae*.

19. **Answer: A.** The clue is gram-negative curved rods with polar flagella often in pairs to give a "seagull" appearance, microaerophilic on special media and growing at 42°C. That description is most compatible with *Campylobacter jejuni*. Poultry are the most important reservoirs, so **choice A** is the correct response.

20. **Answer: A.** The causal agent is *Neisseria meningitidis*. The clues are age, dorm room, petechial rash, and nuchal rigidity. *Neisseria meningitidis* is a gram-negative diplococcus and can ferment maltose. Remember that *Neisseria* **m**eningitidis can ferment **m**altose. Gram-negative coccus, ferments glucose only (**choice B**) describes *Neisseria gonorrhoeae*. Gram-negative coccobacillus, capsular serotype b (**choice C**) describes *Haemophilus influenzae*. Gram-positive coccus, alpha hemolytic, optochin-sensitive (**choice D**) describes *Streptococcus pneumoniae*. Gram-positive rods, growth at 4°C (**choice E**) describes *Listeria monocytogenes*.

21. **Answer: D.** The clues are endocarditis, heart valve replacement, and gram-positive cocci that are catalase-positive and coagulase-negative. Many times *Staphylococcus epidermidis* can be a contaminant, but the fact that it was present in 3 consecutive blood cultures identifies it as the causal agent. *Enterococcus faecalis* (**choice A**) is catalase-negative. *Kingella kingae* (**choice B**) is a gram-negative rod. *Staphylococcus aureus* (**choice C**) is coagulase-positive. *Staphylococcus saprophyticus* (**choice E**) is the causal agent of UTIs, not endocarditis.

22. **Answer: E.** Capsules, cell wall, and cytoplasmic membranes are found in both gram-positive and gram-negative bacteria. Endospores (**choice D**) occur with certain gram-positive bacteria, e.g., *Bacillus* and *Clostridium*. Only gram-negatives have an outer membrane.

23. **Answer: D.** The clues are travel, constipation, which is more common than diarrhea, enlarged spleen, and rose-colored spots on the abdomen. It also is an H₂S producer and motile. Remember, salmon(ella) swim upstream (are motile). EHEC (**choice A**) does not produce H₂S and produces bloody diarrhea. ETEC (**choice B**) does not produce H₂S and produces watery diarrhea. *Salmonella enterica* subsp. *enteritidis* (**choice C**) diarrhea (watery, can be bloody) is associated with consumption of raw or undercooked poultry. *Shigella dysenteriae* (**choice E**) does not produce H₂S and causes bloody diarrhea.

24. **Answer: E.** The disease here is whooping cough, caused by *Bordetella pertussis*. The pertussis toxin (also known as the lymphocytosis-promoting toxin) is not believed to be directly cytotoxic, but stimulates adenylate cyclase by ribosylating regulatory proteins. It causes a variety of effects depending on the cell type involved: insulin secretion, lymphocytosis, and alteration of immune effector cells. Of the distractors: the filamentous hemagglutinin (**choice F**) mediates attachment; the adenylate cyclase toxin (**choice B**) stimulates local edema; the organism produces only a small zone of hemolysis around its colonies, so **choice C** is not true; it is an aerobe and does not grow anaerobically (**choice D**). All systemic manifestations of the disease arise from the circulation of the toxins, not the organism itself (**choice A**).

25. **Answer: B.** In children younger than age 5, the most serious complication of EHEC is hemolytic uremic syndrome, or HUS. This is because the toxin (which inhibits protein synthesis) can also bind to the glomerular epithelial cells. Also, because this toxin is Shiga-like, it is important to remember that *Shigella* can also lead to HUS.

26. **Answer: A.** The causal agent is *Streptococcus pneumoniae*. It is a gram-positive coccus, which is alpha hemolytic and optochin-sensitive, and it is the most common cause of pneumonia in the elderly. It is the capsule of *S. pneumoniae* which protects it against phagocytosis. That is why asplenic individuals have a difficult time clearing infections with *S. pneumoniae*, because a major antibody-producing organ is missing and phagocytosis is inhibited in organisms with capsules. Coagulase (**choice C**) is an anti-phagocytic attribute of *Staphylococcus aureus*. M protein (**choice D**) of *Streptococcus pyogenes* is anti-phagocytic. Catalase (**choice B**) breaks down H₂O₂, and teichoic acids (**choice E**) mediate adherence. Neither protects against phagocytosis.

27. **Answer: B.** The causal agent *E. coli* is gram-negative, and the primary means of developing septic shock with gram-negative organisms is via lipopolysaccharide (endotoxin).

28. **Answer: C.** The causal agent is *Rickettsia rickettsiae*, the disease is Rocky Mountain spotted fever. The clues are North Carolina (located in the tick belt of U.S.), rash that spread from extremities to trunk, conjunctivitis, and proteinuria. Rocky Mountain spotted fever is spread via a tick vector.

29. **Answer: B.** The case diagnosis is poststreptococcal glomerulonephritis caused by group A strep. The Lancefield group is determined by the C carbohydrate and the serotype is determined via the M proteins. This is particularly important in post streptococcal glomerulonephritis, as certain strains, such as the M12 serotype, are more commonly associated with this type of nonsuppurative sequela.

30. **Answer: B.** The causal agent is *Bordetella pertussis*. The clues are severe cough, can't catch breath, vomiting, incomplete vaccination history, conjunctival redness, and gram-negative coccobacilli on Bordet-Gengou medium. Pertussis toxin works by ADP ribosylation of G_i. ADP ribosylation of elongation factor 2 (**choice A**) describes toxins found in *Corynebacterium diphtheriae* and *Pseudomonas aeruginosa*. ADP ribosylation of a GTP-binding protein (**choice C**) describes the toxins found in ETEC and *Vibrio cholerae*. Blocks release of acetylcholine (**choice D**) describes the toxin found in *Clostridium botulinum*. Blocks release of inhibitory transmitters GABA and glycine (**choice E**) describes the toxin found in *Clostridium tetani*.

31. **Answer: D.** The toxin described is tetanus toxin, which would be acquired via some type of penetrating wound. Eating home-canned foods (**choice A**) describes transmission of adult botulism. Fecal-oral, travel to foreign country (**choice B**) describes ETEC, *Vibrio cholerae*, etc. Infant given honey during the first year of life (**choice C**) describes infant botulism. Respiratory, with incomplete vaccination history (**choice E**) describes *Bordetella pertussis*, for example.

32. **Answer: D.** The diagnosis is infant botulism caused by *Clostridium botulinum*. The clues are flaccid paralysis, constipation, difficulty breathing, tox screen of stool, and age. The flaccid paralysis is due to a toxin that blocks the release of acetylcholine. ADP ribosylation of eukaryotic elongation factor 2 (eEF-2; **choice A**) describes toxins found in *Corynebacterium diphtheriae* and *Pseudomonas aeruginosa*. ADP ribosylation of G_i, an inhibitory subunit of the G protein (**choice B**), describes *Bordetella pertussis*. ADP ribosylation of GTP-binding protein (**choice C**) describes the toxins found in ETEC and *Vibrio cholerae*. Blocks release of inhibitory transmitters GABA and glycine (**choice E**) describes the toxin found in *Clostridium tetani*.

33. **Answer: C.** The causal agent is *Corynebacterium diphtheriae*. The clues are incomplete vaccination history and (dirty gray pseudomembrane which causes bleeding when displaced). *C. diphtheriae* are gram-positive rods, and the toxin functions by inhibition of protein synthesis.

34. **Answer: A.** The causal agent is *Vibrio cholerae*. The clues are history of travel and voluminous "rice water" diarrhea. *Vibrio* are gram-negative curved rods, and the toxin functions by increasing intracellular cAMP.

35. **Answer: A.** The causal agent is *Helicobacter pylori*. The clues are midepigastric pain, relief after meals, positive urease test. *H. pylori* is a gram-negative curved rod that is microaerophilic. Gram-negative rod, aerobic (**choice B**) describes *Pseudomonas aeruginosa*, for example. Gram-negative rod, facultative anaerobe (**choice C**) describes *Escherichia coli*, for example. Gram-positive rod, aerobic (**choice D**) describes *Bacillus*, for example. Gram-positive rod, microaerophilic (**choice E**) does not describe a medically relevant genus.

36. **Answer: B.** The causal agent is *Streptococcus pyogenes*. The clues: sore throat, beta hemolytic, gram-positive cocci. To answer this question, you have to know that the agent is gram-positive and that gram-positive organisms have a thick peptidoglycan layer that protects them from osmotic damage. Lipopolysaccharide (**choice A**) is only found on gram-negative organisms and is associated with shock. Phospholipids (**choice C**) are found in the membranes of gram-positive and gram-negative organisms. Polysaccharide (**choice D**) can be found on gram-positive and gram-negative organisms. Teichoic acid (**choice E**) is only found on gram-positives and is used for attachment.

37. **Answer: E.** *Escherichia coli* is the most common cause of cystitis overall and should be assumed to be the cause of any case of cystitis unless contrary culture characteristics are described. It generally reduces nitrates and is also a lactose fermenter. **Choice A** identifies *Neisseria gonorrhoeae*; **choice B**, *Staphylococcus saprophyticus*; **choice C**, *Streptococcus viridans*; **choice D**, *Clostridium*.

38. **Answer: D.** This case history describes botulism (key words: home-canned green beans and visual problems). Foods classically associated are those with a neutral or alkaline pH. *C. botulinum,* the agent of botulism, is an anaerobe and thus has a low oxidation-reduction requirement. **Choice A,** *Staph aureus*; **choice B,** *Bacillus cereus*; **choice C,** *S. viridans*; **choice D,** *C. botulinum*; **choice E,** *E. coli.*

39. **Answer: A.** The disease is most likely *Mycoplasma* pneumonia caused by *Mycoplasma pneumoniae*, which is non-Gram staining and requires cholesterol for growth. **Choice B,** *C. diphtheriae*; **choice C,** *Streptococcus pyogenes*; **choice D,** *Staph aureus*; **choice E,** *Clostridium.*

40. **Answer: C.** The causal agent is *Listeria monocytogenes*. The clues are neonatal meningitis (age), gram-positive rods. The only organism in the list that is a gram-positive rod is *Listeria*. *Escherichia coli* (**choice A**) is a gram-negative rod. *Haemophilus influenzae* (**choice B**) is a gram-negative coccobacillus. *Neisseria meningitidis* (**choice D**) is a gram-negative diplococcus. *Streptococcus agalactiae* (**choice E**) is a gram-positive coccus.

41. **Answer: A.** The agent is viridans streptococcus. The clues are heart valve replacement, gram-positive cocci, alpha hemolytic, and optochin resistant. *Pseudomonas aeruginosa* and *Serratia marcescens* (**choices B and C**) are gram-negative rods. *Staphylococcus aureus* (**choice D**) is a catalase-positive, gram-positive coccus. *Streptococcus pneumoniae* (**choice E**) is a gram-positive, catalase-negative coccus, but it is optochin-sensitive.

42. **Answer: A.** The clues are abscess, polymicrobial, gram-negative anaerobe. *Bacteroides* is the only anaerobe listed.

43. **Answer: D.** The causal agent is *Mycobacterium tuberculosis*. The clues are coughing up blood, acid-fast bacilli, and homeless. Sulfatides are sulfolipids which hydrolyze to form sulfuric acid. The acidic pH of the *M. tuberculosis*-containing phagosome acts to stop lysosomal fusion. Cord factor (**choice A**) is responsible for serpentine growth in vitro. Calcium dipicolinate (**choice B**) is a component of endospores. Peptidoglycan (**choice C**) is a cell wall component. Tuberculin (**choice E**) is a surface protein, which is not involved in protection from phagosome-lysosome fusion.

44. **Answer: A.** The causal agent is *Gardnerella vaginalis*. The clues are malodorous discharge, positive whiff test, thin gray discharge. Gram-negative diplococci in PMNs (**choice B**) is consistent with *Neisseria gonorrhoeae*. Koilocytic cells (**choice C**) is consistent with human papilloma virus. Owl-eye inclusions (**choice D**) are consistent with cytomegalovirus. Tzanck smears (**choice E**) are diagnostic for herpes simplex virus.

45. **Answer: E.** The causal agent is *Bacillus anthracis*. The clues are postal workers, hemoptysis and mediastinal widening. Elementary body and reticulate body (**choices A and D**) are consistent with *Chlamydia*. Endotoxin and periplasmic space (**choices B and C**) are consistent with gram-negative bacteria.

46. **Answer: C.** The clues are fist fight wound, gram-negative rods with bleach-like odor.

47. **Answer: E.** The causal agent is *Proteus vulgaris*. The clues are lower back pain (kidney stones), gram-negative rods, lactose nonfermenter, UTI. Capsules (**choice A**) are antiphagocytic, and *Proteus* does not have a capsule. Catalase (**choice B**) is produced by *Proteus*, but is not a major mechanism of pathogenesis. Coagulase (**choice C**) is produced by *Staphylococcus aureus*. Exotoxins (**choice D**) are secreted toxins.

48. **Answer: A.** The causal agent is *Clostridium difficile*. The clues are clindamycin, loose, mucoid, stools, yellow plaques. Clindamycin and other broad-spectrum antibiotics are associated with pseudomembranous colitis, as they kill off the normal gut flora and *C. difficile* flourishes without competition.

49. **Answer: A.** The patient has inclusion conjunctivitis caused by *Chlamydia trachomatis*. The only form of this bacterium that has the ability to bind to the membranes and infect is the elementary body.

50. **Answer: A.** The causal agent is *Klebsiella pneumoniae*. The clues are gelatinous and bloody sputum, PMNs, and gram-negative rods identified in the sputum. The most likely patient to present with *K. pneumoniae* would be elderly with a preexisting condition, like chronic obstructive pulmonary disease, or an alcoholic.

51. **Answer: D.** Group B *Streptococcus* (GBS) is the most common cause of neonatal meningitis, followed by *E. coli*. *S. pneumoniae* is most common in adults.

52. **Answer: A.** The clues are elderly, catheter, gram-positive cocci, catalase-negative, growth in 6.5% sodium chloride. *Staphylococcus aureus* and *Staphylococcus epidermidis* (**choices B and C**) are catalase-positive. *Streptococcus pyogenes* and viridans streptococci (**choices D and E**) would not grow in a high concentration of salt.

53. **Answer: D.** The clues are immunosuppressed (HIV+), necrotic lesion with black center and erythematous margin (ecthyma gangrenosum). *Bacillus anthracis* (**choice A**) is close because a black eschar can resemble ecthyma gangrenosum, but it usually would appear at the point of contact (probably not on the buttock). *Clostridium perfringens, Enterococcus faecalis,* and *Staphylococcus aureus* (**choices B, C,** and **E**) do not fit the case description.

54. **Answer: B.** The causal agent is *Streptococcus pyogenes*; the disease is scarlet fever. The clues are sore throat for 1 week, rash, red tongue (strawberry tongue). Gram-positive coccus, alpha hemolytic, catalase-negative (**choice A**) is descriptive of *Streptococcus pneumoniae*. Gram-positive coccus, alpha hemolytic, catalase-positive (**choice C**) does not describe an important medical pathogen. Gram-positive coccus, beta hemolytic, catalase positive (**choice D**) is descriptive of *Staphylococcus aureus*. Gram-positive coccus, gamma hemolytic, catalase negative (**choice E**) is descriptive of some strains of *Enterococcus*.

55. **Answer: D.** The causal agent is *Helicobacter pylori*. The clues are ulcer, urease positive, gram-negative curved rod. It is important to know all organisms that are associated with an increased risk of developing cancer.

56. **Answer: D.** The most likely causal agent here is a bacterium. Viral meningitis is usually mild and would not fit the CSF values. Both the age of the patient and the petechial rash suggest it is most likely to be *Neisseria meningitidis*, which is a Gram-negative diplococcus that is oxidase-positive. The overproduction of outer-membrane fragments is what leads to the petechial rash, even prior to antibiotic treatment.

57. **Answer: E.** Transposition or transpositional recombination is a form of site-specific recombination and is largely responsible for the creation of multiple drug resistant plasmids. Chromosomal drug resistance may arise by movement of a plasmid gene to the chromosome, but it is usually just a solitary gene and not a repetitive event. The Hfr chromosome arises through a single site-specific integration of a fertility factor with the bacterial chromosome.

58. **Answer: D.** This question is asking what carries the genetic code for diphtheria toxin, which must be some kind of DNA, which in turn means that the protein eEF-2 can be immediately eliminated. The diphthamide on eEF-2 is actually the substrate for the ADP-ribosylation done by the diphtheria toxin. Genes expressing the diphtheria toxin originally enter *C. diphtheriae* as part of the DNA of the temperate corynephage. Integration of this temperate phage results in a stable prophage, which directs the production of the diphtheria toxin.

59. **Answer: C.** Site-specific recombination of phage DNA into bacterial cell DNA by the process of lysogeny creates a prophage. The *recA* gene product (**choice A**) is necessary for homologous recombination with an exogenote but does not create a prophage. A virulent bacteriophage (**choice B**) causes lysis of the host cell and not the production of prophage. The lambda phage, (**choice D**), is a temperate phage, which can cause lysogeny of infected cells, but the lambda repressor is necessary in such cases to prevent the lytic life cycle. **Choice E** might be the pathway a prophage could choose to reinitiate its lytic lifestyle, but it would not be a means to create a prophage.

60. **Answer: E.** This hypothetical condition describes the mixing of one Hfr cell with 100 F⁻ recipients. Over time, with no cell division occurring, the one Hfr cell would repeatedly conjugate with the F⁻ cells and transfer one strand of its chromosomal DNA in sequence, beginning with oriT and theoretically ending with the tra genes. The most frequently transferred

bacterial genes also have the greatest likelihood of successful recombination; they are those closest to oriT; in this example, the A allele. The entire chromosome is so large that it is virtually never transferred in its entirety and thus, the tra genes would not be transferred. (Even if tra genes were transferred, oriT and tra genes have no homologous regions in the recipient cell chromosome and so would not successfully recombine within.) Thus, the recipient cell acquires only new chromosomal alleles and NOT the whole fertility factor and never changes phenotype to become an Hfr cell. Therefore, any of the answers with cell one (the Hfr parent) as the dominant type would be wrong.

The genes are transferred in linear order, so allele A will always be transferred more frequently than any of the later genes.

Therefore, given sufficient time for conjugation, the cell type that would be most numerous is that of the recipient genotype with a newly acquired allele close to oriT. This means that the best answer is choice F: cell two with a new A gene. The farther from oriT that the allele is, the less likely that it will be successfully transferred. The distractor, choice C, with all 4 alleles transferred in, is less likely.

61. **Answer: A.** The F⁺ cell would contain both the bacterial chromosome and the fertility factor. The other two would just each have the bacterial chromosome (F⁻) or the single DNA molecule of the chromosome with the integrated fertility factor.

62. **Answer: C.** Only F⁺ and Hfr can donate genes to a recipient or F⁻ cell. The F⁺ cell would transfer only plasmid genes. The Hfr would be the only one likely to transfer chromosomal genes.

63. **Answer: F.** In transformation, free DNA from lysed cells is not protected from the environment either by a cell or by a phage coat, but is instead naked and therefore subject to nucleases.

64. **Answer: C.** The DNA is transferred in as a linear piece and must be stabilized by homologous recombination.

65. **Answer: F.** The statement fits the definition of competency required for transformation.

66. **Answer: B.** This is generalized transduction, but what are your clues? First, it says "one phage" rather than all the phage in the cell (as for specialized). Then it also says plasmid DNA could be picked up. For specialized transduction, only episomal plasmid DNA (incorporated into the bacterial chromosome near an attachment site) or chromosomal DNA could be picked up. Finally, it mentions a lytic virus lifecycle. Lytic viruses are only capable of generalized transduction.

67. **Answer: D.** Transpositional movement actually involves a type of recombination called transposition that is a form of site-specific recombination. Site-specific recombination is also involved in integration of a temperate bacteriophage. Both transformation and transduction require homologous recombination as would transfer of Hfr DNA by conjugation. But either F factor or R factor DNA circularizes when it enters a new cell and thus is

stable without recombination since circular DNA is not subject to cellular exonucleases.

68. **Answer: A.** Choice D is a definition of lysogeny but lysogenic conversion is when lysogeny changes the characteristic of the lysogenized organism. In medicine this usually means an increased pathogenicity from the process.

69. **Answer: B.** Choice A would require phage infection with a temperate corynephage. Choice C is most likely to take place through a conjugal transfer. Choice D might occur by specialized transduction.

70. **Answer: D.** Multiple drug resistance is almost always plasmid-mediated, which rules out choices A, B, and E. Transposition is moving a piece of DNA to another molecule of DNA within the cell.

71. **Answer: C.** This is the classic description of a bacteriostatic agent.

72. **Answer: E.** The Kirby-Bauer agar disk diffusion test is a means to compare the functions of several antibiotics against one bacterial isolate. In a general sense, bacteria will be inhibited from growing in close proximity to any disk of antibiotic to which they are sensitive, so the larger the zone of inhibited growth around the filter paper disk, the more sensitive the bacteria are to that drug. Comparison between the disks cannot be accomplished without the key which comes with the kit, however, since the company which prepared the kit has done the clinical trials which correlate the in vitro results with those in human patients.

73. **Answer: E.** The MIC (Minimal Inhibitory Concentration) is the most dilute amount of drug in which no growth of a bacterial isolate will occur. The MBC (Minimal Bactericidal Concentration) of a drug is the most dilute amount of a drug in which there will be no colonial growth after the drug is removed. In some cases the MBC may be equal to the MIC, but the amount of drug necessary to kill all bacteria is never less than the amount required to inhibit their growth temporarily.

74. **Answer: E.** The disease is viral pharyngoconjunctivitis, caused by adenovirus, which is very commonly contracted through swimming pools. (Adenovirus is a naked virus and chlorination of pools does not inactivate it.) Hiking in a heavily wooded area (**choice A**) could be associated with a vector-borne disease, such as Rocky Mountain spotted fever. Eating undercooked shellfish (**choice B**) could be associated with hepatitis A or *Vibrio parahaemolyticus*, for example. Playing with toys in a day care center (**choice C**) and traveling to a developing country (**choice D**) both could begin the infection of a long list of agents.

75. **Answer: D.** The presence of hepatitis B surface antigen and the absence of the surface antibody (anti-HBs) indicate either an acute HBV infection (if patient has had the disease for only a short time) or a chronic carrier state (if the hepatitis has been going on for at least 6 months). Because acute HBV is not a choice, **choice D** then becomes the correct answer. **Choice B** would be a right answer if HBsAg had been negative and HBsAb positive. Core antibodies would not be present if the person is only vaccinated (**choice C**). Also, HBsAg should not be present in a detectable amount

from vaccination. HBeAg and HBeAb are correlated to how contagious the patient might be, and these serologic results were not given (**choice A**).

76. **Answer: A.** The clues are lacy body rash preceded by a facial rash in a school aged child with fever. HHV-6 (**choice B**) is the causal agent of roseola, which is fever, followed by a lacy body rash in infants. Measles (**choice C**) is identified by cough, coryza, and conjunctivitis with photophobia, Koplik spots, and an exanthematous rash beginning below the ears then spreading to the trunk and extremities. Rubella (**choice D**) is the causal agent of German measles, which involves a rash beginning at the forehead and spreading down.

77. **Answer: C.** The *pol* gene codes for reverse transcriptase, integrase, and protease. Reverse transcriptase creates the provirus and integrase allows the proviral DNA to be integrated, apparently at a random site, into a chromosome in the host cell. Of the distractors, both **choices A and B** are accomplished using the host cell's RNA polymerase. **Choice D** is a function of the *gag* gene, and **choice E** is controlled by *tat* and *rev* genes.

78. **Answer: A.** The presence of HBsAg, HBcAb, and HBeAg are all indicators of an acute infection at 2 months postexposure. It is too early to identify a chronic infection (**choice B**), but the presence of HBsAg after 6 months is the main indication of a chronic infection. With a fulminant infection (**choice C**), the patient's symptoms are usually much more serious, likely a superinfection with hepatitis D or the delta agent. If he were immune (**choice D**), he would have had HBsAb in his serum. Since he has hepatitis B viral antigens in his blood, **choice E** is wrong.

79. **Answer: D.** The inmate is immune, as he has a complete complement of anti-viral antibodies.

80. **Answer: B.** This patient has herpes simplex encephalitis, whch typically affects the temporal lobes. California encephalitis (**choice A**) affects older children in the middle and northwestern U.S. The polio virus (**choice C**) causes a flaccid paralysis with no sensory loss, and does not occur in the United States. St. Louis encephalitis (**choice D**) and the West Nile virus (**choice E**) usually affect older individuals.

81. **Answer: B.** The clues are transplant patient with interstitial pneumonia; CMV is the most common cause. Adenovirus (**choice A**) is associated with conjunctivitis and acute respiratory disease in military recruits, among other diseases. Although influenza (**choice C**) can cause pneumonia, there is no mention of season, and CMV is still the most common cause in transplant patients. Respiratory syncytial virus (**choice D**) is usually seen in children (especially premature infants), and rhinovirus (**choice E**) causes the common cold.

82. **Answer: A.** Polio is caused by the poliovirus. The clues are flaccid paralysis and India, and polio is transmitted by the fecal-oral route.

83. **Answer: B.** The clinical presentation is consistent with chickenpox caused by VZV. Exanthem subitum is caused by human herpes virus 6, not by CMV. Herpetic gingivostomatitis refers to herpes simplex type 1, not VZV. Infectious mononucleosis is a lymphadenopathy and herpetic whitlow is a painful herpes infection of the nail bed.

84. **Answer: E.** The only nucleic acid in the composite parental virus is the RNA belonging to poliovirus. Thus, only poliovirus is made. The only role the Coxsackie virus would play in the infection is to bind to the host cell and stimulate the uptake of the composite virus. Once uncoating takes place, the Coxsackie components play no further role. A perfect poliovirus will have been made. The progeny will have the host-cell range of polio (**choice A**) because that is what they'll be. There is no genetic material coding for the Coxsackie components, so you cannot get a composite (**choice B**). No capsid components of Coxsackie will be made; there can be no mixing (**choice C**). There was only one type of RNA; there can never be recombination (**choice D**). Sabin is a polio-specific vaccine, and poliovirus will be produced.

85. **Answer: E.** A common cause of gastroenteritis on cruise ships is the Norovirus. Norovirus is a member of the Caliciviridae family and is a nonenveloped RNA virus. Acid-fast oocysts (**choice A**) refer to persistent diarrhea caused by *Cryptosporidium parvum* or *Isospora belli*, usually seen in AIDS patients. Enveloped DNA and RNA viruses (**choices B and C**) cannot be transmitted via the fecal-oral route or live in the gastrointestinal tract because of the instability of the envelope. A nonenveloped DNA virus (**choice D**) would be consistent with adenoviral gastroenteritis, which is not the most likely cause of cruise ship gastroenteritis.

86. **Answer: B.** Gp120 is the surface antigen of HIV that mediates its attachment to CD4 lymphocytes. Gp41 is a transmembrane glycoprotein, and p24, p17, and nucleocapsid protein are all internal molecules, which would rarely be accessible to the immune response.

87. **Answer: E.** This patient has rabies, which exhibits these neurologic symptoms. In the eastern United States, the primary reservoir is raccoons.

88. **Answer: E.** An infant with difficulty breathing, wheezing, and giant multinucleated cells (syncytia) is likely to have respiratory syncytial virus. B19 (**choice A**) and influenza (**choice B**) would not show giant multinucleated cells, and B19 does not usually cause breathing difficulty. Parainfluenza (**choice C**) causes croup, which exhibits the swelling of the larynx and the seal-like barking cough. There is no mention of rash or Koplik spots, which would indicate the measles (**choice D**).

89. **Answer: E.** The virus is HSV 2, a herpesvirus, which is a dsDNA virus that uses the mechanisms of our own cells to transcribe an RNA strand from its genomic DNA and use the transcribed RNA as a messenger RNA. Of the distractors: **choice A** is the technique used by the negative-sense RNA viruses; **choice B** is used by the positive-sense RNA viruses; **choice C** is used by the retroviruses; **choice D** is used during the genomic duplication of positive sense RNA viruses; **choice F** would not produce RNA; and **choice G** is used in genomic replication by most DNA viruses.

90. **Answer: C.** The disease is mumps. The complication often seen in adult males is orchitis, which can lead to sterility.

91. **Answer: A.** CMV is an extremely common virus and crosses the placenta oftentimes without causing obvious symptoms. Fortunately, rubella, which is highly teratogenic particularly in early pregnancy, is generally prevented

by routine vaccination in childhood or at least 16 weeks prior to pregnancy. A small percentage of hepatitis B infections may occur in utero. HSV 2 will only cross the placenta if the mother acquires herpes for the first time during her pregnancy. RSV and other respiratory viruses will not. Other viruses that can cross the placenta include coxsackie B, HIV, and B19.

92. **Answer: D.** Cytomegalovirus, hepadnavirus, and poxvirus are all dsDNA viruses and not RNA. Retrovirus is an RNA virus but replicates through a dsDNA, so it also is not the correct answer. Toga is a positive RNA virus that replicates through a negative RNA intermediate and has no DNA; therefore, it's the correct answer.

93. **Answer: D.** The monospot is the most commonly used test for the diagnosis of infectious mononucleosis caused by EBV. However, it does not detect EBV-specific antibody. It instead detects heterophile antibody, which is non-specific in that it may be present in different organisms and individuals and it cross-reacts with many animal RBCs. Epstein-Barr nuclear antigen test is not routinely run in the diagnosis of mononucleosis. Atypical lymphocytes are found in mononucleosis caused by EBV and CMV, but CMV is heterophile antibody–negative. Isolation of EBV is cumbersome and laborious, and would not distinguish previous infections from current active ones.

94. **Answer: D.** The segmented influenza viruses may undergo recombination with a similar animal virus. This leads to drastic genetic change and pandemics result from the fact that there is no underlying "herd immunity" to the new viral entity.

95. **Answer: C.** HIV. It is this genetic drift that makes it difficult for the body to fight off HIV and has complicated the development of an effective vaccine. Genetic drift is due to minor mutational change, and is possible with any organism but best described in HIV.

96. **Answer: D.** Both the symptomology, length of infection, and the epidemiological clues (college student, age 19, has given it to his girlfriend) strongly suggest that this is EBV, which is a herpesvirus.

    Choice A = parvo; **choice B** = adeno, papilloma, polyoma; **choice C** = pox; **choice D** = herpes/hepadna because there's no distinction as to circular or partial dsDNA; **choice E** = reovirus; **choice F** = arena, bunya, and orthomyxo; **choice G** = rabies; **choice H** = none; **choice I** = calici, hepe, or picorna; **choice J** = flavi and toga; **choice K** = retro.

97. **Answer: F.** The description fits congenital rubella, a togavirus, which is an enveloped positive-sense RNA virus that is not segmented.

98. **Answer: D.** If you have any trouble, think about which of these viruses has respiratory symptoms (in this case, pneumonia).

99. **Answer: C.** Remember that type 4 strains cause common warts, and these are largely transmitted by fomites or direct contact.

100. **Answer: C.** This describes the typical presentation of molluscum contagiosum, which is commonly acquired through small breaks in the skin in environments where moisture keeps the virus viable (swimming pools, showers).

101. **Answer: B.** CMV is the most common viral cause of death in bone-marrow transplant patients, causing an interstitial pneumonia.

102. **Answer: D.** Perinatal infection with human papilloma virus can cause infantile laryngeal warts.

103. **Answer: B.** Cutaneous candidiasis is a problem in skin folds of obese individuals. It is an even greater problem in diabetic patients because of the high sugar levels. Only the members of the genus *Candida* would produce a creamy surface growth. The erythematous base is due to the production of a cytotoxin. *Aspergillus, Epidermophyton,* and *Microsporum* are all monomorphic filamentous fungi and would not fit the description. *Sporothrix* is found as cigar-shaped budding yeasts but would not clinically present like this. It is traumatically implanted to start subcutaneous infections.

104. **Answer: E.** The causal agent is *Coccidioides immitis.* The clues are southwest U.S., migrant worker (works outside), erythematous skin rash (erythema nodosum). The diagnostic form of *C. immitis* in the sputum is a spherule. Broad-based budding yeast (**choice A**) describes *Blastomyces dermatitidis.* Monomorphic encapsulated yeast (**choice B**) describes *Cryptococcus neoformans.* Nonseptate hyphae with broad angles (**choice C**) describes *Mucor* species. Septate hyphae dichotomously branching at acute angles (**choice D**) describes *Aspergillus fumigatus.*

105. **Answer: C.** The clues here are the geography, weight loss, granulomatous inflammation, and macrophages engorged with oval structures (RES disease). The colonial appearance and tuberculate spores strongly suggest the causal agent to be *Histoplasma capsulatum. Histoplasma* is acquired from dusty environments containing bird (most often chicken or starling) or bat feces. The areas of highest endemicity are in the great central river beds with bat caves, chicken coops, and starling roosts having extremely high levels.

106. **Answer: D.** The causal agent is *Blastomyces dermatitidis.* The clues are southeastern U.S. and a sputum smear revealing thick-walled, refractile, double-contoured yeast cells (another way to say broad-based budding). Remember that the name of the organism contains the site of dissemination.

107. **Answer: A.** The clues are immunocompromised, myocardial infarction, and septate acutely branching hyphae in nearly every tissue. Remember, *Aspergillus* is extremely invasive in immunocompromised individuals.

108. **Answer: D.** The causal agent is *Cryptococcus neoformans.* The clues are HIV, headache and blurred vision, encapsulated organisms in CSF. *C. neoformans* is the number one cause of meningitis in AIDS patients. You should know that it is monomorphic. "Spaghetti and meatballs" KOH (**choice A**) describes *Malassezia furfur.* Branching septate hyphae (**choice B**) describes *Aspergillus.* Mycelial form at room temperature and a yeast at 37°C (**choice C**) describes all of the dimorphic fungi. Nonencapsulated dimorphic yeast that reproduces by budding (**choice E**) describes *Blastomyces.*

109. **Answer: D.** The clues are AIDS patient and atypical pneumonia. *Pneumocystis jirovecii* is the hallmark atypical pneumonia of AIDS.

110. **Answer: C.** This patient is suffering from *Plasmodium falciparum* malaria acquired shortly before her departure from Kenya. Liver stages of *Plasmodium* are not susceptible to chloroquine killing. Because she did not continue the prophylaxis after her return to the States, those parasites were allowed to initiate all of the erythrocytic stages of the life cycle. Any erythrocytic stages generated out of the liver phase of the life cycle while she remained on prophylaxis would have been killed. Thus, the late onset of her symptoms was due to survival of exoerythrocytic stages that had not yet left the liver at the time she ceased prophylaxis. Hypnozoites (**choice A**) are responsible for relapse of symptoms in *P. vivax* and *P. ovale* malarias, but do not exist in *P. falciparum*, and it is clear that she has *falciparum* malaria due to the delicate ring forms multiply infecting erythrocytes and the sausage-shaped gametocytes. Sporozoites (**choice B**) are the infectious forms injected by mosquitoes and would not have been available in this country to initiate the symptoms on the time course described. Erythrocytic schizonts and merozoites (**choices D and E**) would have been killed by prophylaxis before she left Africa and could not be responsible for the late onset of symptoms.

111. **Answer: D.** This child has the typical symptoms of hookworm disease, caused in this country usually by *Necator americanus*. The infection is acquired by penetration of the filariform larvae through the skin of the feet or buttocks, after contamination of soil with the eggs of the agent deposited in human feces. Of the other distractors, **choice A** would be most likely if the infection were due to ascarids, pinworms, or whipworms. **Choice C** would describe infection with either *Taenia* or *Trichinella*, and **choice E** would be the means of infection with *Plasmodium*.

112. **Answer: E.** The described infection could be *Cryptosporidium*, *Isospora*, *Microsporidia*, or *Cyclospora*, which are very difficult infections in AIDS patients even though they are self-resolving in normal noncompromised individuals. In AIDS patients they are most commonly unrelenting, even with treatment. They are usually acquired from water. *Toxoplasma* (**choice D**) is from cats.

113. **Answer: D.** The positive IgM titer arising in the eighth month means that this woman has become acutely infected with *Toxoplasma*. Infections acquired at this time have a high likelihood of infecting the fetus and are most likely to be manifested by the development of retinochoroiditis. A mother can transmit this parasite to her fetus only during an acute infection; therefore, all future fetuses will be protected from the disease (**choice A**). Because IgG antibodies cross the placenta (**choice B**), presence of the anti-*Toxoplasma* antibodies of this class in the neonate may simply reflect the infection of the mother—only a positive IgM response in the neonate is proof of the child's infection, which should therefore be treated. There is no way to reverse major organ damage (**choice E**) when it occurs in utero, but it would not be expected to occur with an acute infection beginning in the third trimester.

114. **Answer: F.** *Leishmania* spp. are transmitted by the bite of sandflies. They cannot be transmitted from person to person by trivial means, so unless organ transplantation is occurring in the barracks, direct human contact (**choice E**) is not a possibility. To survive outside the human host, they must be in the vector (sandfly), so transmission by food or water (**choices A or D**) is not possible. Of the distractors that involve true vectors: *Anopheles*

mosquitoes (**choice B**) transmit malaria; reduviid bugs (**choice C**) transfer American trypanosomiasis (Chagas disease); and tsetse flies (**choice G**) transmit African trypanosomiasis (sleeping sickness).

115. **Answer: C.** *Giardia* is common in mountain streams throughout the U.S., and the presentation of prolonged fatty diarrhea and weight loss is pathognomonic. It causes its pathology by its adherence to the mucosa of the upper small intestine with its ventral sucking disc. No toxic metabolites or lytic enzymes are involved in the pathology, which apparently results from blockage of normal fat digestion. The organism is a flagellate, and thus has flagella, but migration into extraintestinal sites is not a well known problem associated with pathology. And although the organism does encyst as it passes along the intestine, this is not known to produce symptoms.

116. **Answer: B.** The clues are bloody diarrhea, fever, bacterial cultures negative, organisms with RBCs inside them. *Cryptosporidium parvum* (**choice A**) is typically found in AIDS patients. *Giardia lamblia* (**choice C**) is associated with fatty, foul smelling diarrhea. *Toxoplasma gondii* (**choice D**) would likely cause a flu-like illness in this age group if acquired as primary infection; if acquired in utero, might cause blindness later in life. You can rule out *Shigella dysenteriae* (**choice E**), because bacterial cultures were negative.

117. **Answer: C.** The clues are Egypt, blood in urine, eggs with terminal spines, working in rice field (indicates his possible exposure to contaminated water). Also, be aware that in Africa, *S. haematobium* is associated with bladder cancer. *Entamoeba histolytica* (**choice A**) would cause bloody stool, not urine. *Fasciolopsis buski* (**choice B**) is the intestinal fluke; eggs do not have terminal spines. *S. japonicum* and *S. mansoni* (**choices D** and **E**) are intestinal schistosomes and would not cause blood in urine; the egg for *S. mansoni* has a subterminal spine, whereas the egg for *S. japonicum* is fat and oval with one tiny lateral spine.

118. **Answer: D.** The clues are frothy, yellow discharge, itching, organisms identified on wet mount, bacterial cultures were negative. With *Candida albicans* (**choice A**), the discharge would have been white and creamy. *Trichophyton* (**choice B**) causes skin, hair, and nail infections and is a cutaneous fungus. *Chlamydia trachomatis* (**choice C**) would not be visible on wet mount and causes intracellular infection of epithelial cells. *Giardia lamblia* (**choice E**) is associated with diarrhea.

119. **Answer: B.** The clues are missionary, high fever, chills, Africa, multiple ring structures, and crescent-shaped gametes. *Leishmania* (**choice A**) produces amastigotes inside phagocytic cells and causes either visceral, cutaneous, or mucocutaneous pathology. *Plasmodium malariae* (**choice C**) clues might include bar and band forms in RBCs, and 72 hour fever spikes. In *P. ovale* and *P. vivax* (**choices D** and **E**) there will be Schüffner dots in RBCs.

120. **Answer: D.** The clues are perianal itching, irritable during the day, not sleeping at night, eggs with flattened side, and Scotch tape test.

121. **Answer: E.** The clues are tropical country, prolapsed rectum, worms resembling whips, barrel shaped eggs with bipolar plugs. The common name for *Trichuris* is whipworm.

Index

A

A-B component toxins, 222
Abbreviations for infectious diseases, 373
A-B component toxins, 196
Abdominal pain, 252
ABO blood groups, 92, 94, 118
Abortive viral infections, 299
Absidia sp., 355–356
Acanthamoeba sp., 357, 360
Accelerated acute graft rejection, 124
Acetylcholine, 118, 218
Acid alcohol stain reagent, 201
Acid fast organisms, 201, 391
Acinetobacter baumannii, 233
Actinobacillus actinomycetemcomitans, 240
Actinomyces israelii, 223
Actinomyces sp., 201, 214
Actinomycosis, 223
Active immunity, 100–101
Acute abdominal pain, 384
Acute endocarditis, 378
Acute glomerulonephritis, 195, 209
Acute graft rejection, 124
Acute hepatitis B, 304
Acute infection response timeline, 5
Acute inflammatory response, 37–42
Acute lymphoblastic leukemia, 19
Acute otitis media, 376
Acute pneumonia, 379
Acute pulmonary fungal infections, 350, 351, 353
Acute respiratory disease (ARD), 311
Acute respiratory distress (ARD), 325, 342, 379
Acute rheumatic fever, 118
Acute septicemia, 237
Acute viral gastroenteritis, 321
Acyclovir, 314
adaptive. *See* adaptive immunity
Adaptive immunity, 3–4, 4, 6, 31, 35
 autoimmune responses, 4, 22, 22–23, 25
 complement cascade, 74
 effector mechanisms, 62
 lymphoid white blood cells, 11
ADCC (antibody dependent cellular cytotoxicity), 33, 72, 73, 76, 83
Adenovirus, 102, 294, 306, 311
Adherence of pathogens, 194
Adhesins, 194

Aerobic bacteria, 201, 393
Aeromonas spp., 249
Affinity, 21, 22, 25, 67, 72, 100
Agars, , 239
Age groups
 viral infection risk, 300
Age groups affected, 299, 382–383
Agglutination assays
 ABO blood groups, 92, 94
 fungal antigen detection, 347
 positive cold agglutinins, 355, 265
 zone of equivalence, 89–90
AIDS, 328, 331, 344
Albinism, 109
Allelic exclusion, 20
Allergens, 63, 75, 115–116, 117, 349
Allergic bronchopulmonary aspergillosis, 354
Allergic rhinitis, 117
Allogeneic grafts, 123
Allotypes of antibodies, 86
Alphaviruses, 296
Amastigotes, 363
Amebae, 357, 360
Aminoglycoside resistance, 284, 285, 286
Ampicillin resistance, 284, 285
Anaerobic bacteria, 201, 393
Anaplasma phagocytophila, 263
Ancylostoma braziliense, 371
Ancylostoma caninum, 371
Ancylostoma sp., 358
Anemia, 92, 109, 118, 308, 385
 erythropoietin for, 131
 parasitic, 362, 369, 371
 sickle-cell anemia, 389
Anergy via skin test, 348
Animal bites, 375, 398
Animal exposure, 398–399
Anthrax toxin, 214, 245
Antibiotics
 antibiotic-associated diseases, 220
 mechanism of action antibiotics, 190
 R factor genetic map, 284
 susceptibility testing, 287–289
Antibodies
 autoantibodies, 117
 helper T lymphocytes, 62
 idiotypes, 16, 18–26, 67–68, 86–87
 immune feedback, 5, 6

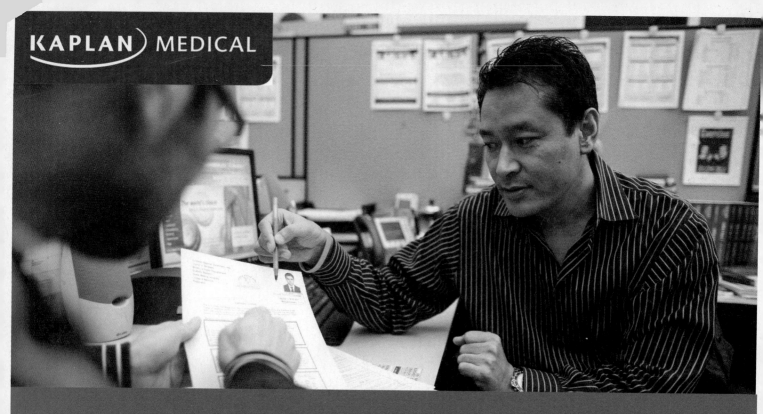